Gastrointestinal Infections

Editors

M. NEDIM INCE
DAVID E. ELLIOTT

GASTROENTEROLOGY CLINICS OF NORTH AMERICA

www.gastro.theclinics.com

Consulting Editor
ALAN L. BUCHMAN

June 2021 • Volume 50 • Number 2

ELSEVIER

1600 John F. Kennedy Boulevard • Suite 1800 • Philadelphia, Pennsylvania, 19103-2899
http://www.theclinics.com

GASTROENTEROLOGY CLINICS OF NORTH AMERICA Volume 50, Number 2
June 2021 ISSN 0889-8553, ISBN-13: 978-0-323-83598-5

Editor: Kerry Holland
Developmental Editor: Karen Solomon

Gastroenterology Clinics of North America (ISSN 0889-8553) is published quarterly by Elsevier Inc., 360 Park Avenue South, New York, NY 10010-1710. Months of issue are March, June, September, and December. Business and Editorial Offices: 1600 John F. Kennedy Blvd., Suite 1800, Philadelphia, PA 19103-2899. Customer Service Office: 6277 Sea Harbor Drive, Orlando, FL 32887-4800. Periodicals postage paid at New York, NY and additional mailing offices. Subscription prices are $365.00 per year (US individuals), $100.00 per year (US students), $945.00 per year (US institutions), $391.00 per year (Canadian individuals), $100.00 per year (Canadian students), $997.00 per year (Canadian institutions), $463.00 per year (international individuals), $220.00 per year (international students), and $997.00 per year (international institutions). Foreign air speed delivery is included in all *Clinics* subscription prices. All prices are subject to change without notice. **POSTMASTER**: Send address changes to *Gastroenterology Clinics of North America*, Elsevier Health Sciences Division, Subscription Customer Service, 3251 Riverport Lane, Maryland Heights, MO 63043. **Telephone: 1-800-654-2452 (U.S. and Canada); 314-447-8871 (outside U.S. and Canada). Fax: 314-447-8029. E-mail: journalscustomerservice-usa@elsevier.com (for print support); journalsonlinesupport-usa@elsevier.com (for online support).**

Reprints. For copies of 100 or more, of articles in this publication, please contact the Commercial Reprints Department, Elsevier Inc., 360 Part Avenue South, New York, New York 10010-1710. Tel. 212-633-3874, Fax: 212-633-3820, E-mail: reprints@elsevier.com.

Gastroenterology Clinics of North America is also published in Italian by Il Pensiero Scientifico Editore, Rome, Italy; and in Portuguese by Interlivros Edicoes Ltda., Rua Commandante Coelho 1085, 21250 Cordovil, Rio de Janeiro, Brazil.

Gastroenterology Clinics of North America is covered in *MEDLINE/PubMed (Index Medicus), Excerpta Medica, Current Contents/Clinical Medicine, Science Citation Index, ISI/BIOMED*, and *BIOSIS*.

Contributors

CONSULTING EDITOR

ALAN L. BUCHMAN, MD, MSPH, FACP, FACN, FACG, AGAF
Professor of Clinical Surgery (Gastroenterology), Medical Director, Intestinal Rehabilitation and Transplant Center, The University of Illinois at Chicago/UI Health, Chicago, Illinois, USA

EDITORS

M. NEDIM INCE, MD
Associate Professor of Medicine, Division of Gastroenterology and Hepatology, Department of Internal Medicine, University of Iowa, Carver College of Medicine, Iowa City Veterans Affairs Medical Center, Iowa City, Iowa, USA

DAVID E. ELLIOTT, MD, PhD
Professor of Medicine, Division of Gastroenterology and Hepatology, Department of Internal Medicine, University of Iowa, Carver College of Medicine, Iowa City Veterans Affairs Medical Center, Iowa City, Iowa, USA

AUTHORS

CYBÉLE LARA R. ABAD, MD
Clinical Associate Professor, Department of Medicine, Section of Infectious Diseases, University of the Philippines-Manila, UP-Philippine General Hospital, Philippines

SAEED ALI, MBBS
Department of Internal Medicine, University of Iowa Healthcare, Iowa City, Iowa, USA

ZHIBO AN, MD, PhD
Division of Gastroenterology and Hepatology, Department of Internal Medicine, University of Iowa Hospitals and Clinics, Iowa City, Iowa, USA

ANTONIO BERUMEN, MD
Division of Gastroenterology and Hepatology, Mayo Clinic, Rochester, Minnesota, USA

ANNIE L. BRASETH, MD
Clinical and Research Fellow, Division of Gastroenterology and Hepatology, Department of Internal Medicine, University of Iowa, Carver College of Medicine, University of Iowa Hospitals & Clinics, Iowa City, Iowa, USA.

DANIEL BUSHYHEAD, MD
Division of Gastroenterology and Hepatology, Lynda K. and David M. Underwood Center for Digestive Disorders, Houston Methodist Hospital, Houston, Texas, USA

ANDREW CHAO, MD
Assistant Professor, Division of Infectious Disease, Department of Medicine, Medical College of Georgia/Augusta University, Augusta, Georgia, USA

JAEHOON CHO, MD
Gastroenterology Fellow, Division of Gastroenterology, Brown University, Providence, Rhode Island, USA

ADAM L. EDWINSON, PhD
Division of Gastroenterology and Hepatology, Mayo Clinic, Rochester, Minnesota, USA

DAVID E. ELLIOTT, MD, PhD
Professor of Medicine, Division of Gastroenterology and Hepatology, Department of Internal Medicine, University of Iowa, Carver College of Medicine, Iowa City Veterans Affairs Medical Center, Iowa City, Iowa, USA.

HALUK ERAKSOY, MD
Professor, Department of Infectious Diseases and Clinical Microbiology, Istanbul Faculty of Medicine, Istanbul University, Istanbul, Turkey

JAMES M. FLECKENSTEIN, MD
Professor, Division of Infectious Diseases, Department of Medicine, Washington University in St. Louis, School of Medicine, Infectious Disease Section, Medicine Service, Veterans Affairs Saint Louis Health Care System, St Louis, Missouri, USA

MADHUSUDAN GROVER, MD
Division of Gastroenterology and Hepatology, Mayo Clinic, Associate Professor, Department of Medicine and Physiology, Enteric NeuroScience Program, Rochester, Minnesota, USA

JENNIFER E. HRABE, MD
Department of Surgery, University of Iowa Hospitals & Clinics, Iowa City, Iowa, USA

DILEK INCE, MD
Associate Professor of Medicine, Division of Infectious Diseases, Department of Internal Medicine, University of Iowa, Carver College of Medicine, Iowa City, Iowa, USA

M. NEDIM INCE, MD
Associate Professor of Medicine, Division of Gastroenterology and Hepatology, Department of Internal Medicine, University of Iowa, Carver College of Medicine, Iowa City Veterans Affairs Medical Center, Iowa City, Iowa, USA

NICOLA L. JONES, MD, PhD, FRCPC
Department of Gastroenterology, Hepatology and Nutrition, The Hospital for

F. MATTHEW KUHLMANN, MD, MSCI
Assistant Professor, Division of Infectious Diseases, Department of Medicine, Washington University in St. Louis, School of Medicine, St Louis, Missouri, USA

STEVEN J. McELROY, MD
Associate Professor, Stead Family Department of Pediatrics, Department of Microbiology and Immunology, University of Iowa, Iowa City, Iowa, USA

JEFFERY L. MEIER, MD
Associate Professor of Medicine, Division of Infectious Diseases, Department of Internal Medicine, University of Iowa Carver College of Medicine, Iowa City Veterans Affairs Healthcare System, Iowa City, Iowa, USA

STEVEN F. MOSS, MD
Professor of Medicine, Division of Gastroenterology, Brown University, Providence, Rhode Island, USA

ARVIND R. MURALI, MD
Division of Gastroenterology-Hepatology, Department of Internal Medicine, University of Iowa Carver College of Medicine, University of Iowa, Iowa City, Iowa, USA

LEMUEL R. NON, MD
Assistant Professor, Division of Infectious Diseases, Department of Internal Medicine, University of Iowa, Carver College of Medicine, Iowa City, Iowa, USA

SAMEER PRAKASH, DO
Department of Internal Medicine, University of Iowa Healthcare, Iowa City, Iowa, USA

AKRITI PRASHAR, PhD
Department of Gastroenterology, Hepatology and Nutrition, Research Fellow, Cell Biology Program, The Hospital for Sick Children, University of Toronto, Toronto, Ontario, Canada

EAMONN M. QUIGLEY, MD, FRCP, FACP, MACG, FRCPI, MWGO
Division of Gastroenterology and Hepatology, Lynda K. and David M. Underwood Center for Digestive Disorders, Houston Methodist Hospital, Houston, Texas, USA

NASIA SAFDAR, MD, PhD
Professor, Department of Medicine, Division of Infectious Diseases, William S. Middleton Memorial Veterans Hospital, University of Wisconsin-Madison, Madison, Wisconsin, USA

NADAV SAHAR, MD
Clinical Assistant Professor, Division of Gastroenterology and Hepatology, Department of Internal Medicine, University of Iowa Hospitals & Clinics, Iowa City, Iowa, USA

ALAULLAH SHEIKH, PhD
Postdoctoral Fellow, Division of Infectious Diseases, Department of Medicine, Washington University in St. Louis, School of Medicine, St Louis, Missouri, USA

DAKOTA T. THOMPSON, MD
Department of Surgery, University of Iowa Hospitals & Clinics, Iowa City, Iowa, USA

JOSE A. VAZQUEZ, MD
Professor of Medicine, Chief, Division of Infectious Disease, Department of Medicine, Medical College of Georgia/Augusta University, Augusta, Georgia, USA

SARAH N. WATSON, MD
Fellow, Department of Obstetrics and Gynecology, University of Iowa, Iowa City, Iowa, USA

Contents

permitting judicious selection of antibiotic use in more severe forms of illness.

Viral acute gastroenteritis (AGE) is common and afflicts people of all ages. Nonviral causes of AGE are less common. Norovirus is a leading cause of sporadic cases and outbreaks of AGE across all ages. Universal rotavirus vaccination of infants has reduced frequency and severity of rotavirus AGE cases in children and indirectly reduced cases in older adults. Severe illness is more likely in persons at age extremes or with immunocompromising conditions. Viral causes of AGE can lead to protracted diarrheal illness in immunocompromised persons. Nucleic acid amplification tests are changing diagnostic testing algorithms.

Antibiotic-associated diarrhea and Clostridioides difficile infection (CDI) occur frequently among adults. The pathophysiology of CDI is related to disruption of normal gut flora and risk factors include hospitalization, use of antibiotic therapy, and older age. Clinical manifestations can range from mild disease to toxic megacolon. Diagnosis is challenging and is based on a combination of clinical symptoms and diagnostic tests. Therapy includes cessation of antibiotics, or use of other agents depending on the severity of illness. Many novel agents for the treatment and prevention of CDI show promise and are under investigation.

Gastrointestinal (GI) tuberculosis (TB) remains a significant problem worldwide, and may involve the luminal GI tract from oral cavity to perianal area in addition to associated viscera and peritoneum. Although GI TB more commonly affects immunocompromised hosts, it can also occur in immunocompetent people. Diagnosis is difficult because it usually mimics a malignancy or inflammatory bowel disease. A high index of clinical suspicion and appropriate use of combined investigative methods help in early diagnosis, and reduce morbidity and mortality. Anti-TB therapy is the same as for pulmonary disease, and invasive and specialized interventions are reserved for selected complications.

Parasites have coevolved with humans. Several of them colonize the human body and establish a symbiotic relationship. Other parasites cause severe and lethal diseases. Prevalence of parasitic infections is decreased in highly industrialized countries, largely due to enforced hygienic practices. In contrast, parasites cause significant morbidity and mortality in parts of the world with barriers to effective public hygiene. Some parasites have emerged as potent pathogens in specific patient populations, such as immune suppressed individuals, regardless of sanitation. This article reviews common parasites encountered in clinical practice and, in the setting of host-parasite symbiosis, discusses their immune regulatory role.

Nonhepatotropic viruses such as adenovirus, herpes simplex virus, flaviviruses, filoviruses, and human herpes virus, and bacteria such as Coxiella burnetii, can cause liver injury mimicking acute hepatitis. Most of these organisms cause a self-limited infection. However, in immunocompromised patients, they can cause severe hepatitis or in some cases fulminant hepatic failure requiring an urgent liver transplant. Hepatic dysfunction is also commonly seen in patients with severe acute respiratory syndrome coronavirus-2 infection. Patients with preexisting liver diseases are likely at risk for severe coronavirus disease 2019 (COVID-19) and may be associated with poor outcomes.

Acute cholangitis, also referred to as ascending cholangitis, is an infection of the biliary tree characterized by fever, jaundice, and abdominal pain, which in most cases is the consequence of biliary obstruction. Diagnosis is commonly made by the presence of clinical features, laboratory tests, and imaging studies. The treatment modalities include administration of intravenous fluids, antimicrobial therapy, and prompt drainage of the bile duct. Early diagnosis and treatment of acute cholangitis are crucial to prevent unwanted clinical outcome of the disease. This article provides an update on early diagnosis and management of acute cholangitis.

Infectious gastroenteritis is common after transplantation and can lead to increased morbidity and mortality. A wide range of organisms can lead to gastroenteritis in this patient population. Clostridioides difficile, cytomegalovirus, and norovirus are the most common pathogens. Newer diagnostic methods, especially multiplex polymerase chain reaction, have increased the diagnostic yield of infectious etiologies. In this review, we describe the epidemiology and risk factors for common infectious pathogens leading to gastroenteritis.

Necrotizing enterocolitis is a serious and yet incompletely understood gastrointestinal disease of infancy that predominately impacts premature neonates. Prevention is a key strategy for the management of necrotizing enterocolitis. Although postnatal risk factors have been the focus of prevention efforts, obstetric complications, including intrauterine inflammation and infection, growth restriction, preeclampsia, and prenatal medications, have been associated with an increased risk of necrotizing enterocolitis. This article reviews the evidence behind the prenatal risk factors for necrotizing enterocolitis, and discusses how these risk factors may elucidate the pathogenesis of necrotizing enterocolitis and provide insight into prevention and treatment.

Epidemiologic data support that acute gastrointestinal infection is one of the strongest risk factors for development of irritable bowel syndrome (IBS). Risk of post-infection IBS (PI-IBS) seems to be greater with bacterial and protozoal than viral enterocolitis. Younger individuals, women, and those with severe enterocolitis are more likely to develop PI-IBS. Disease mechanisms in animal models and humans involve chronic perturbation of intestinal microbiome, epithelial and neuronal remodeling, and immune activation. These mechanisms can lead to luminal (increased proteolytic activity, altered bile acid composition) and physiologic (increased permeability, transit changes, and visceral hypersensitivity) alterations that can mediate PI-IBS symptoms.

The term "small intestinal bacterial overgrowth" (SIBO) has been used to refer to a disorder resulting from the colonization of the small bowel by an increased number of microorganisms or by the presence of bacteria that are not usual constituents of this part of the gastrointestinal tract. Clinical presentations, often in patients with certain risk factors, can range from a full-blown malabsorption syndrome to such "functional" complaints as bloating and flatulence. SIBO is diagnosed by either culture of a small bowel aspirate or one of several breath tests. Treatment of SIBO entails risk factor modification, correction of nutritional deficiencies, and oral antibiotics.

Intra-abdominal and anorectal abscesses are common pathologies seen in both inpatient and outpatient settings. To decrease morbidity and mortality, early diagnosis and treatment are essential. After adequate drainage via a percutaneous or incisional approach, patients need to be monitored for worsening symptoms or recurrence and evaluated for the underlying condition that may have contributed to abscess formation.

GASTROENTEROLOGY CLINICS OF NORTH AMERICA

SERIES OF RELATED INTEREST

Gastrointestinal Endoscopy Clinics of North America
(Available at: https://www.giendo.theclinics.com)
Clinics in Liver Disease
(Available at: https://www.liver.theclinics.com)

THE CLINICS ARE AVAILABLE ONLINE!
Access your subscription at:
www.theclinics.com

GASTROENTEROLOGY
CLINICS OF NORTH AMERICA

Foreword

Gastrointestinal Infections: Forward (or Backward)

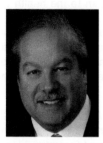

Alan L. Buchman, MD, MSPH
Consulting Editor

Running down the gutter with a piece of bread and butter

Diarrhea, diarrhea

Running down the gutter with a piece of bread and butter

Diarrhea, diarrhea

Some people think it's funny but it's really wet and runny

Diarrhea, diarrhea

Sorry we're late, Bob had diarrhea!

Ew! What? I love you, mom
—*The Diarrhea Song by John Roberts and John Dylan Keith (Fox Music)*

Infections may have saved humanity from extinction at the feet of alien beings in War of the Worlds, but despite our modern technology, anti-infective agents and infection-control practices, infections continue to wreak havoc on the human body, most notably the gastrointestinal (GI) tract. As the only organ system with at least 2 openings to the outside world, the GI tract remains most susceptible to infections. Despite that, GI infections are not often talked about or written about, at least in song. Clearly, GI infections are not as popular among the public as "Cat Scratch Fever."

However, the embarrassment of GI infections aside, some of these infections may cause chronic disease and/or even lead to malignancy and death. They are a cause of significant morbidity as well as mortality for humans and represent common reasons for visits to a clinic or emergency room. In 2013, it was estimated that treatment of GI

Gastroenterol Clin N Am 50 (2021) xiii–xiv
https://doi.org/10.1016/j.gtc.2021.03.002
0889-8553/21/© 2021 Published by Elsevier Inc.

gastro.theclinics.com

infections by medical professionals, not including self-care, amounted to over $2.2 billion USD annually just in Poland.[1] In the United States, the total cost of treatment for GI disease was estimated at $140 billion USD in 2018,[2] although the percentage that consists of treatment for GI infections alone is unclear. In 2004, it was estimated that the cost for treated Salmonella infections in the United States alone was $2.8 billion USD,[3] and in 2016, the cost for just inpatient treatment of *Clostridium difficile* infections was estimated at $6.3 billion USD.[4] Therefore, the diagnosis and treatment of GI infections represent a substantial real and financial burden to the health care system.

Drs Ince and Elliott have assembled a comprehensive group of experts that cover the wide-ranging groups of bacterial, fungal, and viral organisms that adversely affect the human GI tract. The appropriate diagnostics techniques and treatment are discussed, as well as the complications from these infections and their therapy and appropriate management of those complications.

Alan L. Buchman, MD, MSPH
Intestinal Rehabilitation and Transplant Center
Department of Surgery/UI Health
University of Illinois at Chicago
840 South Wood Street
Suite 402 (MC958)
Chicago, IL 60612, USA

E-mail address:
a.buchman@hotmail.com

REFERENCES

1. Czech M, Magdalena R, Rogalska J, et al. Costs of medically attended acute gastrointestinal infections: the Polish Prospective Healthcare Utilization Survey. Value Health Regional Iss 2013;2:210–7.
2. Peery AF, Crockett SD, Murphy CC, et al. Burden and cost of gastrointestinal, liver, and pancreatic diseases in the United States: update 2018. Gastroenterology 2019;156:254–72.
3. Adhikari B, Angulo F, Martin M. Economic burden of Salmonella infections in the United States. Presented at the American Agricultural Economics Association Annual Meeting. Denver, Colorado, August 1–4, 2004.
4. Zhang S, Palazuelos-Munoz S, Balsells EM, et al. Cost of hospital management of *Clostridium difficile* infection in United States—a meta-analysis and modelling study. BMC Infect Dis 2016;16:447.

Preface

Facing an Infection as a Health Care Provider

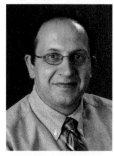 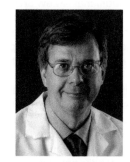

M. Nedim Ince, MD   David E. Elliott, MD, PhD
Editors

In fact mortality among the doctors was the highest of all, since they came more frequently in contact with the sick.
    —*History of the Peloponnesian War by Thucydides (c. 460–400 bc)*

The old-time pandemic described in the *History of the Peloponnesian War* was believed to have started in Africa and reached the Eastern Mediterranean and Europe through Egypt and Libya. It was so devastating that it made the Greek historian Thucydides stop writing about the war and start giving details about the plague. Many centuries later, investigators proposed that the plague had been caused by typhoid fever based on DNA analysis from dental pulp of patients in a mass burial pit,[1] even though there were significant differences between how Thucydides had described the clinical symptoms and how typhoid fever presents itself in patients today. During the Crimean War in the nineteenth century, morbidity and mortality due to dysentery were more dramatic among soldiers treated in the hospital in Üsküdar (Scutari, a district of Istanbul on the Asian side) than the casualties on the battlefield. A similar comparison can be made for dysentery-versus battle-related casualties for soldiers fighting during the American Civil War, which took place only few years after the Crimean War.

Like other contagious illnesses, gastrointestinal infections not only have caused large outbreaks throughout history but also continue to represent a major cause of morbidity and mortality in the modern world. In this issue of the *Gastroenterology Clinics of North America*, 14 groups of experts from health care centers in the United States and other parts of the world share their approach to infectious diseases occurring in different parts of the gastrointestinal tract and the hepatobiliary system. First, several articles review the clinical strategies in contemporary management of

Gastroenterol Clin N Am 50 (2021) xv–xvi
https://doi.org/10.1016/j.gtc.2021.03.001
0889-8553/21/© 2021 Published by Elsevier Inc.   **gastro.theclinics.com**

pathogens known for a long time, like bacteria, viruses, fungi, and parasites. These also include articles on other rare causes of hepatitis, mycobacterial infections, and peptic ulcer disease caused by the relatively more recently recognized pathogen, *Helicobacter pylori*. Second, emerging pathogens in special patient populations, for example, the transplant recipients or individuals infected with the human immunodeficiency virus, are discussed in detail by different experts in other articles. Infectious complications that require management by advanced endoscopists, interventionalists, or surgeons are also covered in 2 additional review articles. Last, a group of articles informs the reader about the clinical management of disorders, which although triggered or driven by gut microorganisms and important for gastroenterologists, are often overlooked as an infectious disease or a complication, such as necrotizing enterocolitis, small intestinal bacterial overgrowth, or postinfectious irritable bowel syndrome.

With the development of public health measures, vaccines, and antibiotics in the twentieth century, the incidence of several gastrointestinal infections and various forms of hepatitis has decreased significantly. These advances made some authorities predict that the era of infectious diseases was over. Unfortunately, this has not proven true. When the assignments were first given to us as guest editors, and the authors were invited to write review articles, a deadly and devastating pandemic had just started. Health care providers needed to update processes and practices to care for patients with COVID-19, while also protect themselves, other personnel, and other patients. This health care crisis mirrored the concerns raised by Thucydides some 2500 years ago and shows that we must always keep these agents in mind. In this context, we would like to thank all the authors who spent their precious and stressful time during the COVID-19 outbreak for sharing and synthesizing contemporary scientific knowledge and writing their articles enriched with their wide experience and expert opinion.

We hope that you enjoy reading this issue of the *Gastroenterology Clinics of North America* on gastrointestinal infections.

M. Nedim Ince, MD
University of Iowa Hospitals and Clinics
4546 JCP, 200 Hawkins Drive
Iowa City, IA 52242, USA

David E. Elliott, MD, PhD
University of Iowa Hospitals and Clinics
4607 JCP, 200 Hawkins Drive
Iowa City, IA 52242, USA

E-mail addresses:
m-nedim-ince@uiowa.edu (M.N. Ince)
david-elliott@uiowa.edu (D.E. Elliott)

REFERENCE

1. Papagrigorakis MJ, Yapijakis C, Synodinos PN, et al. DNA examination of ancient dental pulp incriminates typhoid fever as a probable cause of the plague of Athens. Int J Infect Dis 2006;10(3):206–14.

Fungal Infections of the Gastrointestinal Tract

Andrew Chao, MD, Jose A. Vazquez, MD*

KEYWORDS

- Fungus • Infection • Gastrointestinal tract • Yeast • Mold • Enterocolitis
- Endemic mycosis

KEY POINTS

- Fungi are ubiquitous in nature and commensal organisms on people.
- In the right clinical situations, they can cause invasive disease affecting multiple organ systems often originating from the gastrointestinal tract.
- Diagnosis of many fungal infections remains difficult and frequently prolongs the initiation of antifungal therapy.

Fungi are important members of the diverse array of microorganisms that are omnipresent in nature. People are routinely exposed to fungi through respiratory, cutaneous, and gastrointestinal (GI) routes. Traditionally, fungal organisms of the GI tract were identified via stool culture. However, advances in DNA and rRNA sequencing and serologic testing have led to shifts in how gut fungal microbiota are identified and in diagnosing opportunistic infections. These fungi to which humans are routinely exposed can, in the right circumstances, cause clinical disease. Occurrence of invasive fungal infections is dependent on numerous factors including geographic location and routes of exposure, and host factors, such as predisposing conditions, high-risk medications, or underlying medical comorbidities that modulate overall immune function. This article serves as a review for important causes of fungal GI infections, their epidemiology, clinical presentation, and treatment recommendations.

RISK FACTORS

Specific risk factors predisposing toward infection vary among the different fungal species and between the different individual host factors that are frequently associated with their comorbid conditions. Deficiencies in host immunity, more often in the innate than adaptive immune systems, are predisposing risks for fungal disease. Immune deficiencies encompasses a heterogeneous population that includes people living with human immunodeficiency virus (HIV) and AIDS, people with diabetes,

Division of Infectious Disease, Department of Medicine, Medical College of Georgia/Augusta University, 1120 15th Street, Augusta, GA 30912, USA
* Corresponding author.
E-mail address: jvazquez@augusta.edu

Gastroenterol Clin N Am 50 (2021) 243–260
https://doi.org/10.1016/j.gtc.2021.02.009
0889-8553/21/© 2021 Elsevier Inc. All rights reserved.

people who receive immunosuppressive therapy or who have undergone either solid organ or stem cell transplantations, people with immune cell mutations that impair signaling or other cell function, and people with underlying hematologic malignancies.[1]

Neutropenia is commonly defined as an absolute neutrophil count less than 1500 per mm[3] and severe neutropenia as less than 500 cells per mm[3]. Quantitative deficiencies in neutrophil count, independent of neutrophil function, have long since been recognized as a major predisposing risk factor for all infections including invasive fungal disease.[2] Neutropenia in this setting could be caused by underlying disease and malignancy, or as sequelae from cytotoxic chemotherapy. The overlap between these two groups is best demonstrated in patients undergoing aggressive treatment of hematologic malignancy, where not only severe neutropenia is present but also neutropenia for extended periods of time. Extended durations of neutropenia are associated with an increasing frequency in the number of infectious episodes[2] and an increased risk for infections caused by invasive mold disease.

People with diabetes, especially those with poor glycemic control, are another population at increased risk for invasive fungal infections. Although people with diabetes commonly comprise this group, individuals on corticosteroids also are at risk. This increased risk is attributable to a combination of factors, specifically the role of hyperglycemia in compromising neutrophil function.[3] Hyperglycemia has been demonstrated to have a wide variety of effects on neutrophil function including impaired chemotaxis, blunted phagocytic ability, and reduced oxidative killing.[4,5] In addition to the direct effects on cellular immune function caused by hyperglycemia, the acidemia and iron mobilization resultant from diabetic ketoacidosis is also recognized as major factors promoting fungal proliferation and angioinvasion.[6] Patients receiving systemic corticosteroids have increased risk for fungal disease similar to that seen in people with diabetes. In addition to the compromised neutrophil function caused by secondary hyperglycemia, corticosteroids themselves impair macrophage and neutrophil function with regards to phagocytosis and production of reactive oxygen species. Additional causes of immunosuppression from corticosteroids occur because of the inhibition of proinflammatory cytokines. Risk increases with daily steroid doses in excess of 0.5 mg/kg or duration of therapy greater than 1 week.[7] Fungal infections in these groups tend to be more of a chronic process with less acuity and invasion, although acute fulminant cases have been described.

In patients that are HIV-positive, invasive fungal disease is generally associated with AIDS, when the CD4 count decreases to less than 200 cells per mm3. AS the CD4 count drops, the incidence of fungal infections increase, starting with oropharyngeal and esophageal candidiasis. In general, infections caused by *Pneumocystis jirovecii*, *Aspergillus* spp, or the endemic fungi, including *Histoplasma capsulatum* and *Coccidioides immitis*, tend to be seen with CD4 counts less than 50 cells per mm[3] (**Table 1**).

Although not extremely common, chronic mucocutaneous candidiasis (CMC) may occasional produce recurrent and relapses in oral and esophageal candidiasis. This entity is a heterogeneous complex of immune deficiency diseases characterized by increased infections and recurrent infections primarily caused by *Candida* spp, although other organisms can also be involved. These infections tend to occur in the skin, nails, and mucous membranes. Mutations in several different genes have been associated with CMC, including STAT1, AIRE, CARD-9, and Dectin-1. The most commonly described mutation is in the STAT-1 gene (signal transducer and activator of transcription-1). STAT-1 proteins are essential components of the adaptive immune response to numerous organisms. Mutations in this gene result in either a loss of function or gain of function. The gain of function mutations are associated

Table 1
Fungal infections of the gastrointestinal tract and risk factors

Disease State	Risk Factors
Candidiasis	Antimicrobial therapy Age Radiation therapy Corticosteroids Neutropenia HIV/AIDS Immunosuppressive therapy Chronic mucocutaneous candidiasis
Zygomycosis	Neutropenia Malnutrition Diabetes Acidosis Corticosteroids Malignancy Solid organ and stem cell transplants
Aspergillosis	Corticosteroids Neutropenia HIV/AIDS Immunosuppressive therapy Solid organ and stem cell transplants
Cryptococcosis	Neutropenia HIV/AIDS Chronic liver disease Immunosuppressive therapy Solid organ and stem cell transplants
Histoplasmosis	Residing in endemic area HIV/AIDS Tumor necrosis factor blockers
Blastomycosis	Residing in endemic area HIV/AIDS
Coccidioidomycosis	Residing in endemic area HIV/AIDS Age >50 Immunosuppressive therapy Tumor necrosis factor blockers

with increased bacterial, mycobacterial, and fungal infections. STAT-1 mutations are described in 40% of patients with CMC.

GASTROINTESTINAL CANDIDIASIS

Candida spp are widely acknowledged as the predominant cause of fungal infections in humans and represent a significant contribution to human morbidity and mortality, especially in the health care setting. There are more than 165 species of *Candida*, but more than 90% of invasive candidiasis is caused by one of five *Candida* spp: *Candida albicans*, *Candida glabrata*, *Candida tropicalis*, *Candida parapsilosis*, and *Candida krusei* (**Table 2**).

The yeast *C albicans* is the most commonly isolated fungus in animals and humans. Carriage rates can vary, but it is a common component of the oral mucocutaneous flora and throughout the GI tract[8] and represents the most common pathogen in

Table 2
Candida spp with in vitro susceptibilities

Species	Risk Factors[a]	Colonizing Sites	MIC Susceptibility			
			Fluconazole	Voriconazole	Micafungin	Caspofungin
C albicans		Skin, mouth, GI and GU tracts	≤2	≤0.12	≤0.25	≤0.25
C glabrata	Fluconazole use, parenteral nutrition	Mouth, GI and GU tracts	DDS	N/A	≤0.06	≤0.12
C tropicalis	ICU, malignancy	Skin, GI and GU tracts	≤2	≤0.12	≤0.25	≤0.25
C parapsilosis	Neonates, parenteral nutrition	Skin	≤2	≤0.12	≤2	≤2
C krusei	Fluconazole use, malignancy	N/A	Resistant	≤0.5	≤0.25	≤0.25

Abbreviations: DDS, dose-dependent susceptibility; GU, genitourinary; ICU, intensive care unit; MIC, minimum inhibitory concentration; N/A, not available.
[a] Common risk factors include ICU stay, the use of broad-spectrum antibiotics, recent surgery, immunocompromise, mechanical ventilation, and presence of indwelling catheters.

invasive candidiasis. Risk factors associated with an increased risk of candidiasis include HIV/AIDS, neutropenia, uncontrolled diabetes, increased age, innate immunodeficiency (CMC), local trauma, radiation therapy, steroid use, and antimicrobial therapy. Antimicrobial use is well known to be a frequent and common risk factor associated with mucosal candidiasis and is most likely a sequela caused by the elimination of commensal bacteria flora, allowing for yeast overgrowth. C albicans tends to be fairly susceptible to all forms of treatment, although resistance and relapse of disease can occur, especially in chronic immunosuppressed states, such as advanced HIV and prolonged and persistent neutropenia. In addition, patients that suffer from various forms of CMC are also at risk of developing secondary resistant to antifungals.

In recent years, the incidence of non-*albicans Candida* spp has increased dramatically. The acknowledgment of these species is extremely important in the management of candidiasis, because many of these are intrinsically resistant to commonly used antifungals and their presence in tissues potentially alters the standard therapeutic management. C glabrata is the second-most commonly isolated *Candida* spp. C glabrata have a variable dose-dependent susceptibility to azoles, such as fluconazole and itraconazole, and frequently require empiric antifungal treatment with an alternative class of antifungals, such as echinocandins. C parapsilosis and C tropicalis are the third and fourth most commonly isolates species. Although susceptible to azoles, C parapsilosis may be less susceptible to echinocandins. C krusei is intrinsically resistant to most azoles, including fluconazole, itraconazole, and voriconazole. Isolates of Candida lusitaniae are intrinsically resistant to amphotericin B, as are some isolates of Candida guilliermondii (see **Table 2**).[9] In the past 5 years, an emerging species named Candida auris has been increasing worldwide and is presenting a serious global health problem. C auris presents a clinical challenge because it is the only species that is multidrug-resistant and is frequently misidentified by standard laboratory methods. Although rarely seen as a cause of mucosal candidiasis, it has already caused several health care outbreaks globally. Recommendations for the initial treatment of C auris infections is the use of echinocandins.

Diagnostic Modalities for Candida

Diagnosis of Candida infections is traditionally made by visualization of the organism from infected tissues and the isolation of the organism from cultures. Common examples include blood cultures, direct swab, or biopsy of a suspicious lesion; historically stool cultures were performed as well, although this has fallen into disuse. Blood cultures have previously been demonstrated to have equal, if not superior, sensitivity to modalities, such as polymerase chain reaction for the detection of candidemia.[10] Historically, isolates from blood culture were identified phenotypically; however, this is time-consuming and required expertise. Laboratories are increasingly shifting to the use of matrix-assisted laser desorption ionization/time-of-flight mass spectrometry for the rapid and reliable identification of microorganisms, including fungi.[11,12] However, reliance on blood cultures for the diagnosis of invasive candidiasis comes with its own pitfalls, because the utility of blood cultures is predicated on the presence of secondary candidemia from deep-seated candidiasis.[13] The gold standard diagnosis includes sterile culture growth from tissues, and often requires invasive procedures that may not be readily obtainable in a timely manner. There is an ongoing investigation into alternative testing modalities for rapid and accurate detection of Candida spp, some of which are already commercially available. Many yeasts including Candida and some molds have $(1-3)$-β-D-glucan as a component of their fungal cell wall, which is detected in serum with an estimated sensitivity of 76.8% and specificity of

85.3%.[14,15] Unfortunately, the assay is not effective in diagnosing mucocutaneous candidiasis.

Oropharyngeal Candidiasis

C albicans is the primary cause of oropharyngeal candidiasis (OPC).[16] In addition to previously identified at-risk populations, additional risk factors for OPC include the use of dentures, use of tobacco, and the use of systemic and inhaled corticosteroids.

There are several different clinical forms of OPC. Pseudomembranous candidiasis or thrush has the classic and most common form of OPC. The physical findings include diffuse erythema with scrapeable, patchy, white lesions that may involve the tongue, buccal mucosa, throat, and even gums (**Fig. 1**). In acute atrophic candidiasis patients complain of a burning sensation in their tongue and tend to have a hyperemic tongue. It is seen in association with certain vitamin deficiencies. Chronic atrophic stomatitis (denture stomatitis) produces chronic erythema of the gums and mucosa that are in direct contact with dentures. Chronic hyperplastic candidiasis (candida leukoplakia) has an appearance of speckled or coalescent white lesions on the buccal mucosa and lateral tongue. It is strongly associated with smoking and is also considered a potentially premalignant lesion. Median rhomboid glossitis (midline glossitis) is another chronic atrophic form of oral candidiasis, affecting primarily the midline or the dorsum of the tongue. Risk factors for this form include inhaled steroid use and smoking tobacco, and results in *Candida* proliferation with atrophy and loss of papillae. This form of OPC rarely causes symptoms. Angular cheilitis and cheilosis is characterized by fissuring and cracks of the corner of the mouth with associated pain and erythema (**Fig. 2**). Cheilitis in these circumstances is often present with OPC or chronic atrophic candidiasis and generally responds to topical therapy (**Box 1**).

It should be noted that findings of OPC can be complicated by concomitant processes, such as mucositis secondary to cytotoxic chemotherapy; leukoplakia; or even other infections, such as superimposed bacterial[17] or herpes simplex virus infection. Diagnosis is confirmed by microscopic visualization of yeast with potassium hydroxide preparation. Cultures are not essential for diagnostic purposes, and do not distinguish between colonization and true disease. However, they may be useful in patients with recalcitrant infections to identify resistant organisms and perform in vitro susceptibilities.

Treatment

The available treatments for OPC have not markedly changed over the past decade. Gentian violet, first introduced nearly a century ago, is still used in most of the world.

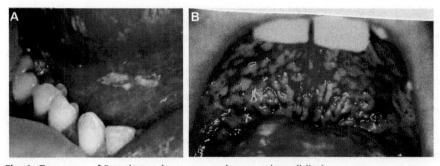

Fig. 1. Two types of Pseudomembranous oropharyngeal candidiasis.

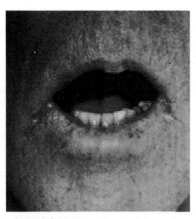

Fig. 2. Atrophic form of oral candidiasis.

Use of gentian violet has long since been superseded by more efficacious antifungals, although it is still available over the counter and is inexpensive. Therapy with topical agents, such as nystatin, remains the classic treatment modality for thrush in immuno-competent children and many adults. Although they have a good safety profile, limitations to use include bitter taste and frequency of dosing. In addition, the efficacy of nystatin has been shown to be less effective than oral azole antifungals in immuno-compromised populations. In HIV-positive patients, the use of nystatin was associated with a higher incidence of relapse rate,[18] whereas some studies in patients with cancer receiving chemotherapy also noted the occurrence of candidemia after treatment with nystatin.[19] For mild disease, we recommend clotrimazole troches, 10 mg five times daily, or miconazole mucoadhesive buccal, 50-mg tablets applied to the mucosal surface daily for 7 to 14 days. Nevertheless, nystatin remains an alternative for mild disease, as a suspension dosed at 4 to 6 mL (100,000 U/mL) four times a day or one to two pastilles (200,000 U) four times a day, for 7 to 14 days. The use of azole antifungals has been the mainstay of OPC for the past few decades. Fluconazole has enjoyed excellent treatment success with cure rates in excess of 90%.[20] Fluconazole dosing for moderate to severe disease is recommended at 100 to 200 mg once a day for 7 to 14 days of treatment. Although uncommon, fluconazole-resistant *C albicans* or the presence of a non-*albicans* species of *Candida* can be treated with itraconazole solution, or newer triazoles, such as posaconazole, 400 mg twice daily for 3 days, followed by daily for up to 28 days or voriconazole, 200 mg twice daily. The use of triazoles does come with its own concerns including side effect profile, cost,

---

Box 1
Clinical manifestations of oral candidiasis

Pseudomembranous candidiasis (thrush)

Angular cheilitis

Denture stomatitis (chronic atrophic stomatitis)

Candida leukoplakia (chronic hyperplastic candidiasis)

Median rhomboid glossitis (midline glossitis)

Acute atrophic candidiasis

Chronic mucocutaneous candidiasis

and drug interactions. Other alternative therapies for use in severe disease include echinocandins (caspofungin, micafungin, anidulafungin) or amphotericin B deoxycholate suspension, 100 mg/mL four times a day.

Esophageal Candidiasis

Although Candida can be cultured in approximately 11% of healthy adults,[21] carriage of *Candida* spp within the esophagus is not as prevalent as in other anatomic sites, such as the skin, oral, and enteric mucosa. Immune suppression in at-risk patients is presumed to facilitate an increased adherence and colonization, and predispose to the development of invasive disease. The presentation of esophageal candidiasis typically includes dysphagia, odynophagia, and retrosternal chest pain, which is quite debilitating. These symptoms may be accompanied by low-grade fever, although this is absent in the immunocompromised population. In patients with prolonged disease, weight loss and anorexia are common. Although OPC is recognized as a risk factor, it may not present concomitantly with esophageal candidiasis and patients may have a normal-appearing oral cavity. In addition to greatly diminished quality of life from the primary infection, long-term and serious sequelae of esophageal candidiasis can include esophageal strictures, esophageal perforation, or esophagotracheal fistula formation. The appearance of esophageal candidiasis on endoscopy can vary in severity, character, and distribution. The classification system developed by Kodsi and colleagues[22] separates *Candida* esophagitis into four types based on endoscopic appearance. Type I disease is described as white plaques up to 2 mm in diameter with hyperemia without edema or ulceration. The plaques seen in type II *Candida* esophagitis are more numerous than type I, with sizes greater than 2 mm with hyperemia and edema but without ulceration. Type III *Candida* esophagitis is described as confluent, linear, and elevated plaques with hyperemia and ulceration (**Fig. 3**). Type IV disease has all the characteristics of type II, with the addition of narrowing of the esophageal lumen and increased friability of the mucosa. There remains significant overlap between atypical cases of esophageal candidiasis with other causes of esophagitis including herpes simplex virus or cytomegalovirus. Therefore, definitive diagnosis of *Candida* esophagitis should be made by histologic evidence of tissue invasion on biopsy. Esophageal brushings, although sensitive for detecting *Candida*, are not able to distinguish invasive disease from colonization, nor do they have utility in evaluation for other causative etiologies.

The current recommendation includes systemic antifungal therapy for a duration of 2 to 3 weeks. Oral fluconazole remains the mainstay of therapy for esophageal candidiasis, dosed at 200 to 400 mg (3–6 mg/kg) for 14 to 21 days. For patients with severe symptoms or if they cannot tolerate oral therapy, fluconazole is administered intravenously at 400 mg (6 mg/kg) daily, or an echinocandin, such as caspofungin, micafungin, or anidulafungin is used. Caspofungin is dosed at 70 mg intravenously on Day 1, followed by 50 mg daily thereafter; micafungin therapy is dosed 150 mg intravenously daily and anidulafungin 200 mg daily. For cases treated initially with intravenous therapy, treatment step-down to oral fluconazole is recommended once the patient is able to tolerate oral intake. For management of fluconazole-refractory disease, it is strongly recommended to perform endoscopy with tissue sampling to confirm the diagnosis. Failure of fluconazole may reflect de novo resistance, new infection with a fluconazole-resistant organism, or a misdiagnosis of an alternative infectious cause. Development of resistance reflects long-term antifungal prophylaxis in patients with neutropenia or immunocompromised patients, or because of repeat treatment of recurrent disease. Treatment recommendations for fluconazole-refractory, confirmed *Candida* esophagitis include itraconazole, 200 mg daily oral solution; voriconazole,

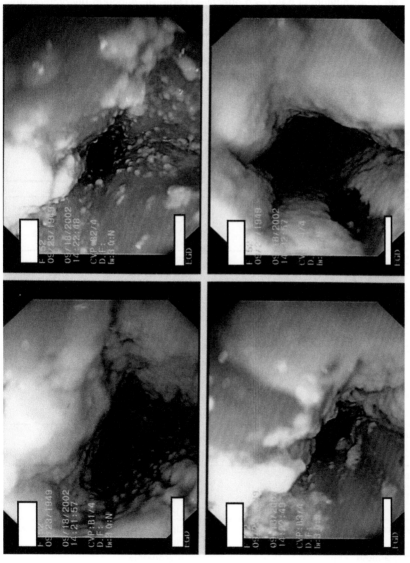

Fig. 3. Severe esophageal candidiasis in an HIV-positive patient.

200 mg orally or intravenously twice a day; or posaconazole, 400 mg oral suspension twice a day or 300 mg once a day of extended-release capsules. Echinocandin therapy at the standard dosing also remains a viable treatment option in these circumstances. It should be cautioned that since their introduction, echinocandin-resistance in some *Candida* spp has been described. Use of parenteral amphotericin B at 0.3 to 0.7 mg/kg daily is typically reserved for treatment-resistant esophageal candidiasis when no other antifungal has been effective (**Table 3**). Although uncommon, there are still cases of chronic or recurrent oropharyngeal and esophageal candidiasis. This is seen primarily in patients with advanced HIV infection with CD4 counts less than 50 and who have had several bouts of mucosal candidiasis. In addition to the management of active fungal infection, attention should be directed to reversing an underlying immunocompromised state. For patients with HIV/AIDS this includes initiating highly active antiretroviral therapy; in stem cell or solid organ transplantation, this may require reduction in the intensity of an immunosuppressive regimen if feasible.[23]

Table 3
Gastrointestinal infections and appropriate antifungal therapy

Disease State	Antifungal Therapy
Candidiasis	
Oral mild–moderate	Nystatin Clotrimazole troches Miconazole mucoadhesive tablets Fluconazole tablets
Oral severe	Fluconazole Itraconazole Posaconazole
Esophageal candidiasis	Fluconazole Itraconazole Voriconazole Posaconazole
Fluconazole-refractory candidiasis	Posaconazole Caspofungin Micafungin Anidulafungin Amphotericin B deoxycholate Liposomal amphotericin B
Mucormycosis	Liposomal amphotericin B Isavuconazonium sulfate Posaconazole
Aspergillosis	Voriconazole Isavuconazonium sulfate Posaconazole Liposomal amphotericin B
Cryptococcosis	Liposomal amphotericin B + flucytosine Fluconazole
Histoplasmosis	Itraconazole Liposomal amphotericin B
Blastomycosis	Itraconazole Liposomal amphotericin B
Coccidioidomycosis	Itraconazole Fluconazole Liposomal amphotericin B

In these high-risk populations with ongoing immunosuppression, secondary prophylaxis with thrice weekly fluconazole, 100 mg, is highly recommended.

Candida Enterocolitis

Infections of the small and large bowel can have drastic implications with regard to morbidity and mortality, particularly in the immunocompromised population.[24,25] Because several Candida spp are routinely found within the gut as commensal organisms, it is easy to underestimate their proclivity to cause invasive disease in these individuals. A meta-analysis of prior studies of patients with neutropenic enterocolitis estimate the pooled frequency of fungal cause to be at least 3.4%, of which Candida spp predominated.[24] Autopsy surveys of healthy adults and those with hematologic malignancies have demonstrated mucosal invasion of the small and large bowel by Candida spp.[26] The frequency of invasive Candida enterocolitis in adult healthy hosts is unknown. In the pediatric population, Candida causing necrotizing enterocolitis in premature neonates is uncommon, but when present is associated with a mortality rate of 27% in patients with severe disease requiring surgery.[27]

MUCORMYCOSIS

Mucormycosis (zygomycosis) comprises a group of infections caused by a wide array of saprophytic molds, the most important genera include Rhizopus, Mucor, and Absidia spp.[7,28] Although rare, mucormycosis is the third most common cause of invasive fungal infections. As with other opportunistic infections, risk factors include neutropenia cancer, solid organ and stem cell transplants, and uncontrolled diabetes, iron overload syndromes, steroids, and defuroxime use.[1,6,29] A key pathogenic feature of mucormycosis is their propensity for angioinvasion with resultant embolic mold-septic complexes, resulting in ischemia and tissue infarction followed by necrosis. Mucormycosis typically presents in five major clinical forms: (1) rhinocerebral, (2) pulmonary, (3) abdominopelvic and gastric, (4) primary cutaneous, and (5) disseminated disease. GI mucormycosis is a rare manifestation of disease and signifies ingestion of organisms in vulnerable patients, whereas the other manifestations represent inhalation or direct inoculation of the respiratory tract and skin. Patients at additional risk for GI mucormycosis include premature neonates and malnourished children.[30] Mucormycosis can occur in any portion of the GI tract, but most commonly affects the stomach, followed by the colon and then ileum.[30,31] The liver, spleen, and pancreas are less commonly involved. Symptoms for GI disease can be nonspecific and include fever and abdominal pain, and marked GI tract bleeding in invasive disease. On further work-up, it may be encountered as a mass or ulceration within the GI tract, with the resultant differential including malignancy, intra-abdominal abscess, or other infectious etiologies. Consequently, diagnosis may be delayed or missed until later in the clinical course or on autopsy. Confirmation of mucormycosis depends on the biopsy demonstration of organism invading tissue, likely in association with findings of thrombosis and tissue infarction. A high clinical suspicion for mucormycosis is needed to facilitate a timely diagnosis by endoscopic biopsy or surgical resection.

Mucormycosis is a rapid and fatal condition unless promptly diagnosed and treated aggressively with a of combination of extensive surgical debridement, reversal of underlying immunosuppression, and antifungal therapy. Antifungal therapy includes either liposomal amphotericin B, 5 to 7 mg/kg daily intravenously, or mold-active triazole antifungals (posaconazole or isavuconazonium sulfate) (see **Table 3**). Note that the triazole voriconazole does not have activity against the organisms of mucormycosis. Despite the use of effective antifungal therapy, 1-year mortality for mucormycosis ranges from 50% to 80%, with better outcomes associated with reversal of the underlying immunocompromise or predisposing condition.[1]

ASPERGILLOSIS

Aspergillus spp are ubiquitous in the environment and have a worldwide distribution. Although typically found as saprophytes in nature, they have been identified as transient and commensal organisms in humans. There are more than 600 species of *Aspergillus* identified including *Aspergillus fumigatus*, *Aspergillus flavus*, *Aspergillus niger*, and *Aspergillus terreus*. Together, *Aspergillus* spp compromise the second most common cause of invasive fungal disease in immunocompromised patients, of which *A fumigatus* is the most commonly identified species. The pathogenicity of *Aspergillus* is correlated to smaller conidial size facilitating inhalation and penetration, and blunting host defenses including opsonization and complement activation.[32] Although rare, upper and lower GI tract infection caused by invasive aspergillosis have been described, as either primary sites of tissue invasion or as sequelae from disseminated disease because of hematogenous spread.[33] Initially, the infection may be asymptomatic or have nonspecific manifestations depending on the site of involvement. Fever can be present, but is often blunted in the immunocompromised setting. Classic manifestations may include abdominal pain/cramps, rectal bleeding or hematemesis, and diarrhea. Autopsies of patients with GI invasive aspergillosis noted mucosal invasion extending to the muscularis and vascular invasion, with resultant thrombosis and infarction. Sequelae include hemorrhage, hollow viscus perforation, and peritonitis, potentially as a polymicrobial infectious process. The diagnosis of GI aspergillosis remains elusive and is difficult to establish. Similar to *Candida* infections, nonculture-based diagnostic tests from the blood are seeing increased use. Serum galactomannan, a fungal cell wall component found in several molds, such as *Aspergillus*, also is detected in the blood and may be useful as an adjunct diagnostic test. Sensitivity and specificity vary markedly between studies, ranging from 91.3% and 71.7%, respectively,[34] to 20% to 60%.

The management of aspergillosis is a combination of medical therapy and surgical control. Triazole antifungals, such as voriconazole, posaconazole, and isavuconazonium sulfate, have excellent activity against *Aspergillus* spp and comprise first-line therapeutic recommendations. Alternative recommendations include the polyene class of antifungals, specifically liposomal amphotericin B formulations dosed at 5 mg/kg/d.[7,35] As with other mold infections, long-term survival is contingent on control of the acute infection and rapid reversal of the underlying immunosuppression (see **Table 3**).

CRYPTOCOCCOSIS

Cryptococcosis remains a clinically important disease in immunocompetent and immunosuppressed individuals. An infection by an encapsulated yeast, it is best recognized by the species *Cryptococcus neoformans*, which remains the second most common fungal infection in patients living with AIDS. *C neoformans* has a worldwide distribution. Cryptococcosis is also increasingly caused by a second species complex, *Cryptococcus gattii*, typically found in tropical and subtropical areas of the world, but more recently (perhaps with global warming) in the oceanic climates of California and the Pacific Northwest. Typically, these fungi are found in soil, decaying biomatter, or bird droppings. Infection is usually acquired through inhalation of the cryptococcal organisms, which then produces a pulmonary infection (pneumonia) or can progress to a more disseminated extrapulmonary disease, the most well-known of which includes meningitis. Cryptococcosis can also occur in immunocompetent hosts, although it is primarily seen in immunosuppressed individuals. Specific risk factors include individuals with AIDS, cirrhotic liver disease, and those who have undergone organ transplantation.[36,37] Isolated GI cryptococcosis is rarely reported in the literature but can occur throughout the GI tract and has manifestations that vary depending on the location of involvement. GI cryptococcosis frequently occurs concomitantly with disseminated disease. Fever and constitutional symptoms are commonly described. Lower GI tract disease can present as chronic abdominal pain with or without diarrhea. Oropharyngeal and esophageal disease is characterized by ulcerations of the mucosa and destructive, tumorlike masses. Gastric, small bowel, and colonic disease may have a mixed appearance of ulcerative lesions and focal, nodular lesions representing cryptococcomas.[38,39] Diagnosis is confirmed by cryptococcal antigen in the serum, peritoneal fluid, or cerebrospinal fluid and is a rapid and useful test with high sensitivity and specificity. It is always important to rule out cryptococcal meningoencephalitis in disseminated disease.

Treatment of GI cryptococcosis typically falls under the category of nonmeningeal and nonpulmonary cryptococcosis and, for all intents and purposes, is treated in the same manner as central nervous system disease. Management involves induction therapy with lipid formulation amphotericin B (5 mg/kg/d) in combination with flucytosine, 100 mg/kg/d divided into four doses. Alternatively, high-dose fluconazole, 800 mg daily, is used in conjunction with flucytosine in situations where amphotericin B intolerance or toxicity occurs. In situations where patients are unable to receive either amphotericin B or flucytosine, higher doses of fluconazole up to 1200 mg per day may also be used.[40] Duration of therapy is dependent on underlying risk factors for each patient. In non-HIV and nontransplant patients the recommendation is a 4-week course of induction. Following induction, the recommended treatment for consolidation is fluconazole, 400 mg daily for 8 weeks, followed by 200 mg daily afterward for long-term maintenance or secondary prophylaxis (see **Table 3**). Discontinuation of maintenance therapy is contingent on reversal of underlying immunosuppression in immunocompromised hosts.

HISTOPLASMOSIS

H capsulatum is a dimorphic fungus with a worldwide distribution and represents one of the most common causes of endemic mycoses within the United States. Its range spans from the Gulf Coast to the Great Lakes and the southeastern United States. It is commonly isolated from soil particularly in association with bird and bat droppings; decaying organic matter and detritus; and caves, chicken coops, and other bird roosts. Both immunocompetent and immunocompromised individuals develop symptomatic disease, although patients with AIDS or other immunocompromise may develop more progressive or disseminated disease.[41] The clinical syndromes described with histoplasmosis include acute self-limited pneumonia, chronic pulmonary histoplasmosis, and disseminated histoplasmosis. Acute symptoms in immunocompetent hosts include fever, headaches, chills, cough, and chest pains. Disseminated disease in the setting of immunocompromise can have a more acute and severe presentation with associated shock, respiratory and renal failure, and disseminated intravascular coagulation.[42] GI involvement is identified in approximately 70% of autopsy studies in the setting of disseminated disease. GI histoplasmosis typically develops as sequelae from hematogenous spread in disseminated disease and may involve any point of the GI tract from the mouth to anus. Additional symptoms associated with GI histoplasmosis include abdominal pain, bleeding, and diarrhea. Manifestations in the oropharynx are characterized by focal granulomatous lesions causing deep ulcerations. In the remainder of the GI tract, the sites commonly involved are the terminal ileum and descending colon.[43] Findings in the lower GI tract include erythema, ulcerations, plaques, strictures, subcentimetric nodular lesions, or large masses. Complications of disease may depend on sites of involvement and can include bowel obstruction, perforation, and peritonitis.[41] Computed tomography scans of the abdomen may also demonstrate hepatosplenomegaly with or without lesions, and generalized lymphadenopathy. Diagnosis of disseminated histoplasmosis depends on visualization of fungus within well-formed granulomas on biopsy and in addition to isolation from culture. Serum and urine antigen testing for *H capsulatum* are noninvasive tests that have a sensitivity of 95% in the setting of disseminated histoplasmosis.[44] Antibody against *H capsulatum* can help diagnose chronic infections, whereas titers greater than or equal to 1:32 or a four-fold rise in antibody titer in acute to convalescent serum are evidence of active infection.

Survival depends on prompt diagnosis and the initiation of effective therapy.[43] Amphotericin B remains the drug of choice for fulminant and disseminated disease, dosed at 3 to 5 mg/kg/d for liposomal formulations and continued for at least 2 weeks. Itraconazole, 200 mg twice a day, remains the standard for long-term maintenance therapy following initial amphotericin B treatment (see **Table 3**). In patients without underlying immunocompromise, total duration of therapy can be as long as 12 months. Because of high rates of relapse in more than 90% of cases, indefinite suppressive therapy with antifungals is recommended in patients with AIDS until CD4 count has recovered to more than 200 cells/μL and has been sustained for more than a year.

BLASTOMYCOSIS

Blastomyces dermatitidis is a dimorphic yeast that is an uncommon cause of endemic mycoses within the United States. As with *H capsulatum*, it is found worldwide and within the eastern half of the United States, particularly the Mississippi and Ohio river valleys and the Great Lakes. Symptomatology of blastomycosis is dependent on immune status because half of immunocompetent hosts with infection have subclinical or mild disease. In contrast, infections in immunocompromised and high-risk persons are prone to developing progressive and disseminated disease. Most cases of blastomycosis are primarily pulmonary or cutaneous disease following inhalation or inoculation of spores. It generally produces symptoms resembling influenza or a community-acquired bacterial pneumonia in the acute setting. GI disease is rare and thought to occur secondary to hematogenous dissemination. GI blastomycosis manifests as ulcerative lesions of the proximal GI tract especially the oropharynx; more distal GI involvement is rare. Diagnosis of GI blastomycosis requires the isolation of *B dermatitidis* by culture or histopathologic evaluation of suspected lesions, visualized as broad-based budding yeast. Adjunctive testing with serologic antibody and serum and urinary antigen testing have sensitivities and specificities of more than 90%.[45] Antifungal treatment should be considered in all infected individuals to prevent disseminated disease, even in immunocompetent patients.[46] Itraconazole capsules are used to treat mild to moderate disease, dosed at 300 mg once or twice daily for a duration of 6 to 12 months (see **Table 3**). For more severe disease, lipid formulations of amphotericin B dosed at 3 to 5 mg/kg/d is recommended for the first 1 to 2 weeks or until clinical improvement, then transitioning to oral itraconazole capsules.

COCCIDIOIDOMYCOSIS

Coccidioidomycosis, or San Joaquin Valley fever, is an infection caused by the dimorphic fungi *C immitis* and *Coccidioides posadasii* and represents the third major endemic mycosis seen in the United States. Distributed throughout the western hemisphere, *Coccidioides* spp in North America are commonly found in the southwestern United States and northern Mexico. The route of exposure and infection is via the inhalation of arthroconidia, initially causing pulmonary disease, which is the primary manifestation. Extrapulmonary or disseminated disease is uncommon and represents less than 5% of infections.[47] Risk factors for dissemination include pregnancy; age older than 50 years; being of Philippine, Asian, or African descent; or with underlying immunosuppression, especially HIV-positive/AIDS. GI coccidioidomycosis is rare and is primarily described in the literature in case reports. Manifestations range from focal inflammation with the presence of nodular lesions on intestinal mucosa, perforation or bowel obstruction, and peritoneal disease.[48] Diagnosis is made after visualization of hyphae in affected tissues or from cultures. Adjunctive tests include serologic assays for *Coccidioides* antibody and antigen testing. Treatment of coccidioidomycosis includes itraconazole, posaconazole, or fluconazole. Fluconazole is administered at dosages of 800 to 1000 mg/d and itraconazole at 200 mg two to three times per day. Liposomal amphotericin B can also be used in cases of disseminated infection at doses of 5 mg/kg daily (see **Table 3**). Treatment courses can range from 3 to 6 months or even longer, depending on extent of disease and concomitant dissemination.

CLINICS CARE POINTS

- Most common fungal infection in humans remains Candida spp.
- The diagnosis of many fungal infections, especially those that are systemic remains hampered due to poor testing and assays.
- In recent years, there has been a shift of susceptible organisms such as C. *albicans*, to the more resistant C. *glabrata*, and more recently C. *auris*.
- Due to diagnostic delays, initiation of approriate antifungal therapy is also delayed, which increases the morbidity and mortality of many fungal infections.

DISCLOSURE

A. Chao: No conflict of interest. J.A. Vazquez: Speaker Bureau for Astellas; Consultant for Cidara, F2G, and Amplyx.

REFERENCES

1. Turner JH, Soudry E, Nayak JV, et al. Survival outcomes in acute invasive fungal sinusitis: a systematic review and quantitative synthesis of published evidence. Laryngoscope 2013;123(5):1112–8.
2. Bodey GP, Buckley M, Sathe YS, et al. Quantitative relationships between circulating leukocytes and infection in patients with acute leukemia. Ann Intern Med 1966;64(2):328–40.
3. Kontoyiannis DP, Lewis RE. Agents of Mucormycosis and Entomophthoramycosis. In: Bennet J, Dolin R, Blaser MJ, editors. Principles and Practice of Infectious Disease, Vol 2, 9th Edition. Philadelphia: Elsevier; 2020. p. 3117–30.
4. Turina M, Fry DE, Polk HC. Acute hyperglycemia and the innate immune system: clinical, cellular, and molecular aspects. Crit Care Med 2005;33(7):1624–33.
5. Hostetter MK. Handicaps to host defense. Effects of hyperglycemia on C3 and *Candida albicans*. Diabetes 1990;39(3):271–5.

6. Liu M, Spellberg B, Phan QT, et al. The endothelial cell receptor GRP78 is required for mucormycosis pathogenesis in diabetic mice. J Clin Invest 2010; 120(6):1914–24.

7. Davoudi S, Kumar VA, Jiang Y, et al. Invasive mould sinusitis in patients with haematological malignancies: a 10 year single-centre study. J Antimicrob Chemother 2015;70(10):2899–905.

8. Auchtung TA, Fofanova TY, Stewart CJ, et al. Investigating colonization of the healthy adult gastrointestinal tract by fungi. mSphere 2018;3(2):e00092-18.

9. Perea S, Patterson TF. Antifungal resistance in pathogenic fungi. Clin Infect Dis 2002;35(9):1073–80.

10. Pfeiffer CD, Samsa GP, Schell WA, et al. Quantitation of *Candida* CFU in initial positive blood cultures. J Clin Microbiol 2011;49(8):2879–83.

11. Marklein G, Josten M, Klanke U, et al. Matrix-assisted laser desorption ionization-time of flight mass spectrometry for fast and reliable identification of clinical yeast isolates. J Clin Microbiol 2009;47(9):2912–7.

12. Pulcrano G, Iula DV, Vollaro A, et al. Rapid and reliable MALDI-TOF mass spectrometry identification of *Candida* non-albicans isolates from bloodstream infections. J Microbiol Methods 2013;94(3):262–6.

13. Clancy CJ, Nguyen MH. Finding the "missing 50%" of invasive candidiasis: how nonculture diagnostics will improve understanding of disease spectrum and transform patient care. Clin Infect Dis 2013;56(9):1284–92.

14. Obayashi T, Yoshida M, Mori T, et al. Plasma (1–>3)-beta-D-glucan measurement in diagnosis of invasive deep mycosis and fungal febrile episodes. Lancet 1995; 345(8941):17–20.

15. Karageorgopoulos DE, Vouloumanou EK, Ntziora F, et al. β-D-glucan assay for the diagnosis of invasive fungal infections: a meta-analysis. Clin Infect Dis 2011;52(6):750–70.

16. Odds FC. Candida and candidosis. London: Bailliere; 1988.

17. Smith JM, Meech RJ. The polymicrobial nature of oropharyngeal thrush. N Z Med J 1984;97(756):335–6.

18. Pons V, Greenspan D, Lozada-Nur F, et al. Oropharyngeal candidiasis in patients with AIDS: randomized comparison of fluconazole versus nystatin oral suspensions. Clin Infect Dis 1997;24(6):1204–7.

19. Meunier F, Aoun M, Gerard M. Therapy for oropharyngeal candidiasis in the immunocompromised host: a randomized double-blind study of fluconazole vs. ketoconazole. Rev Infect Dis 1990;12(Suppl 3):S364–8.

20. Hughes WT, Bartley DL, Patterson GG, et al. Ketoconazole and candidiasis: a controlled study. J Infect Dis 1983;147(6):1060–3.

21. Vermeersch B, Rysselaere M, Dekeyser K, et al. Fungal colonization of the esophagus. Am J Gastroenterol 1989;84(9):1079–83.

22. Kodsi BE, Wickremesinghe C, Kozinn PJ, Iswara K, Goldberg PK. Candida esophagitis: a prospective study of 27 cases. Gastroenterology 1976 Nov; 71(5):715–9.

23. Martins MD, Lozano-Chiu M, Rex JH. Declining rates of oropharyngeal candidiasis and carriage of *Candida albicans* associated with trends toward reduced rates of carriage of fluconazole-resistant *C. albicans* in human immunodeficiency virus-infected patients. Clin Infect Dis 1998;27(5):1291–4.

24. Gorschlüter M, Mey U, Strehl J, et al. Invasive fungal infections in neutropenic enterocolitis: a systematic analysis of pathogens, incidence, treatment and mortality in adult patients. BMC Infect Dis 2006;6:35.

25. Hughes WT. Systemic candidiasis: a study of 109 fatal cases. Pediatr Infect Dis 1982;1(1):11–8.

26. Eras P, Goldstein MJ, Sherlock P. Candida infection of the gastrointestinal tract. Medicine (Baltimore) 1972;51(5):367–79.
27. Coggins SA, Wynn JL, Weitkamp JH. Infectious causes of necrotizing enterocolitis. Clin Perinatol 2015;42(1):133–54, ix.
28. Michael RC, Michael JS, Ashbee RH, et al. Mycological profile of fungal sinusitis: an audit of specimens over a 7-year period in a tertiary care hospital in Tamil Nadu. Indian J Pathol Microbiol 2008;51(4):493–6.
29. Lanternier F, Dannaoui E, Morizot G, et al. A global analysis of mucormycosis in France: the RetroZygo Study (2005-2007). Clin Infect Dis 2012;54(Suppl 1): S35–43.
30. Petrikkos G, Skiada A, Lortholary O, et al. Epidemiology and clinical manifestations of mucormycosis. Clin Infect Dis 2012;54(Suppl 1):S23–34.
31. Neame P, Rayner D. Mucormycosis. A report on twenty-two cases. Arch Pathol 1960;70:261–8.
32. Dagenais TR, Keller NP. Pathogenesis of *Aspergillus fumigatus* in invasive aspergillosis. Clin Microbiol Rev 2009;22(3):447–65.
33. Kami M, Hori A, Takaue Y, et al. The gastrointestinal tract is a common target of invasive aspergillosis in patients receiving cytotoxic chemotherapy for hematological malignancy. Clin Infect Dis 2002;35(1):105–6 [author reply: 106–7].
34. Choi SH, Kang ES, Eo H, et al. Aspergillus galactomannan antigen assay and invasive aspergillosis in pediatric cancer patients and hematopoietic stem cell transplant recipients. Pediatr Blood Cancer 2013;60(2):316–22.
35. Chen CY, Sheng WH, Cheng A, et al. Invasive fungal sinusitis in patients with hematological malignancy: 15 years experience in a single university hospital in Taiwan. BMC Infect Dis 2011;11:250.
36. La Hoz RM, Pappas PG. Cryptococcal infections: changing epidemiology and implications for therapy. Drugs 2013;73(6):495–504.
37. Singh N, Husain S, De Vera M, et al. *Cryptococcus neoformans* infection in patients with cirrhosis, including liver transplant candidates. Medicine (Baltimore) 2004;83(3):188–92.
38. Washington K, Gottfried MR, Wilson ML. Gastrointestinal cryptococcosis. Mod Pathol 1991;4(6):707–11.
39. Park WB, Choe YJ, Lee KD, et al. Spontaneous cryptococcal peritonitis in patients with liver cirrhosis. Am J Med 2006;119(2):169–71.
40. Perfect JR, Dismukes WE, Dromer F, et al. Clinical practice guidelines for the management of cryptococcal disease: 2010 update by the Infectious Diseases Society of America. Clin Infect Dis 2010;50(3):291–322.
41. Wheat J, Hafner R, Korzun AH, et al. Itraconazole treatment of disseminated histoplasmosis in patients with the acquired immunodeficiency syndrome. AIDS Clinical Trial Group. Am J Med 1995;98(4):336–42.
42. Wheat LJ, Slama TG, Zeckel ML. Histoplasmosis in the acquired immune deficiency syndrome. Am J Med 1985;78(2):203–10.
43. Kahi CJ, Wheat LJ, Allen SD, et al. Gastrointestinal histoplasmosis. Am J Gastroenterol 2005;100(1):220–31.
44. Hage CA, Ribes JA, Wengenack NL, et al. A multicenter evaluation of tests for diagnosis of histoplasmosis. Clin Infect Dis 2011;53(5):448–54.
45. Richer SM, Smedema ML, Durkin MM, et al. Development of a highly sensitive and specific blastomycosis antibody enzyme immunoassay using *Blastomyces dermatitidis* surface protein BAD-1. Clin Vaccin Immunol 2014;21(2): 143–6.

46. Chapman SW, Dismukes WE, Proia LA, et al. Clinical practice guidelines for the management of blastomycosis: 2008 update by the Infectious Diseases Society of America. Clin Infect Dis 2008;46(12):1801–12.
47. Kirkland TN, Fierer J. Coccidioidomycosis: a reemerging infectious disease. Emerg Infect Dis 1996;2(3):192–9.
48. Malik U, Cheema H, Kandikatla R, et al. Disseminated coccidioidomycosis presenting as carcinomatosis peritonei and intestinal coccidioidomycosis in a patient with HIV. Case Rep Gastroenterol 2017;11(1):114–9.

Helicobacter pylori Infection

Jaehoon Cho, MD[a,1], Akriti Prashar, PhD[b,c,1],
Nicola L. Jones, MD, PhD, FRCPC[b,c,d], Steven F. Moss, MD[a,*]

KEYWORDS

- *Helicobacter pylori* • Peptic ulcer • Gastric cancer • Microbial pathogenesis
- Diagnosis • Antibiotic resistance

KEY POINTS

- *Helicobacter pylori* infection is the major cause of gastric cancer, gastric lymphoma, and peptic ulcer disease, and is associated with immune thrombocytopenic purpura and iron deficiency anemia.
- *H pylori* is a major public health concern given its high global prevalence.
- The pathogenesis of *H pylori*–related disease involves complex microbial-epithelial interactions affecting epithelial cell function and evasion of host defense mechanisms to allow persistent colonization.
- Increasing antibiotic resistance has led to bismuth-based quadruple therapy becoming the initial treatment of choice for *H pylori* eradication.
- If initial therapy fails, alternative regimens should be selected based on knowledge of population and patient-specific antibiotic susceptibility profiling.

INTRODUCTION

Helicobacter pylori is a common pathogen that is responsible for much gastrointestinal morbidity worldwide. The discovery of the organism and its eradication by combination antibiotic therapy unveiled its crucial role in the development of gastritis and peptic ulcer disease, and subsequently in gastric carcinoma, and gastric mucosal–associated lymphoid tissue (MALT) lymphoma. In 1994, the World Health Organization classified *H pylori* as a definite (class 1) carcinogen because of its strong association with gastric cancer. Gastric cancer is the third leading cause of cancer death and the

Grant support: None.
[a] Division of Gastroenterology, Brown University, 593 Eddy Street, POB 240, Providence, RI 02903, USA; [b] Department of Gastroenterology, Hepatology and Nutrition, University of Toronto, The Hospital for Sick Children, 555 University Avenue, Toronto, Ontario M5G 1X8, Canada; [c] Cell Biology Program, The Hospital for Sick Children, 686 Bay Street, Toronto, Ontario M5G0A4, Canada; [d] Department of Paediatrics, University of Toronto, Toronto, Ontario, Canada
[1] Joint co–first authors.
* Corresponding author.
E-mail address: Steven_Moss@brown.edu

Gastroenterol Clin N Am 50 (2021) 261–282
https://doi.org/10.1016/j.gtc.2021.02.001
0889-8553/21/© 2021 Elsevier Inc. All rights reserved.

fifth most frequently diagnosed cancer.[1] Because most gastric cancers are attributable to H pylori infection, this organism has become an important public health concern, especially in the developing world, where infection is most prevalent.

EPIDEMIOLOGY

The prevalence of H pylori infection exceeds 50% in many developing countries, although it is generally declining in fully developed regions. In a recent meta-analysis, Africa had the highest pooled prevalence (70.1%), followed by Latin America (63.4%), and Asia (54.7%). North America had one of the lowest prevalence rates of 37.1%.[2]

In industrialized nations, H pylori infection is most common in the elderly. This finding is not thought to result from continuing ongoing exposure but from a birth cohort effect back to childhood acquisition at times of very high H pylori transmission.

Within the United States, H pylori infection is more common and most prevalent in Hispanic and Native American people, followed by black people and white people,[3,4] likely related largely to socioeconomic factors. In Canada, indigenous communities have a disproportionate health burden related to H pylori infection.[5] Within more homogenous populations, such as Korea and China, significant declines in prevalence have been associated with improvement in socioeconomic conditions.[6]

TRANSMISSION

Person-to-person infection is the usual route of transmission, given studies showing evidence of increased risk for infection when living in close quarters with those already affected, such as a spouse or a family member.[7,8] Risk of infection is particularly linked to childhood living conditions: it increases with the number of siblings and degree of crowding, especially when children share a bed, and with living in homes lacking a bathroom or indoor toilet.[9]

Person-to-person transmission of H pylori has been postulated to occur by multiple routes. The fecal-oral and oral-oral routes are the most likely because H pylori DNA has been detected in human feces, saliva, and supragingival plaque.[10,11] However, the bacterium has occasionally been identified in untreated water sources and raw vegetables, suggesting that water and uncooked food sources could be an environmental reservoir for the bacterium, especially in countries with suboptimal sanitation.[8]

BASIC MICROBIOLOGY

H pylori are flagellated, gram-negative bacteria with a characteristic spiral shape. However, in culture, they can also exist in a coccoid form, typically associated with a stationary phase of growth or a response to stressful conditions.[12]

H pylori can be isolated from patient biopsies but are not easy to culture. Laboratory-adapted strains grow well at microaerophilic conditions, with optimal growth occurring at 37°C, requiring humidity and a neutral pH.[13] Growth in culture needs specialized media (eg, Columbia or Brucella agar), supplemented with horse or sheep blood. The bacteria grow as small, translucent, smooth colonies that take 3 to 4 days to appear. Liquid media for culturing includes Brucella, Muller-Hinton, and brain heart infusion broth with 2% to 10% serum.[13]

H pylori exhibits high genetic diversity. Strains are subtyped based on the expression of 2 virulence factors: the vacuolating cytotoxin A (VacA) and the cytotoxin-associated gene A (CAGA). All H pylori strains have the vacA gene but genetic differences exist based on variations in the signal (s1/s2), middle (m1/m2), and intermediate (i1/i2) regions of the gene, with s1i1 variants being more pathogenic[14] (**Fig.1**). Significant variation also exists in the 3′ repeat region of the *cagA* gene, which is used to broadly group *H pylori* strains into Western and East Asian subtypes (**Fig.2**). The East Asian subtype is associated with gastric cancer.[15] Unlike the *vacA* gene, not all strains have the *cagA* gene. Presence of both toxins leads to more severe disease outcomes.

CHARACTERISTICS VITAL TO ESTABLISHING PERSISTENT INFECTION
Surviving Harsh Conditions in the Stomach

The central adaptation allowing *H pylori* to survive and persist in the stomach is its ability to synthesize ammonia, which maintains a neutral cytoplasmic and periplasmic pH. The enzyme urease encoded by the *ureA* gene is the most critical component of this response.[16] The hydrogen-gated urea channel, UreI, located in the bacterial inner membrane, transports host-generated urea into the bacterial cytosol, where it gets hydrolyzed into ammonia and carbonate, and buffers the pH.[16] Importantly, presence of both urease and the *ureI* gene is critical for colonization because bacterial strains lacking these are avirulent in animal models.[16] Urease is not only important for early colonization; its continuous expression is also critical for maintaining a chronic infection. Inhibiting urease production after an initial 2 weeks of colonization led to bacterial clearance within 7 days.[17] Furthermore, urease-positive escape mutants were isolated after the long-term infection, showing the strong selective pressure on the bacteria to continue producing urease during colonization.[17] *H pylori* can also produce ammonia using urea-independent mechanisms by hydrolyzing amides to ammonia.[18]

 H pylori acid responsiveness is also controlled by metal ion transcription regulators (nickel response regulator NikR and ferric uptake regulator Fur), and an acid response 2-component system (ArsRS).[18] Recent work with fluorescent *ureA* transcriptional reporters showed that a both NikR and ArsRS are required for the maximal transcription of *ureA*.[19] NikR maintains nickel homeostasis and regulates bacterial uptake of nickel, a cofactor for urease activity. It also directly controls the expression of urease, causing a NikR-dependent upregulation of *ureA* transcription in response to low pH.[20] ΔNikR strains are impaired in colonizing mice. In addition to iron uptake, Fur also acts as a

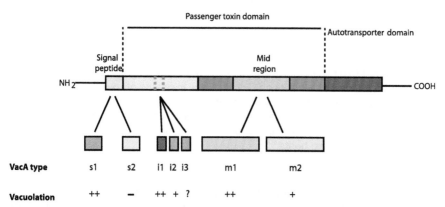

Fig. 1. *vacA* gene structure and allelic diversity. The signal peptide and the autotransporter domain allow the toxin to cross the bacterial inner and outer membranes, respectively. The passenger toxin domain encodes for the 2 subunits of the VacA toxin. Significant genetic diversity exists in the signal (s), intermediate (i) and middle regions (m) regions of the gene. Different variants are associated with different vacuolating abilities and clinical outcomes.

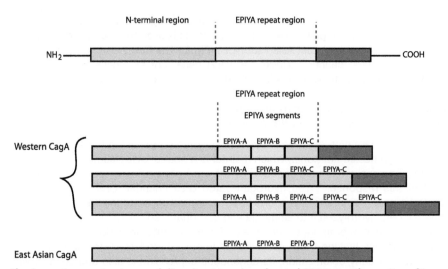

Fig. 2. *cagA* gene structure and diversity. C terminus–located EPIYA motifs are sites of tyrosine phosphorylation. The EPIYA repeat region contains the conserved EPIYA-A and EPIYA-B segments and the EPIYA-D segment specific to the East Asian CagA variant. The Western CagA strains contain variable numbers of EPIYA-C segments.

major regulator of acid-responsive gene expression, including *ureA* expression[21] and ArsRS transcription,[22] and is important for *H pylori* infection in mice and gerbils.[23]

Morphology and Motility

In the gastric environment, *H pylori* must rapidly move to more neutral gastric mucosa, usually within 15 μm of the gastric epithelium, or deep within the gastric glands.[24] A characteristic helical shape, along with flagellar motility, allows *H pylori* to quickly move through the mucus layer by a corkscrew mechanism.[25] Spiral shape is achieved by the coordinated activity of several cell shape–determining proteins that modify the bacterial peptidoglycan, or act as scaffolding proteins. A recent genome-wide screen of *H pylori* shape mutants identified 28 genes that regulate different parameters of bacterial shape.[26] Loss of helical shape decreases swimming speed, and increases the number of immobilized bacteria, facilitating their clearance during mucin removal.[27]

H pylori has 1 to 6 flagella, localized at one of the bacterial poles, allowing rapid bacterial penetration of the mucus layer. The increase in gastric pH by urease activity aids in this process by reducing the viscoelasticity of mucins, decreasing the resistance to bacterial movement. *H pylori* speed correlates with flagella numbers.[27] Compared with *H pylori* mutant strains with no or nonfunctional flagella, motile bacteria are more efficient in infecting hosts.[27]

Chemotaxis

Movement of *H pylori* from lumen to mucosa occurs when chemotactic signals are sensed through the transducerlike chemoreceptor proteins (TlpA, TlpB, TlpC, TlpD).[24] These then transmit signals to the Che histidine kinase family members that regulate flagellar movement. *H pylori* strains lacking tlpA/D receptors have a 100-fold decreased survival in mouse models.[28] TlpB also senses hydrochloric acid, and ΔtlpB strains are impaired in colonizing mice.[29] Interestingly, TlpB also senses a chemoattractant. It binds to urea with high affinity and can recognize nanomolar concentrations of urea released by epithelial cells.[28] Mice infected with Δ*tlpB* strains do not show a defect in colonization; however, they are impaired at 6 weeks, suggesting that this TlpB-urea chemoattractant response is important for bacterial persistence.[28] Supporting this, TlpB-dependent migration of *H pylori* to sites of damage in murine gastric organoids was recently shown to limit damage repair.[30]

Attachment and Invasion Mechanisms

Once the bacteria penetrate the mucus layer, attachment to the gastric epithelial cells allows *H pylori* to escape removal by host clearance mechanisms and use the type IV secretion system (T4SS) to inject bacterial proteins directly into host cells. Attachment occurs through binding of bacterial cell surface proteins with their cognate receptors on the host cell membranes. The blood group antigen binding adhesin (BabA) and the sialic acid-binding adhesin (SabA) bind to Lewis b, and Lewis X and Lewis a antigens, respectively.[15] Other *H pylori* surface proteins important for adhesion include the adherence-associated lipoproteins AlpA and AlpB and the outer inflammatory protein A (OipA).[15] Although both AlpA and AlpB bind to laminin in vitro, the host cell ligands of these adhesins are not yet known. *H pylori* attachment is also mediated by the outer membrane adhesin, *Helicobacter* outer membrane protein Q (HopQ), binding to host epithelial carcinoembryonic antigen (CEA)–related cell adhesion molecules (CEA-CAMs).[31] This HopQ-CEACAM interaction allows cytotoxin-associated gene A (CagA) translocation into epithelial cells, resulting in secretion of inflammatory cytokine interleukin (IL)-8.[31] HopQ-deficient *H pylori* strains cannot colonize or produce inflammation.

PATHOGENESIS
Virulence Determinants

Vacuolating cytotoxin A (VacA)

VacA is a multifunctional toxin secreted by *H pylori* (**Fig.3**) that oligomerizes on the host cell membrane and forms a chloride-selective ion channel, which gets internalized and trafficked to the lysosomes. There it impairs lysosomal maturation, causing enlarged lysosomes.[14] Lysosomal impairment also causes defects in the cellular degradation process of autophagy, which is known to be impaired in several cancers. In addition to effects on endolysosomal machinery, VacA also causes mitochondrial dysfunction.[14] VacA causes a reduction in cellular amino acids, which is sensed by mammalian target of rapamycin complex 1, leading to activation of cellular autophagy.[32] More recently, a direct role for VacA in promoting persistence has been reported. Using mouse-adapted *H pylori* strains expressing the vacuolating s1i1 variant of VacA, intracellular bacteria were observed in vacuoles inside parietal cells where they were protected from antimicrobial treatment, causing infection recrudescence. VacA inhibited the lysosomal calcium channel (TRPML1 (transient receptor potential mucolipin 1)) to cause the formation of this intracellular compartment. Furthermore, treatment with TRPML1 agonists reversed these effects.[33]

Cytotoxin-associated gene A

CagA is the most well-studied *H pylori* virulence factor and targets multiple host pathways to effect cell proliferation, migration, and transformation, all events associated with pathogenesis (**Fig.4**). Its transgenic expression in mice leads to gastric disorder and adenocarcinoma, making it the only known bacterial oncogene. The *cagA* gene is located on a segment of DNA known as the cag pathogenicity island (cagPAI) that also encodes the T4SS, required for toxin translocation. Interaction between the

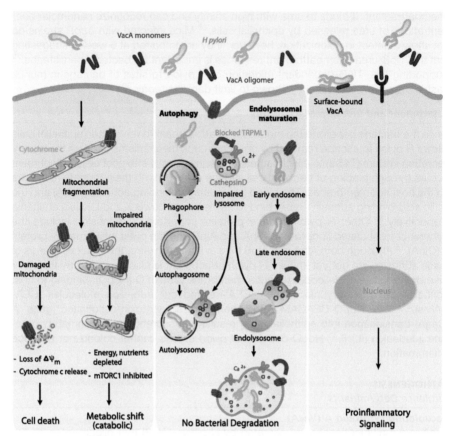

Fig. 3. Effects of VacA on host epithelial cells. Secreted VacA enters host cells, where it causes mitochondrial dysfunction leading to loss of mitochondrial membrane potential and cytochrome c release, leading to apoptotic cell death. Intracellular VacA also impairs the activity of lysosomal calcium channel, TRPML1, and causes the formation of nonfunctional lysosomes, which fail to degrade intracellular bacteria that are targeted by autophagy or by endocytic trafficking. Surface-bound VacA can also trigger proinflammatory immune responses.

T4SS pilus localized CagL and host integrin receptors, namely the $\alpha_5\beta_1$ integrin and a higher affinity interaction with $\alpha_v\beta_6$ facilitate this process.[34] However, interaction with integrins is not essential because CagA translocation was still observed in cells lacking integrin receptors.[35,36] CagA translocation requires HopQ-CEACAM attachment.[32,37] Once injected into host cells via the T4SS, CagA C terminus–located EPIYA (glutamic acid-proline-isoleucine-tyrosine-alanine) motifs are phosphorylated by Src and Abl-c family kinases.[15] Phosphorylated CagA acts as a signaling hub and interacts with host cell proteins, altering host intracellular signaling, rearranging the actin cytoskeleton to cause cell elongation (the characteristic hummingbird phenotype).[15] Cytoskeletal changes also induce cell detachment and motility. Interactions with Crk adaptor protein family members also alters cell motility, proliferation, and spreading.[38] Intracellular CagA also exerts phosphorylation-independent effects. It interacts with proteins responsible for maintaining cellular barrier functions and polarity and causes their mislocalization (described later in relation to damage to the gastric epithelium).

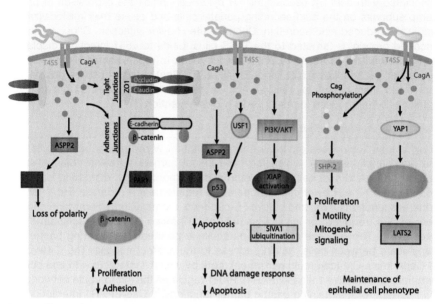

Fig. 4. Effects of CagA on host epithelial cells. *H pylori* translocates CagA directly into the host cells via the T4SS. Intracellular CagA alters multiple cellular pathways in a tyrosine phosphorylation–dependent and tyrosine phosphorylation–independent manner. CagA activity interferes with host cell pathways regulating cell morphology, proliferation, cell polarity, and apoptosis.

CagA also alters cellular stress responses. CagA-dependent downregulation of the proapototic protein Siva1 was observed in animal and infected human tissue.[39] CagA activated the E3 ubiquitin ligase XIAP via the phosphoinositide 3-kinase (PI3K)/AKT pathway, leading to an increase in Siva1 ubiquitination and its subsequent degradation by the proteasome.[39] *H pylori* also impairs cellular DNA damage repair responses by downregulating the expression of the tumor suppressor p53 and one of its main stabilizers, the upstream stimulating factor 1 (USF1), a basic helix-loop-helix transcription factor.[40] *H pylori* infection caused the mislocalization of USF1 away from the nucleus where it is required for DNA damage repair. Severe gastric lesions were observed in USF1-deficient mice after *H pylori* infection, showing its role in carcinogenesis.[41] *H pylori* infection can induce cell proliferation, migration, and epithelial to mesenchymal transition (EMT) by altering the expression of the proto-oncogene lysosomal-associated protein transmembrane 4β (LAPTM4B).[42] *H pylori* also stimulates the Hippo tumor suppressor pathway to interfere with cellular homeostasis. CagA was shown to cause an upregulation of Hippo pathway members, large tumor suppressor 2 (LATS2), and Yes-associated protein 1 (YAP1).[43] Interestingly, activation of this pathway was protective, helping maintain the identity of gastric epithelial cells by controlling the EMT associated with cancer development.

Effect on Acid Secretion

Acute *H pylori* infection causes a usually asymptomatic hypochlorhydria. Chronic infection with an antrum-predominant phenotype is associated with gastrin-dependent acid hypersecretion, whereas a corpus-predominant phenotype is associated with acid hyposecretion.[44] H $pylori$ can inhibit the expression of proton pump subunits on the acid-secreting parietal cells and cause their mislocalization, leading to reduced acid secretion. During acute H $pylori$ infection, CagL, a cagPAI-encoded protein, is targeted to the T4SS pilus, binds to α5β1 integrins, displacing and activating the protease ADAM17, which leads to repression of H+/K+ATPase via activation of nuclear factor kappa B (NF-κB).[45] CagL also binds to the gastrin promoter and alters gastrin expression. Acid secretion is also inhibited by inflammatory cytokine IL-1β produced in response to H $pylori$ infection.[44]

Damage to the Gastric Epithelium

H $pylori$ infection causes gastric barrier dysfunction. H $pylori$ attaches to cells near the tight junctions (TJs), which form the apical barriers between adjacent cells, and uses CagA to alter cell cytoskeleton and cell morphology, disrupting junctional complexes.[46] The H $pylori$ high-temperature requirement A protease (HtrA) targets adherens junctions (AJs) and cleaves E-cadherin, a critical transmembrane component of AJs, required for initial assembly of TJ protein complexes (claudin-8 and occludin).[47] This process increases paracellular permeability, allowing bacteria to translocate between cells, gaining access to the gastric mucosa. The C terminus of CagA has a CM (cag multimerization) motif by which it interacts with and inhibits partitioning-defective 1 kinase (PAR1). PAR1 regulates the microtubule network and is important for maintaining gastric barrier functions.[15] CagA-PAR1 interaction impairs this, leading to cell extrusion from the epithelial monolayer, which can then undergo changes resembling pathogenic EMT. PAR1 also regulates the mitotic spindle in dividing cells, and CagA-dependent effects have been associated with defects in cell division and chromosomal instability. Recently, CagA was shown to interact with apoptosis-stimulating protein of p53 2 (ASPP2), which causes PAR remodeling and loss of cell polarity.[48]

Effect on Stem Cells

H $pylori$ manipulates gastric stem cells and progenitor cells to cause pathogenic transformation. Several studies have reported a CagA-dependent cell dedifferentiation with EMT.[15] CagA can activate Wnt-β catenin-dependent transcription factors that induce cell stemness-associated factors. Studies in infected humans and mice have identified H $pylori$ deep in gastric glands, where they can attach at sites near progenitor or stem cells and grow as surface-associated microcolonies. Here they can stimulate proliferation of Lgr5 (leucine-rich-repeat-containing G-protein-coupled receptor 5)+ stem cells.[49] Interestingly, CagA mutants colonized the glands but did not induce hyperproliferation.[49] Increased oxidative DNA damage, which can lead to pathogenic mutants and cellular reprogramming, has also been reported in Lgr5+ cells in human and mouse tissue infected with H $pylori$. Recent work has shown that this Lrg5 response depends on the R-spondin-3-Wnt signaling pathway in gastric stromal cells, and an intact cag-PAI.[50] H $pylori$ infection also promotes Lrg5+ stem cells differentiation into secretory cells, which produce antimicrobials during infection.[51] In mice, chronic H $pylori$ infection can also stimulate the proliferation of Lrig1 (leucine rich-repeats and immunoglobulin like domain 1)-expressing stem cells in a CagA-dependent manner.[52] These cells form a small subset of stem cells that, in gastric tissue, proliferate in response to injury.[53]

Immune Responses

Activation of NF-κB and downstream IL-8 secretion is one of the hallmarks of the immune response associated with H $pylori$.[15] Several other NF-κB–regulated cytokines, including IL-1β, IL-6, IL-10, and tumor necrosis factor alpha (TNF-α), are also produced during the course of *H pylori* infection. However, some prototypical bacterial ligands that trigger NF-κB activation do not lead to this response in *H pylori* infection. The first line of defense against *H pylori* is the pattern recognition receptors, including Toll-like receptors (TLRs) and nucleotide-binding oligomerization domain (NOD)–like receptors (NLRs) on epithelial and innate immune cells, which recognize pathogen-associated molecular patterns (PAMPS). PAMPS that commonly trigger immune responses include lipopolysaccharide (recognized by TLR4), bacterial flagellin (by TLR5), and bacterial DNA (by TLR9). However, *H pylori* antigens trigger weak TLR responses compared with many other pathogens, with resultant low-level inflammatory responses.[54] Modifications in *H pylori* LPS render it less bioactive than other gram-negative pathogens, with less negative charge so it does not get detected by antimicrobial peptides and escapes TLR detection. *H pylori* flagellin has a mutation in N-terminal TLR5 binding sites, evading detection.[54] However, a TLR5 upregulation in epithelial and immune cells in response to *H pylori* has been reported with CagL acting as a TLR5 activator to control infection, possibly via NF-κB activation.[55]

It was widely accepted that *H pylori*–dependent NF-κB activation was mediated by the recognition of T4SS by NOD1, which is a bacterial peptidoglycan (PG) sensor located in the cytosol of epithelial and immune cells.[15] NOD1 expression is upregulated in gastric epithelial cells in patients with *H pylori*–associated gastritis, and NOD1 polymorphisms are associated with gastric cancer and an increased risk for *H pylori* therapy failure.[56] *H pylori* PG delivered by the T4SS in cagPAI+ strains or by outer membrane vesicles independently of cagPAI activates NOD1.[56] Activated NOD1 interacts with downstream effector RIP2, causing proinflammatory signaling dependent on NF-κB and mitogen-activated protein kinase (MAPK) activation, as well as IRF3/IRF7-dependent type I interferon (IFN) secretion.[56] Interestingly, it was recently shown that, although loss of NOD1 causes a reduction in NF-κB activation and IL-8 production, cytokine production was not eliminated, suggesting the role for an additional pathway.[57] Multiple recent studies have elaborated on the mechanism of *H pylori*–dependent NF-κB activation and identified the *H pylori* ligand necessary for this process. Metabolites produced during the synthesis of the LPS inner heptose core, namely heptose-1,7-bisphosphate (HBP) and β-ADP-heptose, are translocated via the T4SS.[57] These metabolites bind to and activate host α-kinase1 (ALPK1) kinase, which in turn phosphorylates TRAF (tumor necrosis factor receptor associated factor)-interacting protein with forkhead-associated domain (TIFA), causing multimerization and formation of the TIFAsome. This HBP/β-ADP-heptose-ALPK1-TIFA axis activates NF-κB, leading to the canonical downstream signaling, including IL-8 production.[58–60] Collectively, these studies have led to a model where the initial activation of NF-κB by *H pylori* occurs by the ALPK1-TIFA axis, followed by NOD1-dependent signaling.

Chronic *H pylori* infection leads to gastric inflammation mediated by helper type 1 (Th1) and helper type 17 (Th17) T cells, which produce IFN-γ and IL-17 respectively, and T-regulatory cells (Tregs), which promote tolerance.[54] An increase in proinflammatory cytokines (IL-8, IL-1β, TNF-α and IL-6, IL-12) in response to *H pylori* is seen in human biopsy and cell culture models.[56] Studies using murine models have reported higher gastric colonization by *H pylori* when IFN-γ and IL-17 responses are impaired.[56] Collectively, these studies show that proinflammatory cytokines contribute to T-cell response and disorder during *H pylori* infection. NOD1-dependent type I IFN signaling pathways are also involved in generating the Th1 response.

Immune responses are also directly modulated by secreted virulence factors VacA and γ-glutamyl transpeptidase (GGT), which impair T-cell proliferation and differentiation and skew the immune response toward Tregs.[54] GGT prevents T-cell proliferation by regulating cell cycle via cyclin-dependent kinase activity. VacA binds to β2 integrin on T cells and becomes internalized. Cytosolic VacA prevents Ca^{2+}/calmodulin phosphatase calcineurin-dependent nuclear translocation of the transcription factor NFAT (nuclear factor of activated T-cells), blocking IL-2 production.[61] VacA also acts as an immunomodulator by targeting myeloid cells to favor Treg differentiation. It causes an increase in IL-10 and IL-1β expression by macrophages, and a decrease in dendritic cell IL-23. In addition, both VacA and GGT cause a dendritic cell–dependent increase in IL-10 level, leading to differentiation of T cells to Tregs while inhibiting their differentiation to Th1 or Th17 types.[54]

CLINICAL CONSEQUENCES OF *HELICOBACTER PYLORI* INFECTION

Initial infection in childhood is usually asymptomatic, although children may present with nausea, vomiting, and abdominal pain. In almost all cases, this asymptomatic phase is associated with intense gastric inflammation (gastritis) that then persists over a lifetime unless specific antibacterial combination therapy is given. Although most infected individuals do not develop obvious clinical sequelae, peptic ulcers develop in about 10% of infected individuals, and gastric neoplasms eventually result from 1% to 2% of infections, usually consequent to a slowly progressive sequence of gastric mucosal preneoplastic changes marked by atrophic gastritis, intestinal metaplasia, and dysplasia.

The determinants of disease progression in persons infected by *H pylori* are imperfectly understood. Expression of the virulence factors described earlier, CagA and VacA, are linked with increased disease risk. Variations in the geographic distribution of bacterial colonization within the stomach may also determine outcome. For example, an antral-predominant infection is the usual phenotype associated with duodenal ulcer disease, whereas a severe corpus-predominant pangastritis increases the risk of gastric cancer development.[62] Dietary and other environmental cofactors, as well as polymorphisms in cytokine genes and other genes that modulate the gastric inflammatory response to infection, are also of importance in contributing to disease susceptibility following initial infection.[63]

Peptic Ulcers

H pylori is responsible for most cases of peptic (gastric, and especially duodenal) ulcers. *H pylori* eradication is a superior treatment of *H pylori*–positive duodenal ulcers compared with ulcer-healing drugs alone. However, there was no statistically significant difference in gastric ulcer healing between *H pylori* eradication versus ulcer-healing drugs alone.[64] More importantly, *H pylori* infection is responsible for ulcer recurrence. In a meta-analysis of the early randomized studies performed in the 1980s and 1990s, the rate of ulcer recurrence 1 year after initial diagnosis was about 5% in subjects in whom *H pylori* was successfully eradicated, versus about 60% with persistent infection.[65] These convincing results led to the widespread promulgation of clinical guidelines mandating that *H pylori* be tested for, and, if present, eradicated, in all patients with peptic ulcers.[66]

The mechanisms by which *H pylori* predisposes to ulcer formation and recurrence are different in duodenal compared with gastric ulcer disease. In patients with duodenal ulcers, the underlying pathophysiology involves *H pylori* inhibiting gastric antral somatostatin secretion, leading to increased release of the acid-stimulating hormone gastrin and subsequent acid hypersecretion. In contrast, acid secretion tends to be normal or even low in patients with gastric ulcers, compared with uninfected individuals. Interference with host mucosal defenses by the bacterium and/or the associated inflammatory response and direct epithelial cell damage are thought to underlie gastric ulcer pathogenesis.

Gastric Cancer

H pylori is the leading infectious cause of cancer worldwide. Estimates from the World Health Organization in 2018 were that 812,000 new cases of gastric malignancy were attributable to *H pylori* infection, with *H pylori* responsible for 90% of adenocarcinomas arising in the distal (noncardia) stomach, 20% of cardia cancers, and 72% of cases of gastric non-Hodgkin lymphoma.[67] The pathogenesis of *H pylori*–induced gastric cancer involves oxidative stress, DNA damage, apoptosis, and interactions with gastric stem and progenitor cells, as described earlier.

Many clinical trials have been conducted to determine whether eradicating *H pylori* from persons at increased gastric cancer risk will prevent cancer development. In a meta-analysis, *H pylori* eradication has been shown to decrease subsequent gastric cancer development by about 40%, with the greatest benefit seen in populations with the highest *H pylori* prevalences.[68] It should be noted that almost all these trials were conducted in the western Pacific or Central America, where gastric cancer is most prevalent, and it is unclear whether similar benefits would be observed in other regions. However, in a recent retrospective observational study of the United States veterans population, patients who were treated for *H pylori* and had confirmed eradication had a 76% lower incidence of developing noncardia gastric cancer compared with untreated individuals.[69]

H pylori eradication is also beneficial when given after endoscopic mucosal resection of early gastric cancer, decreasing the odds of metachronous cancer development by about 50%.[68] Furthermore, eradicating *H pylori* from first-degree family members of patients with gastric cancer resulted in a 55% reduction in gastric cancer development in a randomized controlled trial from Korea.[70]

Taken together, over the last decade, there has been increasing evidence for the beneficial effects of *H pylori* eradication for the prevention of gastric cancer, at least in populations with high gastric cancer prevalence. This finding has led to the consideration of *H pylori* screening programs in some Asian-Pacific countries. In a pilot program, a mass *H pylori* eradication program was conducted in the Matsu Islands of Taiwan. Adults more than 30 years of age underwent urea breath testing starting in 2004, and eradication therapy was given to those who tested positive. The most recent analysis of this intervention showed a 53% reduction in gastric cancer incidence and 25% reduction in mortality compared with the historical control period (1995–2003), without any obvious detrimental changes.[71]

Gastric Lymphoma

Lymphocytes comprise a large proportion of the inflammatory infiltrate recruited to the stomach by *H pylori* infection. Gastric lymphocyte transformation can give rise to a rare B-cell tumor termed MALT lymphoma. The presenting symptoms may be similar to those of other gastric malignancies (abdominal pain, bleeding, and weight loss). Almost all gastric MALT lymphomas are associated with *H pylori* infection; the standard treatment of the lymphoma is *H pylori* eradication.[72,73] Remarkably, complete remission of the lymphoma after successful eradication of *H pylori* is the norm for low-grade tumors confined to the stomach, the exception being for MALT lymphomas with an AP12-MALT1 fusion protein, which are not responsive to *H pylori* eradication. In patients with MALT lymphoma with negative *H pylori* testing, complete remission of lymphoma has been reported to be achieved with empiric *H pylori* treatment in most patients,[74] suggesting that this should be given for gastric MALT lymphoma regardless of *H pylori* infection status.

Hematological Consequences of Chronic Infection

Iron deficiency is a common adverse health condition, especially in the developing world, and is another clinical manifestation of chronic *H pylori* infection.[75] Eradication of *H pylori* together with oral iron leads to significantly increased hemoglobin, iron, and ferritin levels compared with iron therapy alone.[76] *H pylori* can cause iron deficiency through multiple pathways, including chronic occult bleeding caused by erosions, competition with *H pylori* for dietary iron, hypochlorhydria from destruction of parietal cells, and upregulation of hepcidin from the associated gastric inflammatory response.[77]

Immune thrombocytopenic purpura (ITP) is an autoimmune-mediated acquired disorder characterized by antibody-mediated platelet destruction. An association between *H pylori* and ITP was initially reported in 1998 when significant numbers of patients with ITP who were also infected with *H pylori* had improvements in their platelet count after *H pylori* treatment.[78] This observation has been confirmed in case series and in a recent meta-analysis of a small number of randomized trials.[79] Based on these data, the American Society for Hematology recommends screening for *H pylori* in adults with ITP and treating it in those found to be positive.[80] However, they do not recommend this for children, in whom the benefit seems much weaker.

Other Conditions

A wide variety of diseases and conditions have been studied in relationship to *H pylori* infection, suggesting a possible positive association, including colon, pancreatic, and hepatobiliary cancers; Parkinson disease; diabetes; metabolic syndrome; coronary atherosclerosis; and fatty liver disease.[81] In general, the results of such studies have been inconsistent and with a low level of biological plausibility, but this remains an area of active research.

In Western populations, inverse relations have been described between *H pylori* and certain immune-mediated conditions, including inflammatory bowel disease, celiac disease, eosinophilic esophagitis, and asthma. A postulated underlying mechanism is that *H pylori*–associated gastritis normally promotes regulatory T-cell expansion, with migration of regulatory immune cell populations to extragastric sites, a gastric version of the hygiene hypothesis. These inverse associations and their mechanisms remain controversial. Less controversial, and more consistent, is the inverse relationship described between infection with *H pylori* and reduced risk of esophageal adenocarcinoma.[82] An explanation for how *H pylori* might protect against this cancer is not obvious, because esophageal adenocarcinoma is normally considered a consequence of long-term esophageal acid exposure, with Barrett's esophagus as a precursor lesion.

DIAGNOSIS

Several diagnostic tests are used in clinical practice, each with advantages and disadvantages, depending on the clinical situation (**Table 1**).

Invasive

Invasive tests depend on gastric tissue biopsy and are used when investigating gastric symptoms by upper endoscopy. Endoscopic features of the gastric mucosa, including erythema, nodularity, and ulcers, may suggest underlying infection,[83] but they are not

Table 1
Helicobacter pylori diagnostic tests

Test Modality	Sensitivity (%)	Specificity (%)	Can Assess Antibiotic Sensitivity?	Can Evaluate Virulence Factors?	Accurate in Gastrointestinal Bleeding?
Invasive					
Histology: hematoxylin-eosin	91–100	100	—	—	—
Histology: immunohistochemistry	97–100	100	—	—	—
Rapid urea test	80–100	95–100	—	—	—
Culture	85–95	100	Yes	—	—
Polymerase chain reaction	>95	>95	Yes	Yes	Yes
Noninvasive					
Urea breath test	95	95	—	—	—
Stool antigen	94	97	—	—	—
Serology	91	86	—	Yes	Yes

reliable, and in many instances the endoscopic appearances are entirely normal when there is active infection.

Histology

Histology is the most common initial invasive test for *H pylori* infection in the United States.[84] At least 2 biopsy specimens should be taken from antrum and corpus to maximize the diagnostic yield, especially for patients taking proton pump inhibitors (PPIs), which decrease bacterial numbers and redistribute the bacteria from the antrum to the corpus.[85] Specific histologic features (neutrophil and lymphoplasma-cytic infiltration) suggest the diagnosis, and *H pylori* infection may be confirmed by identifying the organism using standard hematoxylin-eosin staining. However, in many cases, silver stains or immunohistochemistry may be needed to make a definitive diagnosis and increase sensitivity to close to 100%.[86]

Rapid urease test

The rapid urease test (RUT) tests for the presence of *H pylori* in gastric biopsies indirectly, by identification of its urease enzyme activity. Urease hydrolyzes urea to produce ammonia, which increases the pH of the medium and is detected by the RUT. This test is inexpensive, easy to perform, and fast (it can turn positive within minutes) However, it is less sensitive than histology on biopsies with fewer than 10^5 bacteria, such as can occur with antibiotic or acid-suppressive medication usage. False-negative tests are more frequent than false-positive tests for RUT, thus a negative test should not be used to exclude *H pylori*.[87]

Culture

Culturing of *H pylori* has high specificity (close to 100%) but low sensitivity, around 80% in practice. Success can be compromised by environmental factors such as delayed transport, poorly controlled culture temperature, and exposure of the medium to the aerobic environment. Similar to other tests mentioned earlier, culture is affected by use of acid-suppressing medication and low bacterial load. Although it is time consuming and expensive, a major advantage of culturing is the ability to also assess antibiotic sensitivity. With the increase in prevalence of antibiotic-resistant strains, culture may be an important tool in guiding appropriate management after failed H pylori treatment.[88]

Polymerase chain reaction and other molecular tests

Polymerase chain reaction has high sensitivity and specificity (>90%) for diagnosing H pylori in gastric biopsies and is also applicable to saliva, stool, gastric juice, and other specimens. Furthermore, it can potentially evaluate the expression of specific H pylori genes, such as virulence factors and mutations in antibiotic target genes, as indicators of antibiotic sensitivity. Unlike most of the other tests, its sensitivity is not diminished by active gastrointestinal bleeding. Evaluating antibiotic resistance–associated mutations is also now available via next-generation sequencing. With the increased availability and competitive costs of molecular testing for H pylori, and the increased recognition of the importance of resistance testing, it is likely that molecular testing will be increasingly used.

Noninvasive

Diagnosing H pylori can also be done without the cost and inconvenience of endoscopy in adults.

Urea breath test

This is an indirect test of intragastric urease activity via the release of exhaled labeled CO_2. It has high sensitivity and specificity, but it is affected by gastrointestinal bleeding, acid-suppression medication, and antibiotics.[89] Therefore, it is recommended that PPIs be stopped 2 weeks before and antibiotics be discontinued 4 weeks before analysis.

Stool antigen test

This test also has high sensitivity and specificity, especially for the monoclonal antibody–based tests.[90] Similar to breath testing, the diagnostic accuracy of stool antigen testing is influenced by antibiotic and PPI usage, and gastrointestinal bleeding. Similar caveats apply regarding medication cessation before testing. Both the breath and stool test are reliable tests of active infection that can be used to assess the efficacy of H pylori eradication therapy. Both of these tests are noninvasive and convenient enough to be used in pediatric patients, although an aversion to stool handling may make the breath test more attractive for some.

Serology

IgG antibody serology tests are unique among the noninvasive tests in that their accuracy is not affected by gastrointestinal bleeding, antibiotics, or acid-suppression medications. Their major disadvantage is that, after successful treatment of H pylori, antibody levels can remain for a prolonged time. Therefore, they cannot determine active versus past infection. Furthermore, many of the serologic tests in commercial use have low sensitivity and specificity, such that their use is no longer recommended in current clinical guidelines.[91] Antibody testing has the potential to identify the presence of specific H pylori antigens in adults, although this has not yet proved clinically valuable.

Indications for Testing and Treating

H pylori infection is associated with significant clinical comorbidities, as described earlier, although the risk of developing such complications is not predictable.

Therefore, consensus guidelines recommend treating all *H pylori* infection at diagnosis, unless there are extenuating circumstances.[92] In the absence of universal *H pylori* screening, clinicians should be aware of which patients are most likely to benefit from *H pylori* detection and treatment. **Box 1** lists the current indications for *H pylori* testing, based on an amalgamation of 2 recent US guidelines.[91,93]

TREATMENT

Because of its unique intragastric niche and tendency to persistent colonization, successful eradication of *H pylori* requires combination antibiotic therapy, aided by potent acid suppression.[94] Current therapies have mainly been developed empirically, because in vitro susceptibility does not always translate to in vivo effectiveness for this organism.[94]

The standard treatment of *H pylori* infection for many years was a triple therapy consisting of a PPI, clarithromycin, and amoxicillin or metronidazole, given for 7 to 14 days. However, growing resistance to clarithromycin in most regions around the world[95] has reduced the efficacy of this regimen markedly over the last 20 years,[96] such that it is no longer recommended, unless clarithromycin resistance rates are known to be low.[91,97]

Current guidelines recommend using a bismuth-based quadruple therapy for 14 days as first-line therapy, comprising bismuth subsalicylate or subcitrate, tetracycline, metronidazole, and a PPI.[97] This therapy provides greater than 80% successful eradication in clinical practice.[98] If tetracycline is not available or affordable, doxycycline should not be used in its place, because this gives inferior eradication rates. Instead, amoxicillin can be substituted.

Selecting a treatment to prescribe should bismuth quadruple therapy fail is not so straightforward. Levofloxacin-based therapies were initially promising but are now threatened by increasing levofloxacin resistance in many countries.[95] Rifabutin triple therapy (with amoxicillin and a PPI) is a promising alternative[97] because, unlike metronidazole, clarithromycin, and levofloxacin, in vitro resistance to rifabutin (and

---

Box 1
Indications for *Helicobacter pylori* testing

Definite

Current or past gastric/duodenal ulcer

Uninvestigated dyspepsia

Functional (nonulcer) dyspepsia

Gastric mucosa–associated lymphoid tissue lymphoma

After early gastric cancer

First-degree relatives of patients with gastric cancer

Idiopathic thrombocytopenic purpura

Iron deficiency anemia (after exclusion of other causes)

Possible

First-generation immigrants from high-prevalence region

Ethnic groups at high risk for infection

Patients on long-term aspirin/nonsteroidal antiinflammatory drugs

tetracycline and amoxicillin) is rare currently. Resistance to metronidazole, clarithromycin, and levofloxacin is associated with prior use of these drugs in individuals and consumption rate of the antibiotics regionally,[99] so the choice of second-line and subsequent therapy should also take antibiotic history into account.[91] Penicillin allergy is also an important issue because amoxicillin is included in most regimens for refractory cases. Penicillin allergy testing can allow the delisting of this contraindication, because, in most cases, the allergy turns out to be fictional.[91]

Additional information from local and regional antibiotic susceptibility data is also of great help in selecting second-line empiric therapy, although it is rarely available in North America. It is likely that resistance testing for individual patients will become more common in the future, especially after 1 or more failed treatments. Because resistance testing can also be performed from stool samples, this could provide a more affordable and easier alternative to repeating endoscopy to obtain gastric biopsies for this purpose.

Despite appropriate treatment plans with suitable regimens, treatment failures still occur. With these multidrug regimens, the most common cause for failure (if not caused by antibiotic resistance) is from suboptimal adherence to the medications in these complex regimens. Explaining to the patient the rationale for therapy, likely side effects, and emphasizing the need for adherence to the entire regimen are important elements in achieving successful eradication.

In addition, because improvement in symptoms is not a predictable measure of success, and with declining success rates of most treatments, it is recommended to test for cure with a breath or stool test performed at least 1 month after the end of treatment (and off PPIs) to document successful eradication and retreat if necessary.[91]

PEDIATRIC CONSIDERATIONS
Diagnosis

Clinical manifestations of H pylori infection differ between children and adults. Therefore,[100] biopsy-based testing is indicated instead of noninvasive testing for initial diagnosis. Noninvasive testing is only recommended in the setting of chronic immune thrombocytopenia. According to the most recent pediatric guidelines, at least 6 gastric biopsies for bacterial culture, histopathology, RUT, or molecular biopsy-based techniques (eg, real-time polymerase chain reaction) are recommended.[100]

Treatment

Current recommendations are tailored based on the antibiotic resistance in the infecting strains and emphasize adherence to therapy. Therefore, antibiotic sensitivity testing is recommended to tailor treatment, if available. Otherwise, bismuth-based quadruple therapy as first-line therapy is recommended. Triple therapy is restricted for use when infecting strains are sensitive to specific antibiotics. A high-dose PPI, amoxicillin, metronidazole regimen is recommended in cases of bismuth unavailability.[100]

SUMMARY

H pylori infection remains one of the most prevalent infections worldwide, responsible for considerable morbidity and mortality. It is highly adapted to persistently colonize the human stomach and has developed numerous mechanisms to evade host immune responses. The management of H pylori continues to evolve in the face of growing antimicrobial resistance from antibiotic use and overuse. There is growing interest in developing new therapies and incorporating susceptibility testing into treatment algorithms for local and national adoption.

CLINICS CARE POINTS

- The eradication of *H pylori* reduces the risk of gastric cancer development, peptic ulcer recurrence, and also cures most cases of gastric MALT lymphoma.
- *H pylori* can be readily diagnosed through endoscopic biopsies, or non-invasively by urea breath testing or fecal antigen detection. Serology is less accurate, and not recommended.
- Consensus guidelines recommend treating all *H pylori* infection at diagnosis.
- First line therapy comprises 14 days of bismuth subsalicylate or subcitrate, tetracycline, metronidazole, and a proton pump inhibitor.
- Second line therapies should be guided by knowledge of regional or patient-specific antimicrobial resistance patterns. Since clarithromycin and levofloxacin resistance are quite common, these antibiotics should no longer be included in empirically-selected regimens.

DISCLOSURE

S.F. Moss has served on the advisory boards of Redhill Biopharma and Phathom Pharmaceuticals, performs research sponsored by American Molecular Labs, and is a consultant to Takeda. The other authors have nothing to disclose.

REFERENCES

1. Bray F, Ferlay J, Soerjomataram I, et al. Global cancer statistics 2018: GLOBO-CAN estimates of incidence and mortality worldwide for 36 cancers in 185 countries. CA Cancer J Clin 2018;68(6):394–424.
2. Hooi JKY, Lai WY, Ng WK, et al. Global prevalence of helicobacter pylori infection: systematic review and meta-analysis. Gastroenterology 2017;153(2): 420–9.
3. Huerta-Franco MR, Banderas JW, Allsworth JE. Ethnic/racial differences in gastrointestinal symptoms and diagnosis associated with the risk of Helicobacter pylori infection in the US. Clin Exp Gastroenterol 2018;11:39–49.
4. Everhart JE, Kruszon-Moran D, Perez-Perez GI, et al. Seroprevalence and ethnic differences in Helicobacter pylori infection among adults in the United States. J Infect Dis 2000;181(4):1359–63.
5. Colquhoun A, Hannah H, Corriveau A, et al. Gastric cancer in northern canadian populations: a focus on cardia and non-cardia subsites. Cancers (Basel) 2019; 11(4):534.
6. Leja M, Grinberga-Derica I, Bilgilier C, et al. Review: epidemiology of helicobacter pylori infection. Helicobacter 2019;24(Suppl 1):e12635.
7. Weyermann M, Rothenbacher D, Brenner H. Acquisition of Helicobacter pylori infection in early childhood: independent contributions of infected mothers, fathers, and siblings. Am J Gastroenterol 2009;104(1):182–9.
8. Kayali S, Manfredi M, Gaiani F, et al. Helicobacter pylori, transmission routes and recurrence of infection: state of the art. Acta Biomed 2018;89(8-s):72–6.
9. Webb PM, Knight T, Greaves S, et al. Relation between infection with Helicobacter pylori and living conditions in childhood: evidence for person to person transmission in early life. BMJ 1994;308(6931):750–3.

10. Ibrahim A, Ali YBM, Abdel-Aziz A, et al. Helicobacter pylori and enteric parasites co-infection among diarrheic and non-diarrheic Egyptian children: seasonality, estimated risks, and predictive factors. J Parasit Dis 2019;43(2):198–208.

11. Iwai K, Watanabe I, Yamamoto T, et al. Association between Helicobacter pylori infection and dental pulp reservoirs in Japanese adults. BMC Oral Health 2019; 19(1):267.

12. Ierardi E, Losurdo G, Mileti A, et al. The puzzle of coccoid forms of helicobacter pylori: beyond basic science. Antibiotics (Basel) 2020;9(6):293.

13. Kusters JG, van Vliet AH, Kuipers EJ. Pathogenesis of Helicobacter pylori infection. Clin Microbiol Rev 2006;19(3):449–90.

14. Cover TL, Blanke SR. Helicobacter pylori VacA, a paradigm for toxin multifunctionality. Nat Rev Microbiol 2005;3(4):320–32.

15. Takahashi-Kanemitsu A, Knight CT, Hatakeyama M. Molecular anatomy and pathogenic actions of Helicobacter pylori CagA that underpin gastric carcinogenesis. Cell Mol Immunol 2020;17(1):50–63.

16. Sachs G, Weeks DL, Melchers K, et al. The gastric biology of Helicobacter pylori. Annu Rev Physiol 2003;65:349–69.

17. Debowski AW, Walton SM, Chua EG, et al. Helicobacter pylori gene silencing in vivo demonstrates urease is essential for chronic infection. PLoS Pathog 2017;13(6):e1006464.

18. Ansari S, Yamaoka Y. Survival of Helicobacter pylori in gastric acidic territory. Helicobacter 2017;22(4). https://doi.org/10.1111/hel.12386.

19. Carpenter BM, West AL, Gancz H, et al. Crosstalk between the HpArsRS two-component system and HpNikR is necessary for maximal activation of urease transcription. Front Microbiol 2015;6:558.

20. Jones MD, Li Y, Zamble DB. Acid-responsive activity of the Helicobacter pylori metalloregulator NikR. Proc Natl Acad Sci U S A 2018;115(36):8966–71.

21. Lee JS, Choe YH, Lee JH, et al. Helicobacter pylori urease activity is influenced by ferric uptake regulator. Yonsei Med J 2010;51(1):39–44.

22. Roncarati D, Pelliciari S, Doniselli N, et al. Metal-responsive promoter DNA compaction by the ferric uptake regulator. Nat Commun 2016;7:12593.

23. Gancz H, Censini S, Merrell DS. Iron and pH homeostasis intersect at the level of Fur regulation in the gastric pathogen Helicobacter pylori. Infect Immun 2006; 74(1):602–14.

24. Johnson KS, Ottemann KM. Colonization, localization, and inflammation: the roles of H. pylori chemotaxis in vivo. Curr Opin Microbiol 2018;41:51–7.

25. Sycuro LK, Wyckoff TJ, Biboy J, et al. Multiple peptidoglycan modification networks modulate Helicobacter pylori's cell shape, motility, and colonization potential. PLoS Pathog 2012;8(3):e1002603.

26. Yang DC, Blair KM, Taylor JA, et al. A genome-wide helicobacter pylori morphology screen uncovers a membrane-spanning helical cell shape complex. J Bacteriol 2019;201(14):e00724-18.

27. Martínez LE, Hardcastle JM, Wang J, et al. Helicobacter pylori strains vary cell shape and flagellum number to maintain robust motility in viscous environments. Mol Microbiol 2016;99(1):88–110.

28. Huang JY, Sweeney EG, Sigal M, et al. Chemodetection and destruction of host urea allows helicobacter pylori to locate the epithelium. Cell Host Microbe 2015; 18(2):147–56.

29. Croxen MA, Sisson G, Melano R, et al. The Helicobacter pylori chemotaxis receptor TlpB (HP0103) is required for pH taxis and for colonization of the gastric mucosa. J Bacteriol 2006;188(7):2656–65.

30. Hanyu H, Engevik KA, Matthis AL, et al. Helicobacter pylori uses the TlpB receptor to sense sites of gastric injury. Infect Immun 2019;87(9):e00202-19.
31. Javaheri A, Kruse T, Moonens K, et al. Helicobacter pylori adhesin HopQ engages in a virulence-enhancing interaction with human CEACAMs. Nat Microbiol 2016;2:16189.
32. Kim IJ, Lee J, Oh SJ, et al. Helicobacter pylori infection modulates host cell metabolism through VacA-dependent inhibition of mTORC1. Cell Host Microbe 2018;23(5):583–93.e588.
33. Capurro MI, Greenfield LK, Prashar A, et al. VacA generates a protective intracellular reservoir for Helicobacter pylori that is eliminated by activation of the lysosomal calcium channel TRPML1. Nat Microbiol 2019;4(8):1411–23.
34. Buß M, Tegtmeyer N, Schnieder J, et al. Specific high affinity interaction of Helicobacter pylori CagL with integrin α(V) β(6) promotes type IV secretion of CagA into human cells. FEBS J 2019;286(20):3980–97.
35. Zhao Q, Busch B, Jiménez-Soto LF, et al. Integrin but not CEACAM receptors are dispensable for Helicobacter pylori CagA translocation. PLoS Pathog 2018;14(10):e1007359.
36. Tegtmeyer N, Backert S. Different roles of integrin-β1 and integrin-αv for type IV secretion of CagA versus cell elongation phenotype and cell lifting by Helicobacter pylori. PLoS Pathog 2020;16(7):e1008135.
37. Behrens IK, Busch B, Ishikawa-Ankerhold H, et al. The HopQ-CEACAM interaction controls caga translocation, phosphorylation, and phagocytosis of helicobacter pylori in neutrophils. mBio 2020;11(1):e03256-19.
38. Suzuki M, Mimuro H, Suzuki T, et al. Interaction of CagA with Crk plays an important role in Helicobacter pylori-induced loss of gastric epithelial cell adhesion. J Exp Med 2005;202(9):1235–47.
39. Palrasu M, Zaika E, El-Rifai W, et al. Bacterial CagA protein compromises tumor suppressor mechanisms in gastric epithelial cells. J Clin Invest 2020;130(5):2422–34.
40. Bouafia A, Corre S, Gilot D, et al. p53 requires the stress sensor USF1 to direct appropriate cell fate decision. PLoS Genet 2014;10(5):e1004309.
41. Costa L, Corre S, Michel V, et al. USF1 defect drives p53 degradation during Helicobacter pylori infection and accelerates gastric carcinogenesis. Gut 2020;69(9):1582–91.
42. Zhou S, Chen H, Yuan P, et al. Helicobacter pylori infection promotes epithelial-to-mesenchymal transition of gastric cells by upregulating LAPTM4B. Biochem Biophys Res Commun 2019;514(3):893–900.
43. Molina-Castro SE, Tiffon C, Giraud J, et al. The Hippo Kinase LATS2 Controls Helicobacter pylori-induced epithelial-mesenchymal transition and intestinal metaplasia in gastric mucosa. Cell Mol Gastroenterol Hepatol 2020;9(2):257–76.
44. Yao X, Smolka AJ. Gastric parietal cell physiology and helicobacter pylori-induced disease. Gastroenterology 2019;156(8):2158–73.
45. Saha A, Backert S, Hammond CE, et al. Helicobacter pylori CagL activates ADAM17 to induce repression of the gastric H, K-ATPase alpha subunit. Gastroenterology 2010;139(1):239–48.
46. Naumann M, Sokolova O, Tegtmeyer N, et al. Helicobacter pylori: a paradigm pathogen for subverting host cell signal transmission. Trends Microbiol 2017;25(4):316–28.
47. Zarzecka U, Modrak-Wójcik A, Figaj D, et al. Properties of the HtrA protease from bacterium helicobacter pylori whose activity is indispensable for growth under stress conditions. Front Microbiol 2019;10:961.

48. Buti L, Ruiz-Puig C, Sangberg D, et al. CagA-ASPP2 complex mediates loss of cell polarity and favors H. pylori colonization of human gastric organoids. Proc Natl Acad Sci U S A 2020;117(5):2645–55.

49. Sigal M, Rothenberg ME, Logan CY, et al. Helicobacter pylori activates and expands Lgr5(+) stem cells through direct colonization of the gastric glands. Gastroenterology 2015;148(7):1392–404.e1321.

50. Sigal M, Logan CY, Kapalczynska M, et al. Stromal R-spondin orchestrates gastric epithelial stem cells and gland homeostasis. Nature 2017;548(7668): 451–5.

51. Sigal M, Reinés MDM, Müllerke S, et al. R-spondin-3 induces secretory, antimicrobial Lgr5(+) cells in the stomach. Nat Cell Biol 2019;21(7):812–23.

52. Wroblewski LE, Choi E, Petersen C, et al. Targeted mobilization of Lrig1(+) gastric epithelial stem cell populations by a carcinogenic Helicobacter pylori type IV secretion system. Proc Natl Acad Sci U S A 2019;116(39):19652–8.

53. Schweiger PJ, Clement DL, Page ME, et al. Lrig1 marks a population of gastric epithelial cells capable of long-term tissue maintenance and growth in vitro. Sci Rep 2018;8(1):15255.

54. Zhang X, Arnold IC, Müller A. Mechanisms of persistence, innate immune activation and immunomodulation by the gastric pathogen Helicobacter pylori. Curr Opin Microbiol 2020;54:1–10.

55. Pachathundikandi SK, Tegtmeyer N, Arnold IC, et al. T4SS-dependent TLR5 activation by Helicobacter pylori infection. Nat Commun 2019;10(1):5717.

56. Minaga K, Watanabe T, Kamata K, et al. Nucleotide-binding oligomerization domain 1 and Helicobacter pylori infection: a review. World J Gastroenterol 2018;24(16):1725–33.

57. Gall A, Gaudet RG, Gray-Owen SD, et al. TIFA signaling in gastric epithelial cells initiates the cag type 4 secretion system-dependent innate immune response to helicobacter pylori infection. mBio 2017;8(4):e01168-17.

58. Zimmermann S, Pfannkuch L, Al-Zeer MA, et al. ALPK1- and TIFA-dependent innate immune response triggered by the helicobacter pylori type IV secretion system. Cell Rep 2017;20(10):2384–95.

59. Stein SC, Faber E, Bats SH, et al. Helicobacter pylori modulates host cell responses by CagT4SS-dependent translocation of an intermediate metabolite of LPS inner core heptose biosynthesis. PLoS Pathog 2017;13(7):e1006514.

60. Pfannkuch L, Hurwitz R, Traulsen J, et al. ADP heptose, a novel pathogen-associated molecular pattern identified in Helicobacter pylori. FASEB J 2019; 33(8):9087–99.

61. Salama NR, Hartung ML, Müller A. Life in the human stomach: persistence strategies of the bacterial pathogen Helicobacter pylori. Nat Rev Microbiol 2013; 11(6):385–99.

62. Amieva MR, El-Omar EM. Host-bacterial interactions in Helicobacter pylori infection. Gastroenterology 2008;134(1):306–23.

63. Moss SF. The clinical evidence linking helicobacter pylori to gastric cancer. Cell Mol Gastroenterol Hepatol 2017;3(2):183–91.

64. Ford AC, Gurusamy KS, Delaney B, et al. Eradication therapy for peptic ulcer disease in Helicobacter pylori-positive people. Cochrane Database Syst Rev 2016;4(4):Cd003840.

65. Hopkins RJ, Girardi LS, Turney EA. Relationship between Helicobacter pylori eradication and reduced duodenal and gastric ulcer recurrence: a review. Gastroenterology 1996;110(4):1244–52.

66. NIH Consensus Conference. Helicobacter pylori in peptic ulcer disease. NIH consensus development panel on helicobacter pylori in peptic ulcer disease. JAMA 1994;272(1):65–9.
67. de Martel C, Georges D, Bray F, et al. Global burden of cancer attributable to infections in 2018: a worldwide incidence analysis. Lancet Glob Health 2020; 8(2):e180–90.
68. Lee YC, Chiang TH, Chou CK, et al. Association between helicobacter pylori eradication and gastric cancer incidence: a systematic review and meta-analysis. Gastroenterology 2016;150(5):1113–24.e1115.
69. Kumar S, Metz DC, Ellenberg S, et al. Risk factors and incidence of gastric cancer after detection of helicobacter pylori infection: a large cohort study. Gastroenterology 2020;158(3):527–36.e527.
70. Choi IJ, Kim CG, Lee JY, et al. Family history of gastric cancer and helicobacter pylori treatment. N Engl J Med 2020;382(5):427–36.
71. Chiang TH, Chang WJ, Chen SL, et al. Mass eradication of Helicobacter pylori to reduce gastric cancer incidence and mortality: a long-term cohort study on Matsu Islands. Gut 2020. https://doi.org/10.1136/gutjnl-2020-322200.
72. Nakamura S, Sugiyama T, Matsumoto T, et al. Long-term clinical outcome of gastric MALT lymphoma after eradication of Helicobacter pylori: a multicentre cohort follow-up study of 420 patients in Japan. Gut 2012;61(4):507–13.
73. Zucca E, Arcaini L, Buske C, et al. Marginal zone lymphomas: ESMO Clinical Practice Guidelines for diagnosis, treatment and follow-up. Ann Oncol 2020; 31(1):17–29.
74. Gong EJ, Ahn JY, Jung HY, et al. Helicobacter pylori eradication therapy is effective as the initial treatment for patients with h. pylori-negative and disseminated gastric mucosa-associated lymphoid tissue lymphoma. Gut Liver 2016; 10(5):706–13.
75. Muhsen K, Cohen D. Helicobacter pylori infection and iron stores: a systematic review and meta-analysis. Helicobacter 2008;13(5):323–40.
76. Yuan W, Li Y, Yang K, et al. Iron deficiency anemia in Helicobacter pylori infection: meta-analysis of randomized controlled trials. Scand J Gastroenterol 2010; 45(6):665–76.
77. Tsay FW, Hsu PIH. pylori infection and extra-gastroduodenal diseases. J Biomed Sci 2018;25(1):65.
78. Gasbarrini A, Franceschi F, Tartaglione R, et al. Regression of autoimmune thrombocytopenia after eradication of Helicobacter pylori. Lancet 1998; 352(9131):878.
79. Kim BJ, Kim HS, Jang HJ, et al. Helicobacter pylori Eradication in idiopathic thrombocytopenic purpura: a meta-analysis of randomized trials. Gastroenterol Res Pract 2018;2018:6090878.
80. Neunert C, Terrell DR, Arnold DM, et al. American society of hematology 2019 guidelines for immune thrombocytopenia. Blood Adv. 2019;3(23):3829-3866. Blood Adv 2020;4(2):252.
81. Goni E, Franceschi F. Helicobacter pylori and extragastric diseases. Helicobacter 2016;21(Suppl 1):45–8.
82. Xie FJ, Zhang YP, Zheng QQ, et al. Helicobacter pylori infection and esophageal cancer risk: an updated meta-analysis. World J Gastroenterol 2013;19(36): 6098–107.
83. Kato T, Yagi N, Kamada T, et al. Diagnosis of Helicobacter pylori infection in gastric mucosa by endoscopic features: a multicenter prospective study. Dig Endosc 2013;25(5):508–18.

84. Wang YK, Kuo FC, Liu CJ, et al. Diagnosis of Helicobacter pylori infection: current options and developments. World J Gastroenterol 2015;21(40):11221–35.

85. Lash JG, Genta RM. Adherence to the Sydney System guidelines increases the detection of Helicobacter gastritis and intestinal metaplasia in 400738 sets of gastric biopsies. Aliment Pharmacol Ther 2013;38(4):424–31.

86. Batts KP, Ketover S, Kakar S, et al. Appropriate use of special stains for identifying Helicobacter pylori: recommendations from the Rodger C. Haggitt gastrointestinal pathology society. Am J Surg Pathol 2013;37(11):e12–22.

87. Uotani T, Graham DY. Diagnosis of helicobacter pylori using the rapid urease test. Ann Transl Med 2015;3(1):9.

88. Shah SC, Iyer PG, Moss SF. AGA Clinical Practice Update on the management of refractory Helicobacter pylori infection: expert review. Gastroenterology 2021 (in press).

89. Ferwana M, Abdulmajeed I, Alhajiahmed A, et al. Accuracy of urea breath test in Helicobacter pylori infection: meta-analysis. World J Gastroenterol 2015;21(4):1305–14.

90. Gisbert JP, de la Morena F, Abraira V. Accuracy of monoclonal stool antigen test for the diagnosis of H. pylori infection: a systematic review and meta-analysis. Am J Gastroenterol 2006;101(8):1921–30.

91. Chey WD, Leontiadis GI, Howden CW, et al. ACG clinical guideline: treatment of helicobacter pylori infection. Am J Gastroenterol 2017;112(2):212–39.

92. Sugano K, Tack J, Kuipers EJ, et al. Kyoto global consensus report on Helicobacter pylori gastritis. Gut 2015;64(9):1353–67.

93. El-Serag HB, Kao JY, Kanwal F, et al. Houston consensus conference on testing for helicobacter pylori infection in the United States. Clin Gastroenterol Hepatol 2018;16(7):992–1002.e1006.

94. Matsumoto H, Shiotani A, Graham DY. Current and future treatment of Helicobacter pylori infections. Adv Exp Med Biol 2019;1149:211–25.

95. Savoldi A, Carrara E, Graham DY, et al. Prevalence of antibiotic resistance in helicobacter pylori: a systematic review and meta-analysis in world health organization regions. Gastroenterology 2018;155(5):1372–82.e1317.

96. Puig I, Baylina M, Sánchez-Delgado J, et al. Systematic review and meta-analysis: triple therapy combining a proton-pump inhibitor, amoxicillin and metronidazole for Helicobacter pylori first-line treatment. J Antimicrob Chemother 2016;71(10):2740–53.

97. Fallone CA, Moss SF, Malfertheiner P. Reconciliation of recent helicobacter pylori treatment guidelines in a time of increasing resistance to antibiotics. Gastroenterology 2019;157(1):44–53.

98. Alsamman MA, Vecchio EC, Shawwa K, et al. Retrospective analysis confirms tetracycline quadruple as best helicobacter pylori regimen in the USA. Dig Dis Sci 2019;64(10):2893–8.

99. Kenyon C. Population-level macrolide consumption is associated with clarithromycin resistance in Helicobacter pylori: an ecological analysis. Int J Infect Dis 2019;85:67–9.

100. Jones NL, Koletzko S, Goodman K, et al. Joint ESPGHAN/NASPGHAN guidelines for the management of helicobacter pylori in children and adolescents (Update 2016). J Pediatr Gastroenterol Nutr 2017;64(6):991–1003.

Acute Bacterial Gastroenteritis

James M. Fleckenstein, MD[a,b],*, F. Matthew Kuhlmann, MD, MSCI[a],
Alaullah Sheikh, PhD[a]

KEYWORDS

- Diarrhea • Bacteria • Gastroenteritis • Pathogens

KEY POINTS

- Bacterial gastroenteritis syndromes are exceedingly common globally and in the United States, where most infections are foodborne, and food distribution networks can lead to widespread outbreaks.
- Nationwide reporting and strain characterization efforts are in place to mitigate these outbreaks.
- Pathogens continue to evolve through genetic exchange of virulence traits and antibiotic resistance genes.
- Culture-independent molecular-based diagnostic testing provides some advantages compared with traditional microbiologic approaches. However, cultures remain important to provide antibiotic sensitivity data and to archive bacteria for outbreak investigations by public health authorities.
- Most bacterial infections associated with acute gastroenteritis resolve spontaneously with supportive treatment, and antibiotic use may promote resistance and alteration of the microbiota, providing strong impetus for judicious antibiotic use.

INTRODUCTION

Acute gastroenteritis (AGE) is one of the most common bacterial infectious diseases that clinicians face in daily practice. Worldwide, bacterial enteric pathogens cause billions of infections each year with tremendous morbidity. In the United States alone it is estimated that there are nearly 200 million cases of AGE annually.[1]

Funded by: National Institutes of Health (NIH), National Institute of Allergy and Infectious Diseases (NIAID); R01AI089894 (jmf); R01AI126887 (jmf); K23AI1300389 (fmk) and Department of Veterans Affairs 1 I01 BX004825-01 (jmf).
[a] Department of Medicine, Division of Infectious Diseases, Washington University in Saint Louis, School of Medicine, Campus Box 8051, 660 South Euclid Avenue, Saint Louis, MO 63110, USA; [b] Infectious Disease Section, Medicine Service, Veterans Affairs Saint Louis Health Care System, 915 North Grand Boulevard, Saint Louis, MO 63106, USA
* Corresponding author.
E-mail address: jfleckenstein@wustl.edu
Twitter: @eteclab (J.M.F.)

Gastroenterol Clin N Am 50 (2021) 283–304
https://doi.org/10.1016/j.gtc.2021.02.002
0889-8553/21/Published by Elsevier Inc.

gastro.theclinics.com

EPIDEMIOLOGY

Surveillance data provided by the National Outbreak Reporting System (NORS; https://www.cdc.gov/nors/index.html), established by the Centers for Disease Control and Prevention (CDC) in 2009, show the magnitude of the problem, with thousands of outbreaks, and more than 100,000 cases of AGE recorded in the first year of its operation.[2] Foodborne illnesses, estimated at more than 9 million cases each year in the United States,[3,4] are largely caused by bacterial pathogens (**Table 1**). Although sporadic cases of illness occur frequently with improper food handling, the nature of food processing and distribution in the United States can lead to widespread dissemination of a single bacterial pathogen to large numbers of people. More than 200,000 cases of AGE are thought to have been caused by *Salmonella enteritidis* distributed nationwide in ice cream prepared by a single company.[5] Multistate outbreaks of nontyphoidal salmonellae (NTS)[6–13] and Shiga toxin–producing *Escherichia coli* (STEC)[14,15] are common and have occurred repeatedly in the United States. However, public health resources such as FoodNet can facilitate containment of these outbreaks through whole-genome sequencing that links isolates from what would otherwise seem to be sporadic cases of illness.[16,17]

The incidence of bacterial gastroenteritis tends to vary considerably during the year. In contrast with noroviruses, the leading viral causes of AGE, bacterial enteric pathogens tend to predominate during warmer weather, and are more frequently foodborne.

Although the overall incidence of most infections transmitted by food has remained relatively stable, the epidemiology of these illnesses is not necessarily static. For instance, among the *Salmonella enterica* serotypes, *typhimurium* was previously the most common but has continued to decline in incidence, perhaps because of vaccination of chickens.[17] It is now surpassed by serotype *enteritidis* in the United States, commonly transmitted by consumption of eggs or chicken.[18]

In addition, bacteria associated with AGE continue to evolve through acquisition of antimicrobial resistance traits as well as additional virulence factors. This trend is exemplified by the emergence of a novel STEC in Germany in association with an outbreak of more than 4000 illnesses related to sprout consumption[19,20] that resulted in 800 cases of hemolytic uremic syndrome and 50 deaths. Diarrheagenic *E coli* have classically been

---

Table 1
Epidemiology of major foodborne pathogens in the United States

Pathogens	Cases	Hospitalizations	Deaths	References
Campylobacter spp	~850,000–1.5 million	8500	80	3,142
Nontyphoidal *Salmonella* spp	~1.4 million	20,000–26,000	400	3,142,159
Clostridium perfringens	~1 million	450	30	3
STEC[a]	~176,000–250,000	2500	20	3,15
Shigella spp	~130,000	1500	10	3
Yersinia enterocolitica	~95,000–117,000	500–640	35	3
Noncholera *Vibrio* spp	~36,000–52,000	300	50	3,142
ETEC[b]	~18,000–80,000	12	0	3
Other DECs[c]	~12,000	8	0	3

Abbreviations: DECs, diarrheagenic pathovars of *Escherichia coli*; ETEC, enterotoxigenic *E coli*; STEC, Shiga toxin–producing *E coli*.
  [a] Shiga toxin producing *E coli* (includes O157:H7 and other serotypes).
  [b] Enterotoxigenic *E coli*; https://www.cdc.gov/ecoli/diarrheagenic-ecoli.html.
  [c] Diarrheagenic *E coli* (Enteropathogenic and enteraggregative *E coli*).

divided into pathovars determined by the presence of specific virulence genes, such as Shiga toxin (*stx*) genes in STEC. However, the *E coli* strain from the German outbreak had acquired not only *stx* (*stx1*, *stx2*) genes but also virulence genes from other pathovars of diarrheagenic *E coli* in addition to extended-spectrum beta lactamase resistance. A similar trend has been observed in outbreaks of shigellosis in California in which strains gained virulence genes and enhanced resistance to fluoroquinolones.[21] Altogether, the lines separating different species and individual pathovars are expected to continue to become less distinct as these genetically plastic organisms inevitably recombine.[22]

CHARACTERISTICS OF MAJOR BACTERIAL PATHOGENS ASSOCIATED WITH ACUTE GASTROENTERITIS
Campylobacter

Campylobacter are gram-negative, microaerophilic, somewhat fastidious pathogens that are responsible for a large burden of disease both in the United States and abroad. More than 5 species of *Campylobacter* (*Campylobacter jejuni*, *Campylobacter coli*, *Campylobacter upsaliensis*, *Campylobacter fetus*, *Campylobacter lari*, and others) are known to infect humans. *C jejuni* infections are the major cause of disease world-wide, although microbiologic techniques have likely been optimized for *C jejuni*,[23] perhaps biasing its selection to some extent. In the United States, a strong association with chicken consumption[24,25] is predictable given that 40% to 95% of chicken available in grocery stores is infected with *C jejuni*.[26,27] *Campylobacter* is also a major pathogen associated with diarrhea in travelers, particularly in parts of Asia where antibiotic resistance is also increasingly common.[25,28–30]

Illness associated with *C jejuni* is most common during summer months, and may present with diarrhea (often bloody), fever, and abdominal pain with nausea and/or vomiting (**Table 2**). When a college student spending the summer in Arizona (the nephew of one of the authors) prepared chicken on the grill for the first time, and was later hospitalized with fever and bloody diarrhea, *Campylobacter* enteritis was highly likely. Although infection with any of the species that infect humans may be complicated by bacteremia, the incidence is strikingly higher in *C fetus* infections, and infected individuals are more likely to be hospitalized.[23]

Nontyphoidal Salmonella

Worldwide, the NTS (*S enterica* serovars other than *Salmonella typhi* and *paratyphi*) are exceedingly common causes of gastroenteritis, causing in excess of 90 million cases globally,[31] and more than 1 million cases each year in the United States. Most transmission by these diverse pathogens is foodborne, although infection of humans also occurs via animal contact with reptiles and amphibians[32] or poultry.[33] Unlike Typhi, NTS are not human host-restricted pathogens, perhaps accounting for their prevalence as foodborne pathogens. Within the more than 20 different NTS serovars that infect humans, *typhimurium* and *enteritidis* are overall the dominant serovars[34] in most regions.

Fever, abdominal pain, and nonbloody diarrhea typically begin within several days of ingestion and most cases resolve spontaneously within the first week, without the need for antimicrobial therapy.[35,36] Some antibiotics fail to affect the duration of symptomatic gastroenteritis but prolong fecal carriage.[37] Some individuals, particularly the elderly[38] or immunosuppressed, are at higher risk for invasive infection, and some serovars of *Salmonella enterica* (*Salmonella* Dublin) are more commonly reported from bloodstream infections in the United States. Serovars *typhimurium* and *enteritidis* are common causes of invasive disease in Africa,[39–41] which flourishes in malnourished infants and young children.[42–44]

Table 2
Summary of common bacterial enteropathogens associated with acute gastroenteritis syndromes

Pathogens	Exposures	Clinical Presentation	Culture	CIDT	References
			Diagnostic Tests		
Campylobacter spp	Poultry; unpasteurized dairy products, travel abroad, puppies, reptiles, contaminated water	Abdominal pain, fever, nausea, vomiting, diarrhea (often bloody), rarely bacteremia	Yes	Yes	25,160–163
Nontyphoidal *Salmonella* spp	Eggs, chicken, multiple foods, backyard flocks, broad range of pets, including amphibians and reptiles	Abdominal pain, fever, nausea, vomiting, diarrhea, bacteremia more frequent with some serotypes[a]	Yes	Yes	40,164
STEC	Numerous foodborne outbreaks with multiple vehicles of transmission including beef (particularly ground), sprouts, salad greens, cookie dough; petting zoos, childcare centers	Diarrhea, abdominal pain, vomiting > bloody diarrhea (~90%) → HUS (~15%)	Yes	Yes	14,49,165
Shigella spp	Foodborne, travel abroad, homeless, easily transmitted person to person, day care, MSM	1–2-d incubation period; serotype *sonnei* causes most disease in United States. Typically milder illness. Watery/bloody/mucoid stool, fever, abdominal pain, nausea	Yes	Yes	56–58,62,166–168
Y enterocolitica	Pork, pork intestines (chitlins); unpasteurized milk/dairy	Abdominal pain (may mimic appendicitis) diarrhea/bloody persistent diarrhea; bacteremia, particularly with iron-overload states; metastatic infections	Yes	Yes	169,170

(continued on next page)

Table 2
(continued)

| Pathogens | Exposures | Clinical Presentation | Diagnostic Tests | | References |
			Culture	CIDT	
C perfringens	Beef, poultry; catered, prewarmed foods; restaurants	Diarrhea and cramps within 6–24 h (median 11 h) of ingestion. Fever and/or vomiting are infrequent	No	No[b]	86
Bacillus cereus	Rice/fried rice; meat; restaurants	2–12 h (median 5 h), vomiting, diarrhea	No	No[b]	86
Staphylococcus aureus	Diverse vehicles; restaurants	Sudden-onset nausea, vomiting, abdominal pain, diarrhea within 30 min to 8 h (median 4 h) of ingestion. Self-limited	No	No[b]	86,88

Abbreviations: CIDTs, culture-independent molecular diagnostic tests; EAEC, enteroaggregative *E coli*; EPEC, enteropathogenic *E coli*; HIV, human immunodeficiency virus; HUS, hemolytic uremic syndrome; MSM, men who have sex with men.

[a] Dublin > Cholerasuis > Schwarzengrund > Heidelberg > *enteriditis* ~ *typhimurium*.
[b] Preformed toxin detection by reference/public health laboratory.

Shiga Toxin–Producing Escherichia coli

E coli that produce Shiga toxins stx1 and/or stx2 are collectively known as STEC, or previously enterohemorrhagic *E. coli* (EHEC). These pathogens typically require a low inoculum of bacteria to cause illness (as few as 10 colony forming units) and hence are associated with a wide range of transmission vehicles from sprouts to ground beef, as well as person-to-person spread in day care. In the United States, a particular *E coli* serotype, O157:H7, has predominated; however, other serotypes are increasingly common and more easily identified with toxin-based culture-independent testing.

Although many different routes of transmission have been reported, food vehicles often have contamination with the fecal matter of ruminant animals, particularly cattle, as the ultimate source. Cattle lack the globotriaosylceramide (GB_3) endothelial receptor for Shiga toxins[45]; therefore, although their intestinal tracts become colonized with O157:H7 and other strains and cattle shed vast amounts of STEC bacteria in their stool, they do not become ill. Ground beef prepared at an industrial scale has posed a particular risk because of collective processing of meat from multiple animals into single lots. However, municipal water, and many foods, particularly foods consumed raw (eg, leafy green vegetables[15,46] and sprouts [20,47]) have repeatedly been linked to large regional or multistate outbreaks of STEC. Enteric pathogens, including STEC, can persist on the surface of vegetables and seeds for extended periods of time, and the pathogens can be internalized by the growing plants, making them difficult to sterilize simply by washing.[48]

Following ingestion of the organisms, patients typically begin to experience diarrhea within days (median 3 days), which begins as watery stool that becomes bloody in most cases within several days. Abdominal pain and tenderness, and symptoms of pain on defecation, are common, whereas fever is not.[49] Although most cases resolve spontaneously, ~15% of patients who develop bloody diarrhea go on to develop hemolytic uremic syndrome (HUS), characterized by microangiopathic hemolytic anemia, thrombocytopenia, and acute kidney injury. Antibiotics have been shown to accelerate release or production of Stx from lysogenic phages, and treatment with antimicrobial therapy significantly increases the risk for HUS.[50] Therefore, antibiotics should be avoided in initial treatment of patients with bloody diarrhea pending definitive identification of alternative pathogens such as *Campylobacter* or *Shigella*, whereas confirmed STEC infections should be managed supportively with volume expansion.

Shigellosis

Worldwide, shigellae cause tremendous morbidity and are a leading cause of diarrheal mortality in young children of low and middle income countries (LMICs), where they have also been closely associated with nondiarrheal sequelae, including stunting and malnutrition.[51–54] In the United States, these pathogens cause more than 100,000 cases of illness each year.

Four main species of *Shigella*, defined by their oligosaccharide antigens, infect humans. *Shigella dysenteriae*, *Shigella flexneri*, *Shigella sonnei*, and *Shigella boydii* have specific epidemiologic niches, with *S flexneri* being the predominant cause of disease in LMICs and *S sonnei* the main cause of illness in the United States and other high-income regions.

Like STEC, these organisms are easily transmissible, requiring few organisms to cause infection.[55] Unlike NTS, STEC, *Campylobacter*, and *Yersinia*, humans are the only known natural host for *Shigella*. Person-to-person transmission, with high rates of secondary spread, can occur in day care and other settings.[56,57] Outbreaks have also emanated from restaurants, where food may be inadequately prepared or served by infected food handlers.[58] Shigella infections, along with those caused by STEC and NTS, are over-represented in lower socioeconomic communities.[59–61] Notably, drug-resistant *S flexneri*, as well as *S sonnei* transmitted internationally and domestically among men who have sex with men (MSM),[62–66] have emerged repeatedly in outbreaks in recent years. Clinicians caring for MSM, as well as travelers, should be alert to treatment-resistant shigellosis.

After an incubation period of 1 to 4 days, infected individuals may manifest fever, anorexia, vomiting, and watery diarrhea that may resolve without further progression in many healthy hosts. Alternatively, a proportion of cases, particularly with *S dysenteriae* infection, then progress to dysentery symptoms of abdominal pain and tenesmus accompanied by frequent small-volume stools containing blood and mucus.

Diarrheagenic Escherichia coli

In addition to STEC, several other types of *E coli* can cause acute gastrointestinal illness. These types include the enteropathogenic (EPEC), enteroinvasive (EIEC), enteroaggregative (EAEC), and enterotoxigenic *E coli* (ETEC) pathovars, which are defined by specific genes that differentiate these pathovars from one another and from commensal *E coli*. Until recently, these pathogens were not easily distinguished in clinical microbiology laboratories, and only reached recognition during the course of large outbreaks that prompted the involvement of state health departments and/or the CDC. All of these pathogens are more common in LMICs, where they contribute to the large burden of diarrheal morbidity, which is concentrated among young children. Although each of these organisms can be isolated on occasion from travelers returning with diarrhea, ETEC is by far the predominant pathogen perennially associated with diarrhea in travelers.[67]

Interestingly, although classically thought of as a pathogen in LMICs and travelers, foodborne outbreaks of ETEC have occurred repeatedly in the United States[68–80] and have been linked to vehicles as diverse as sushi[75] and potato salad.[70] Although the incidence of ETEC infections in the United States is not certain, recent studies conducted by the Minnesota Department of Health (MDOH) suggest that ETEC is not only the most common cause of diarrhea in travelers but perhaps a common cause of domestically acquired AGE.[73,74] Only ~40% of the documented cases of ETEC in the MDOH study were from international travelers, raising the possibility that many domestic cases have gone unrecognized.

Most of these infections are self-limited and do not require anything beyond replacement fluids in the form of oral rehydration. However, ETEC is occasionally severe and cholera-like, requiring hospitalization and intravenous hydration.[81] Indeed, the initial recognition of the ETEC pathovar came from patients presenting with severe, cholera-like illness in whom *Vibrio cholerae* could not be identified.[82–85]

Preformed Enterotoxin Syndromes

Three bacterial pathogens associated with acute gastroenteritis, *Staphylococcus aureus*, *Bacillus cereus*, and *Clostridium perfringens* (see **Table 2**), have in common the rapid onset of illness caused by toxins elaborated in inappropriately prepared or preserved foods before ingestion.[86] Each of the enterotoxins produced by these pathogens induce diarrhea, whereas vomiting is a predominant manifestation of *S aureus* and *B cereus* intoxications but not that related to *C perfringens*. The food vehicles involved are often diverse. In the case of staphylococcal food poisoning, they simply need to support production of any of the more than 20 different enterotoxins produced by *S aureus* strains.[87,88] The incubation time from ingestion of the contaminated food to onset of symptoms is short (typically within hours). Fortunately, these are self-limited ailments that resolve with supportive treatment within 24 to 48 hours.

PREDISPOSING FACTORS

Medications that counter fundamental host defenses against invading enteric pathogens can put patients at increased risk. Proton pump[89] inhibitors may increase the risk for symptomatic infection[90] with several enteric pathogens, including NTS and *Campylobacter*,[91,92] by reducing gastric acidity, an essential first line of host defense. Similarly, prior antibiotic use has been shown to promote infection by both of these pathogens, presumably by removing the colonization resistance of competing normal flora or by fostering the selection of resistant organisms.[24,93]

Understanding of human host genetic predisposition to enteric pathogens is still evolving. *S typhimurium* has been studied extensively in molecular pathogenesis and susceptibility studies in mice, but parallel confirmation of the importance of individual genes in humans is generally absent.[94] Nevertheless, relapsing *S typhimurium* infection reported in a patient with a mutation in the nuclear factor kappa-B signaling pathway, critical to both innate and adaptive immune responses to pathogens, highlights the potential importance of host genetics to susceptibility.[95] The outcome of enteric infections can also be determined by host factors that permit more efficient colonization by enteric pathogens. For instance, recent studies of enterotoxigenic *E coli* show that a common ETEC extracellular adhesin preferentially binds to A blood group glycans on enterocytes to promote host engagement and toxin delivery.[96] In addition, human volunteers challenged with ETEC were more likely to develop severe illness if they were blood group A, recapitulating earlier studies in Bangladesh[97] that showed that A+ young children were predisposed to develop symptomatic illness following ETEC infection compared with those in B or O blood groups.

COMPLICATIONS AND SEQUELAE OF ACUTE BACTERIAL ENTERITIS

It is important to recognize that, although most cases of bacterial gastroenteritis resolve spontaneously, they are occasionally followed by important sequelae (**Table 3**). Acute infections caused by invasive enteric pathogens, particularly NTS, can be complicated by early dissemination of the pathogen to distant extraintestinal sites. Bacteremia with metastatic foci of infection, including aortitis, and bone and joint infections are well described.[98] Remarkably, ingestion of vehicles not regulated by the US Food and Drug Administration (FDA), such as rattlesnake capsules, has on occasion resulted in serious extraintestinal NTS infections, particularly in immuno-suppressed patients[99,100] seeking remedies outside of traditional medicine.

Campylobacter bacteremia infrequently complicates AGE,[101,102] typically in the setting of underlying chronic illness. Likewise, *Yersinia enterocolitica* is an infrequent cause of bacteremia and extraintestinal infection, and tends to occur in the setting of underlying iron-overload states, including hemochromatosis.[103–105]

Importantly, there is a large burden of invasive NTS (iNTS) in LMICs, particularly in Africa, where large populations of young, often malnourished infants and children, as well as immunocompromised adults, are at substantial risk.[106] However, although iNTS infections far exceed cases of bacteremia complicating AGE in developed countries, iNTS dissemination tends to be more typhoidlike in presentation without clear antecedent gastroenteritis.

Nonsuppurative sequelae that evolve after resolution of the acute infection include reactive arthritis (including a subset of patients with the triad of arthritis, urethritis, and conjunctivitis), and erythema nodosum. These sequelae have been linked to varying degrees to *Campylobacter, Salmonella, Shigella, and Yersinia* infections. Curiously, the incidence of reactive arthritis following AGE has ranged from 2 per 100,000 overall to remarkably high rates of 19% following a well-documented foodborne outbreak of *S enteritidis*[107] gastroenteritis, perhaps suggesting that some pathogens are more likely to be involved in molecular mimicry of the host.

Shigella infections, particularly those caused by *S dysenteriae*, can infrequently be complicated by toxic megacolon, rectal prolapse, and intestinal obstruction or perforation. On occasion, *S dysenteriae* and *S sonnei*[108,109] have been linked to development of HUS, although not with the frequency of STEC.[110] Likewise, although HUS has been reported following antibiotic treatment of *S dysenteriae* with antibiotics,[111] the risk seems to be low relative to STEC infections.[112]

Guillain-Barré syndrome (GBS), closely linked to antecedent *Campylobacter jejuni* gastroenteritis, tends to manifest ~3 weeks after the infection. Infection with *C jejuni* is thought to elicit production of antibodies against lipooligosaccharide (LOS) glycans that cross react with host gangliosides present in peripheral nerves. Because fewer than 1 in 1000 individuals develop GBS following *C jejuni* enteritis, investigators have sought host factors that may be required for effective molecular mimicry between LOS and gangliosides.

Sequelae in Low and Middle Income Countries

Additional potential sequelae of these infections are seen almost exclusively in LMICs. These sequelae include tropical sprue in adults and environmental enteric dysfunction

Table 3
Complications and sequelae of gastroenteritis

Condition	Associated Pathogens	High Risk/Predispositions	References
Bacteremia; extraintestinal infections	Nontyphoidal Salmonella > Campylobacter, Yersinia	Elderly, immunosuppressed Infants, young children, mutations in TLR genes, immunocompromised adults in LMICs	94
Intestinal perforation, toxic megacolon	S dysenteriae, infrequently complicates infection with other Shigella serotypes and other causes of colitis	Typically, S dysenteriae infections	51,177
Nonsuppurative Complications			
Reactive arthritis	Campylobacter, Salmonella, Shigella, Yersinia	Women, severe illness ± HLA-B27, ?PPI, ? antibiotic administration, SNP in INFG, duration of diarrhea	105–107,178–182
Guillain-Barré syndrome	Campylobacter jejuni	Men ~1.5 × women. Molecular mimicry of lipopolysaccharides of some strains and host gangliosides. SNPs in some host genes may contribute	183
Erythema nodosum	Yersinia, Shigella, Salmonella	—	89,184,185
Sequelae of Enteric Infections in LMICs			
Tropical sprue	?Toxin-producing E coli/ Enterobacteriaceae	Expatriates with extended exposure (eg, Peace Corp volunteers) and residents of LMICs	113–115,118,123,124
Environmental enteric dysfunction	ETEC and DEC pathovars, Shigella, Campylobacter	Young children in LMICs	132,133,136,138

Abbreviations: HLA, human leukocyte antigen; INFG, interferon gamma gene; PPI, proton pump inhibitor; SNP, single nucleotide polymorphism; TLR, Toll-like receptor.

(EED) in young children. Both conditions share features of altered nutrient absorption and alteration of the small intestinal architecture.

Tropical sprue most clearly manifests in expatriates[113–115] living for extended periods of time in areas highly endemic for diarrheal diseases (eg, Peace Corp volunteers),[116] who typically present with weight loss, periodic diarrhea, steatorrhea, and vitamin deficiencies.[113,114,117–122] Tropical sprue remains the most common cause of malabsorption in some areas of Asia.[118,123,124] Studies in the 1970s revealed the presence of toxin-producing Enterobacteriaceae, including E coli, in small-intestinal aspirates of patients with tropical sprue[125–129]; however, Koch postulates clearly linking individual pathogens to these illnesses have yet to be established. Importantly, antibiotic therapy combined with folate administration has been shown to ameliorate tropical sprue.[130,131]

EED, or environmental enteropathy,[132,133] is a complex condition of young children in LMICs characterized by growth faltering, and nutrient malabsorption.[134–136] EED has also been epidemiologically linked to prior exposures to enteric pathogens, including ETEC,[137,138] other diarrheagenic E coli, shigellae, and Campylobacter.[139] Similar to tropical sprue, the precise role of these pathogens in the molecular pathogenesis of EED is still not well defined. Unlike tropical sprue, EED has not been shown to be reversed by administration of antibiotics and folate supplementation.

ADVANCES IN DIAGNOSTIC TESTING AND THE IMPACT OF MOLECULAR CULTURE-INDEPENDENT METHODS

Previously, most cases of AGE and foodborne illness never received a pathogen-specific diagnosis, in part because of limitations of culture-dependent methodologies.[1] The recent and expanding deployment of syndromic culture-independent molecular diagnostic tests (CIDTs) for acute gastroenteritis to clinical microbiology laboratories has already had an appreciable impact on the approach to these illnesses.[140] Although the FDA-cleared platforms currently in use vary in the breadth of pathogens that can be detected, they generally share high degrees of sensitivity and specificity and offer some advantages compared with traditional culture-dependent methodologies, including:

1. The detection of pathogens such as the diarrheagenic E coli (other than STEC), for which there were no reliable culture-based methods. Overall, diagnosis of ETEC and other diarrheagenic pathovars of E coli (DECs), enteropathogenic (EPEC), enteroaggregative (EAEC), and more fastidious pathogens such as Campylobacter spp are among the pathogens most likely to benefit from CIDTs.
2. CIDTs permit more rapid diagnosis, typically within hours relative to culture-dependent methods, which may take days.
3. The sensitivity relative to culture-based methods is typically superior. Nevertheless, many cases of AGE do not receive a causal diagnosis even with the improved detection relative to conventional tests.
4. CIDTs may foster more frequent targeted therapy (by excluding viruses) compared with conventional testing.
5. In contrast, CIDTs may also prevent inappropriate empiric antibiotic administration[140] (e.g. in cases of STEC, which can be exacerbated by antibiotic administration[50]).

However, CIDTs in their current state, when used without cultures, also have significant limitations,[141] including inability to provide antimicrobial sensitivity data, and impairment of outbreak investigations caused by lack of isolates for molecular typing and characterization.[142] Therefore, positive CIDTs should be complemented by cultures to generate antibiotic sensitivity data and to preserve the isolate when appropriate.

THERAPY

Treatment of acute gastroenteritis has been reviewed extensively in recently published guidelines.[141,143,144] Therefore, this article summarizes salient developments that may affect patient care since these were released. It is important to recognize that most cases of AGE, both viral and bacterial, resolve without specific antimicrobial therapy.

However, many of the bacterial pathogens associated with AGE have become increasingly resistant to antibiotics.[145,146] *Campylobacter*, NTS, and *Shigella* have all been cited recently by the CDC as posing serious threats as multidrug-resistant pathogens.[147] The rapid exchange of genetic information between gram-negative pathogens and their surroundings will continue to confound a strictly empiric approach to antibiotic treatment of AGE, and necessitate confirmatory sensitivity testing to modify therapy. Antibiotic resistance in *Shigella* has been particularly alarming, and has now emerged in many communities.[148] Heavy use of antibiotics is likely to exacerbate this problem because plasmids encoding extensive drug resistance seem to be easily transferred from commensal *E coli* to *Shigella*.[149] Both use of antibiotics and traveler's diarrhea have been independently associated with colonization by ESBL-producing *Enterobacteriaceae*.[150]

Antibiotic administration can clearly be lifesaving in patients with moderate to severe illness, particularly in the setting of extraintestinal infection. However, it has become increasing appreciated that antibiotics may exert negative effects on the microbiota,[151,152] leading to consequences to human health that persist well beyond the acute infection.[153,154] In addition, fluoroquinolones, widely used for treatment of AGE in the past, have been linked to substantial side effects that should limit their use to more severe infections.[155] Collectively, these developments argue for judicious use of antibiotics to treat what are most often self-limited infections.

DISCUSSION

Foodborne illness and acute gastroenteritis caused by bacterial pathogens is likely to present a continued challenge for clinicians. Although much of the foodborne illness caused by live bacteria could be mitigated by more extensive food irradiation,[156] this strategy has been slow to be adopted in the United States despite the repeated recommendations of multiple public health agencies.[157,158] Although networked public health laboratories can now extinguish outbreaks by investigating the relatedness of isolated pathogens by whole-genome sequencing, it is likely that bacterial gastroenteritis will pose a continued threat for the foreseeable future. Moreover, these pathogens will inexorably evolve through acquisition of virulence traits and resistance determinants posing additional challenges. Only interruption of food contamination at the source is likely to decrease the perennial onslaught of acute bacterial gastroenteritis.

CLINICS CARE POINTS

- AGE is predominantly caused by bacterial pathogens during warmer months, whereas noroviruses predominate in winter.
- CIDTs can accelerate diagnosis and tailor treatment options in most instances. However, in their current state, complementary cultures are recommended to obtain susceptibility data and to provide isolates for analysis in the event of an outbreak.
- Most acute gastroenteritis can be managed supportively. Antimicrobial resistance profiles continue to evolve rapidly, and many pathogens, including some *Shigella* strains, are now extensively multidrug resistant, limiting effective empiric treatment options.

DISCLOSURE

The authors have nothing to disclose.

REFERENCES

1. Scallan E, Griffin PM, Angulo FJ, et al. Foodborne illness acquired in the United States–unspecified agents. Emerg Infect Dis 2011;17(1):16–22.
2. Hall AJ, Wikswo ME, Manikonda K, et al. Acute gastroenteritis surveillance through the National Outbreak Reporting System, United States. Emerg Infect Dis 2013;19(8):1305–9.
3. Scallan E, Hoekstra RM, Angulo FJ, et al. Foodborne illness acquired in the United States–major pathogens. Emerg Infect Dis 2011;17(1):7–15.
4. Dewey-Mattia D, Manikonda K, Hall AJ, et al. Surveillance for Foodborne Disease Outbreaks - United States, 2009-2015. MMWR Surveill Summ 2018; 67(10):1–11.
5. Hennessy TW, Hedberg CW, Slutsker L, et al. A national outbreak of *Salmonella enteritidis* infections from ice cream. The Investigation Team. N Engl J Med 1996;334(20):1281–6.
6. Sheth AN, Hoekstra M, Patel N, et al. A national outbreak of *Salmonella* serotype Tennessee infections from contaminated peanut butter: a new food vehicle for salmonellosis in the United States. Clin Infect Dis 2011;53(4):356–62.
7. Mba-Jonas A, Culpepper W, Hill T, et al. A Multistate outbreak of human *Salmonella agona* infections associated with consumption of fresh, whole papayas imported from Mexico-United States, 2011. Clin Infect Dis 2018;66(11):1756–61.
8. Jain S, Bidol SA, Austin JL, et al. Multistate outbreak of *Salmonella* Typhimurium and Saintpaul infections associated with unpasteurized orange juice–United States, 2005. Clin Infect Dis 2009;48(8):1065–71.
9. Hassan R, Whitney B, Williams DL, et al. Multistate outbreaks of *Salmonella* infections linked to imported Maradol papayas - United States, December 2016-September 2017. Epidemiol Infect 2019;147:e265.
10. Centers for Disease Contro and Prevention. Multistate outbreaks of *Salmonella* infections associated with raw tomatoes eaten in restaurants–United States, 2005-2006. MMWR Morb Mortal Wkly Rep 2007;56(35):909–11.
11. Mahon BE, Ponka A, Hall WN, et al. An international outbreak of *Salmonella* infections caused by alfalfa sprouts grown from contaminated seeds. J Infect Dis 1997;175(4):876–82.
12. Dechet AM, Scallan E, Gensheimer K, et al. Outbreak of multidrug-resistant *Salmonella enterica* serotype Typhimurium Definitive Type 104 infection linked to commercial ground beef, northeastern United States, 2003-2004. Clin Infect Dis 2006;42(6):747–52.
13. Miller EA, Elnekave E, Flores-Figueroa C, et al. Emergence of a novel *Salmonella enterica* serotype Reading clonal group is linked to its expansion in commercial turkey production, resulting in unanticipated human illness in North America. mSphere 2020;5(2). e00056-20.
14. Neil KP, Biggerstaff G, MacDonald JK, et al. A novel vehicle for transmission of *Escherichia coli* O157:H7 to humans: multistate outbreak of *E. coli* O157:H7 infections associated with consumption of ready-to-bake commercial prepackaged cookie dough–United States, 2009. Clin Infect Dis 2012;54(4):511–8.
15. Marshall KE, Hexemer A, Seelman SL, et al. Lessons Learned from a Decade of Investigations of Shiga Toxin-Producing *Escherichia coli* Outbreaks Linked to

Leafy Greens, United States and Canada. Emerg Infect Dis 2020;26(10): 2319–28.

16. Slayton RB, Turabelidze G, Bennett SD, et al. Outbreak of Shiga toxin-producing *Escherichia coli* (STEC) O157:H7 associated with romaine lettuce consumption, 2011. PLoS One 2013;8(2):e55300.

17. Tack DM, Ray L, Griffin PM, et al. Preliminary incidence and trends of infections with pathogens transmitted commonly through food - foodborne diseases active surveillance network, 10 U.S. Sites, 2016-2019. MMWR Morb Mortal Wkly Rep 2020;69(17):509–14.

18. Kimura AC, Reddy V, Marcus R, et al. Chicken consumption is a newly identified risk factor for sporadic *Salmonella enterica* serotype Enteritidis infections in the United States: a case-control study in FoodNet sites. Clin Infect Dis 2004; 38(Suppl 3):S244–52.

19. Buchholz U, Bernard H, Werber D, et al. German outbreak of *Escherichia coli* O104:H4 associated with sprouts. N Engl J Med 2011;365(19):1763–70.

20. Frank C, Werber D, Cramer JP, et al. Epidemic profile of Shiga-toxin-producing *Escherichia coli* O104:H4 outbreak in Germany. N Engl J Med 2011;365(19): 1771–80.

21. Kozyreva VK, Jospin G, Greninger AL, et al. Recent Outbreaks of Shigellosis in California caused by two distinct populations of *Shigella sonnei* with either increased virulence or fluoroquinolone resistance. mSphere 2016;1(6). e00344-16.

22. Denamur E, Clermont O, Bonacorsi S, et al. The population genetics of pathogenic *Escherichia coli*. Nat Rev Microbiol 2020;19(1):37–54.

23. Patrick ME, Henao OL, Robinson T, et al. Features of illnesses caused by five species of *Campylobacter*, foodborne diseases active surveillance network (FoodNet) - 2010-2015. Epidemiol Infect 2018;146(1):1–10.

24. Effler P, Ieong MC, Kimura A, et al. Sporadic *Campylobacter jejuni* infections in Hawaii: associations with prior antibiotic use and commercially prepared chicken. J Infect Dis 2001;183(7):1152–5.

25. Friedman CR, Hoekstra RM, Samuel M, et al. Risk factors for sporadic *Campylobacter* infection in the United States: A case-control study in FoodNet sites. Clin Infect Dis 2004;38(Suppl 3):S285–96.

26. Williams A, Oyarzabal OA. Prevalence of *Campylobacter spp.* in skinless, boneless retail broiler meat from 2005 through 2011 in Alabama, USA. BMC Microbiol 2012;12:184.

27. Willis WL, Murray C. *Campylobacter jejuni* seasonal recovery observations of retail market broilers. Poult Sci 1997;76(2):314–7.

28. Gallardo F, Gascon J, Ruiz J, et al. *Campylobacter jejuni* as a cause of traveler's diarrhea: clinical features and antimicrobial susceptibility. J Trav Med 1998; 5(1):23–6.

29. Mason CJ, Sornsakrin S, Seidman JC, et al. Antibiotic resistance in *Campylobacter* and other diarrheal pathogens isolated from US military personnel deployed to Thailand in 2002-2004: a case-control study. Trop Dis Trav Med Vaccin 2017;3:13.

30. Hoge CW, Gambel JM, Srijan A, et al. Trends in antibiotic resistance among diarrheal pathogens isolated in Thailand over 15 years. Clin Infect Dis 1998;26(2): 341–5.

31. Majowicz SE, Musto J, Scallan E, et al. The global burden of nontyphoidal *Salmonella* gastroenteritis. Clin Infect Dis 2010;50(6):882–9.

32. Mermin J, Hutwagner L, Vugia D, et al. Reptiles, amphibians, and human *Salmonella* infection: a population-based, case-control study. Clin Infect Dis 2004; 38(Suppl 3):S253–61.

33. Outbreaks of *Salmonella* infections linked to Backyard poultry. Available at: https://www.cdc.gov/salmonella/backyardpoultry-05-20/index.html. Accessed October 6, 2020, 2020.

34. Cheng RA, Eade CR, Wiedmann M. Embracing diversity: differences in virulence mechanisms, disease severity, and host adaptations contribute to the success of nontyphoidal *Salmonella* as a foodborne pathogen. Front Microbiol 2019;10:1368.

35. Saphra I, Winter JW. Clinical manifestations of salmonellosis in man; an evaluation of 7779 human infections identified at the New York Salmonella Center. N Engl J Med 1957;256(24):1128–34.

36. Leung DT, Das SK, Malek MA, et al. Non-typhoidal *Salmonella* gastroenteritis at a diarrheal hospital in Dhaka, Bangladesh, 1996-2011. Am J Trop Med Hyg 2013;88(4):661–9.

37. Asperilla MO, Smego RA Jr, Scott LK. Quinolone antibiotics in the treatment of *Salmonella* infections. Rev Infect Dis 1990;12(5):873–89.

38. Chen PL, Lee HC, Lee NY, et al. Non-typhoidal *Salmonella* bacteraemia in elderly patients: an increased risk for endovascular infections, osteomyelitis and mortality. Epidemiol Infect 2012;140(11):2037–44.

39. Feasey NA, Dougan G, Kingsley RA, et al. Invasive non-typhoidal *Salmonella* disease: an emerging and neglected tropical disease in Africa. Lancet 2012; 379(9835):2489–99.

40. Vugia DJ, Samuel M, Farley MM, et al. Invasive *Salmonella* infections in the United States, FoodNet, 1996-1999: incidence, serotype distribution, and outcome. Clin Infect Dis 2004;38(Suppl 3):S149–56.

41. Jones TF, Ingram LA, Cieslak PR, et al. Salmonellosis outcomes differ substantially by serotype. J Infect Dis 2008;198(1):109–14.

42. Sigauque B, Roca A, Mandomando I, et al. Community-acquired bacteremia among children admitted to a rural hospital in Mozambique. Pediatr Infect Dis J 2009;28(2):108–13.

43. Berkley JA, Lowe BS, Mwangi I, et al. Bacteremia among children admitted to a rural hospital in Kenya. N Engl J Med 2005;352(1):39–47.

44. Enwere G, Biney E, Cheung YB, et al. Epidemiologic and clinical characteristics of community-acquired invasive bacterial infections in children aged 2-29 months in The Gambia. Pediatr Infect Dis J 2006;25(8):700–5.

45. Pruimboom-Brees IM, Morgan TW, Ackermann MR, et al. Cattle lack vascular receptors for *Escherichia coli* O157:H7 Shiga toxins. Proc Natl Acad Sci U S A 2000;97(19):10325–9.

46. Bottichio L, Keaton A, Thomas D, et al. Shiga toxin-producing *E. coli* infections associated with romaine lettuce - United States, 2018. Clin Infect Dis 2019; 71(8):e323–30.

47. Taormina PJ, Beuchat LR, Slutsker L. Infections associated with eating seed sprouts: an international concern. Emerg Infect Dis 1999;5(5):626–34.

48. Lynch MF, Tauxe RV, Hedberg CW. The growing burden of foodborne outbreaks due to contaminated fresh produce: risks and opportunities. Epidemiol Infect 2009;137(3):307–15.

49. Tarr PI, Gordon CA, Chandler WL. Shiga-toxin-producing *Escherichia coli* and haemolytic uraemic syndrome. Lancet 2005;365(9464):1073–86.

50. Wong CS, Jelacic S, Habeeb RL, et al. The risk of the hemolytic-uremic syndrome after antibiotic treatment of *Escherichia coli* O157:H7 infections. N Engl J Med 2000;342(26):1930–6.
51. Kotloff KL, Riddle MS, Platts-Mills JA, et al. Shigellosis. Lancet 2018;391(10122): 801–12.
52. Khalil I, Troeger CE, Blacker BF, et al. Capturing the true burden of *Shigella* and ETEC: The way forward. Vaccine 2019;37(34):4784–6.
53. Anderson JDt, Bagamian KH, Muhib F, et al. Burden of enterotoxigenic *Escherichia coli* and *shigella* non-fatal diarrhoeal infections in 79 low-income and lower middle-income countries: a modelling analysis. Lancet Glob Health 2019;7(3): e321–30.
54. Lanata CF, Black RE. Estimating the true burden of an enteric pathogen: enterotoxigenic *Escherichia coli* and *Shigella spp.* Lancet Infect Dis 2018;18(11): 1165–6.
55. DuPont HL, Levine MM, Hornick RB, et al. Inoculum size in shigellosis and implications for expected mode of transmission. J Infect Dis 1989;159(6):1126–8.
56. Arvelo W, Hinkle CJ, Nguyen TA, et al. Transmission risk factors and treatment of pediatric shigellosis during a large daycare center-associated outbreak of multidrug resistant *Shigella sonnei*: implications for the management of shigellosis outbreaks among children. Pediatr Infect Dis J 2009;28(11):976–80.
57. Hines JZ, Jagger MA, Jeanne TL, et al. Heavy precipitation as a risk factor for shigellosis among homeless persons during an outbreak - Oregon, 2015-2016. J Infect 2018;76(3):280–5.
58. Nygren BL, Schilling KA, Blanton EM, et al. Foodborne outbreaks of shigellosis in the USA, 1998-2008. Epidemiol Infect 2013;141(2):233–41.
59. Libby T, Clogher P, Wilson E, et al. Disparities in Shigellosis Incidence by Census Tract Poverty, Crowding, and Race/Ethnicity in the United States, FoodNet, 2004-2014. Open Forum Infect Dis 2020;7(2):ofaa030.
60. Hadler JL, Clogher P, Huang J, et al. The relationship between census tract poverty and shiga toxin-producing *E. coli* Risk, Analysis of FoodNet Data, 2010-2014. Open Forum Infect Dis 2018;5(7):ofy148.
61. Hadler JL, Clogher P, Libby T, et al. Relationship between census tract-level poverty and domestically acquired *Salmonella* incidence: analysis of foodborne diseases active surveillance network data, 2010-2016. J Infect Dis 2020;222(8): 1405–12.
62. Baker KS, Dallman TJ, Ashton PM, et al. Intercontinental dissemination of azithromycin-resistant shigellosis through sexual transmission: a cross-sectional study. Lancet Infect Dis 2015;15(8):913–21.
63. Liao YS, Liu YY, Lo YC, et al. Azithromycin-Nonsusceptible *Shigella flexneri* 3a in Men Who Have Sex with Men, Taiwan, 2015-2016. Emerg Infect Dis 2016;23(2): 345–6.
64. Yousfi K, Gaudreau C, Pilon PA, et al. Genetic mechanisms behind the spread of reduced susceptibility to azithromycin in *Shigella* strains isolated from men who have sex with men in Quebec, Canada. Antimicrob Agents Chemother 2019; 63(2). e01679-18.
65. Eikmeier D, Talley P, Bowen A, et al. Decreased Susceptibility to Azithromycin in Clinical *Shigella* Isolates Associated with HIV and Sexually Transmitted Bacterial Diseases, Minnesota, USA, 2012-2015. Emerg Infect Dis 2020;26(4):667–74.
66. Ingle DJ, Easton M, Valcanis M, et al. Co-circulation of multidrug-resistant *Shigella* among men who have sex with men in Australia. Clin Infect Dis 2019; 69(9):1535–44.

67. Jiang ZD, DuPont HL. Etiology of travellers' diarrhea. J Trav Med 2017; 24(suppl_1):S13–6.
68. Devasia RA, Jones TF, Ward J, et al. Endemically acquired foodborne outbreak of enterotoxin-producing *Escherichia coli* serotype O169:H41. Am J Med 2006; 119(2):168.e1-10.
69. Beatty ME, Adcock PM, Smith SW, et al. Epidemic diarrhea due to enterotoxigenic *Escherichia coli*. Clin Infect Dis 2006;42(3):329–34.
70. Beatty ME, Bopp CA, Wells JG, et al. Enterotoxin-producing *Escherichia coli* O169:H41, United States. Emerg Infect Dis 2004;10(3):518–21.
71. Roels TH, Proctor ME, Robinson LC, et al. Clinical features of infections due to *Escherichia coli* producing heat-stable toxin during an outbreak in Wisconsin: a rarely suspected cause of diarrhea in the United States. Clin Infect Dis 1998; 26(4):898–902.
72. Pattabiraman V, Katz LS, Chen JC, et al. Genome wide characterization of enterotoxigenic *Escherichia coli* serogroup O6 isolates from multiple outbreaks and sporadic infections from 1975-2016. PLoS One 2018;13(12):e0208735.
73. Buuck S, Smith K, Fowler RC, et al. Epidemiology of Enterotoxigenic *Escherichia coli* infection in Minnesota, 2016-2017. Epidemiol Infect 2020;148:e206.
74. Medus C, Besser JM, Juni BA, et al. Long-term sentinel surveillance for enterotoxigenic *Escherichia coli* and non-o157 shiga toxin-producing *E. coli* in Minnesota. Open Forum Infect Dis 2016;3(1):ofw003.
75. Jain S, Chen L, Dechet A, et al. An outbreak of enterotoxigenic *Escherichia coli* associated with sushi restaurants in Nevada, 2004. Clin Infect Dis 2008; 47(1):1–7.
76. Dalton CB, Mintz ED, Wells JG, et al. Outbreaks of enterotoxigenic *Escherichia coli* infection in American adults: a clinical and epidemiologic profile. Epidemiol Infect 1999;123(1):9–16.
77. Centers for Disease Control and Prevention. Foodborne outbreaks of enterotoxigenic *Escherichia coli*–Rhode Island and New Hampshire, 1993. MMWR Morb Mortal Wkly Rep 1994;43(5):87–9.
78. Yoder JS, Cesario S, Plotkin V, et al. Outbreak of enterotoxigenic *Escherichia coli* infection with an unusually long duration of illness. Clin Infect Dis 2006;42(11): 1513–7.
79. Naimi TS, Wicklund JH, Olsen SJ, et al. Concurrent outbreaks of *Shigella sonnei* and enterotoxigenic *Escherichia coli* infections associated with parsley: implications for surveillance and control of foodborne illness. J Food Prot 2003;66(4): 535–41.
80. Rosenberg ML, Koplan JP, Wachsmuth IK, et al. Epidemic diarrhea at Crater Lake from enterotoxigenic *Escherichia coli*. A large waterborne outbreak. Ann Intern Med 1977;86(6):714–8.
81. Finkelstein RA, Vasil ML, Jones JR, et al. Clinical cholera caused by enterotoxigenic *Escherichia coli*. J Clin Microbiol 1976;3(3):382–4.
82. Sack RB, Gorbach SL, Banwell JG, et al. Enterotoxigenic *Escherichia coli* isolated from patients with severe cholera-like disease. J Infect Dis 1971;123(4): 378–85.
83. Gorbach SL, Banwell JG, Chatterjee BD, et al. Acute undifferentiated human diarrhea in the tropics. I. Alterations in intestinal microflora. J Clin Invest 1971; 50(4):881–9.
84. Carpenter CC, Barua D, Wallace CK, et al. Clinical and physiological observations during an epidemic outbreak of non-vibrio cholera-like disease in Calcutta. Bull World Health Organ 1965;33(5):665–71.

85. Sack DA, McLaughlin JC, Sack RB, et al. Enterotoxigenic *Escherichia coli* isolated from patients at a hospital in Dacca. J Infect Dis 1977;135(2):275–80.

86. Bennett SD, Walsh KA, Gould LH. Foodborne disease outbreaks caused by *Bacilluscereus*, *Clostridium perfringens*, and *Staphylococcus aureus*–United States, 1998-2008. Clin Infect Dis 2013;57(3):425–33.

87. Holmberg SD, Blake PA. Staphylococcal food poisoning in the United States. New facts and old misconceptions. JAMA 1984;251(4):487–9.

88. Hennekinne JA, De Buyser ML, Dragacci S. *Staphylococcus aureus* and its food poisoning toxins: characterization and outbreak investigation. FEMS Microbiol Rev 2012;36(4):815–36.

89. Tami LF. Erythema nodosum associated with *Shigella colitis*. Arch Dermatol 1985;121(5):590.

90. Bavishi C, Dupont HL. Systematic review: the use of proton pump inhibitors and increased susceptibility to enteric infection. Aliment Pharmacol Ther 2011; 34(11–12):1269–81.

91. Neal KR, Scott HM, Slack RC, et al. Omeprazole as a risk factor for campylobacter gastroenteritis: case-control study. BMJ 1996;312(7028):414–5.

92. Garcia Rodriguez LA, Ruigomez A, Panes J. Use of acid-suppressing drugs and the risk of bacterial gastroenteritis. Clin Gastroenterol Hepatol 2007;5(12): 1418–23.

93. Pavia AT, Shipman LD, Wells JG, et al. Epidemiologic evidence that prior antimicrobial exposure decreases resistance to infection by antimicrobial-sensitive *Salmonella*. J Infect Dis 1990;161(2):255–60.

94. Gilchrist JJ, MacLennan CA, Hill AVS. Genetic susceptibility to invasive *Salmonella* disease. Nat Rev Immunol 2015;15(7):452–63.

95. Janssen R, van Wengen A, Hoeve MA, et al. The same IkappaBalpha mutation in two related individuals leads to completely different clinical syndromes. J Exp Med 2004;200(5):559–68.

96. Kumar P, Kuhlmann FM, Chakraborty S, et al. Enterotoxigenic *Escherichia coli*-blood group A interactions intensify diarrheal severity. J Clin Invest 2018;128(8): 3298–311.

97. Qadri F, Saha A, Ahmed T, et al. Disease burden due to enterotoxigenic *Escherichia coli* in the first 2 years of life in an urban community in Bangladesh. Infect Immun 2007;75(8):3961–8.

98. Cohen JI, Bartlett JA, Corey GR. Extra-intestinal manifestations of *Salmonella* infections. Medicine (Baltimore) 1987;66(5):349–88.

99. Bottichio L, Webb LM, Leos G, et al. Notes from the field: *Salmonella oranienburg* infection linked to consumption of rattlesnake pills - Kansas and Texas, 2017. MMWR Morb Mortal Wkly Rep 2018;67(17):502–3.

100. Noskin GA, Clarke JT. *Salmonella arizonae* bacteremia as the presenting manifestation of human immunodeficiency virus infection following rattlesnake meat ingestion. Rev Infect Dis 1990;12(3):514–7.

101. O'Hara GA, Fitchett JRA, Klein JL. *Campylobacter* bacteremia in London: A 44-year single-center study. Diagn Microbiol Infect Dis 2017;89(1):67–71.

102. Ben-Shimol S, Carmi A, Greenberg D. Demographic and clinical characteristics of *Campylobacter* bacteremia in children with and without predisposing factors. Pediatr Infect Dis J 2013;32(11):e414–8.

103. Coppens L, Sztern B, Korman D, et al. *Yersinia enterolitica* bacteremia with intracranial extension. Scand J Infect Dis 1995;27(4):409–10.

104. Vadillo M, Corbella X, Pac V, et al. Multiple liver abscesses due to *Yersinia enterocolitica* discloses primary hemochromatosis: three cases reports and review. Clin Infect Dis 1994;18(6):938–41.

105. Collazos J, Guerra E, Fernandez A, et al. Miliary liver abscesses and skin infection due to *Yersinia enterocolitica* in a patient with unsuspected hemochromatosis. Clin Infect Dis 1995;21(1):223–4.

106. Balasubramanian R, Im J, Lee JS, et al. The global burden and epidemiology of invasive non-typhoidal *Salmonella* infections. Hum Vaccin Immunother 2019; 15(6):1421–6.

107. Locht H, Molbak K, Krogfelt KA. High frequency of reactive joint symptoms after an outbreak of *Salmonella enteritidis*. J Rheumatol 2002;29(4):767–71.

108. Adams C, Vose A, Edmond MB, et al. *Shigella sonnei* and hemolytic uremic syndrome: A case report and literature review. IDCases 2017;8:6–8.

109. Koster F, Levin J, Walker L, et al. Hemolytic-uremic syndrome after shigellosis. Relation to endotoxemia and circulating immune complexes. N Engl J Med 1978;298(17):927–33.

110. Blaser MJ. Bacteria and diseases of unknown cause: hemolytic-uremic syndrome. J Infect Dis 2004;189(3):552–5.

111. Al-Qarawi S, Fontaine RE, Al-Qahtani MS. An outbreak of hemolytic uremic syndrome associated with antibiotic treatment of hospital inpatients for dysentery. Emerg Infect Dis 1995;1(4):138–40.

112. Bennish ML, Khan WA, Begum M, et al. Low risk of hemolytic uremic syndrome after early effective antimicrobial therapy for *Shigella dysenteriae* type 1 infection in Bangladesh. Clin Infect Dis 2006;42(3):356–62.

113. Klipstein FA, Falaiye JM. Tropical sprue in expatriates from the tropics living in the continental United States. Medicine (Baltimore) 1969;48(6):475–91.

114. Klipstein FA. Tropical sprue in travelers and expatriates living abroad. Gastroenterology 1981;80(3):590–600.

115. Lindenbaum J, Gerson CD, Kent TH. Recovery of small-intestinal structure and function after residence in the tropics. I. Studies in Peace Corps volunteers. Ann Intern Med 1971;74(2):218–22.

116. Lindenbaum J, Kent TH, Sprinz H. Malabsorption and jejunitis in American Peace Corps volunteers in Pakistan. Ann Intern Med 1966;65(6):1201–9.

117. Tomkins AM, James WP, Walters JH, et al. Malabsorption in overland travellers to India. Br Med J 1974;3(5927):380–4.

118. Brown IS, Bettington A, Bettington M, et al. Tropical sprue: revisiting an underrecognized disease. Am J Surg Pathol 2014;38(5):666–72.

119. Sheehy TW, Cohen WC, Wallace DK, et al. Tropical sprue in North Americans. JAMA 1965;194(10):1069–76.

120. Banwell JG, Gorbach SL, Chatterjee B, et al. Tropical sprue: a study of small intestinal function and the changes resulting from vitamin B12, folate, and tetracycline therapy. Gut 1968;9(6):725.

121. Ghitis J, Tripathy K, Mayoral G. Malabsorption in the tropics. 2. Tropical sprue versus primary protein malnutrition: vitamin B12 and folic acid studies. Am J Clin Nutr 1967;20(11):1206–11.

122. Ramirez I, Santini R, Corcino J, et al. Serum vitamin E levels in children and adults with tropical sprue in Puerto Rico. Am J Clin Nutr 1973;26(10):1045.

123. Dutta AK, Balekuduru A, Chacko A. Spectrum of malabsorption in India–tropical sprue is still the leader. J Assoc Physicians India 2011;59:420–2.

124. Pipaliya N, Ingle M, Rathi C, et al. Spectrum of chronic small bowel diarrhea with malabsorption in Indian subcontinent: is the trend really changing? Intest Res 2016;14(1):75–82.

125. Bhat P, Shantakumari S, Rajan D, et al. Bacterial flora of the gastrointestinal tract in southern Indian control subjects and patients with tropical sprue. Gastroenterology 1972;62(1):11–21.

126. Dickman MD, Schaedler RW. Letter: *Escherichia coli* and tropical sprue. Ann Intern Med 1974;81(1):128.

127. Klipstein FA, Engert RF, Short HB. Enterotoxigenicity of colonising coliform bacteria in tropical sprue and blind-loop syndrome. Lancet 1978;2(8085):342–4.

128. Klipstein FA, Holdeman LV, Corcino JJ, et al. Enterotoxigenic intestinal bacteria in tropical sprue. Ann Intern Med 1973;79(5):632–41.

129. Klipstein FA, Short HB, Engert RF, et al. Contamination of the small intestine by enterotoxigenic coliform bacteria among the rural population of Haiti. Gastroenterology 1976;70(6):1035–41.

130. Rickles FR, Klipstein FA, Tomasini J, et al. Long-term follow-up of antibiotic-treated tropical sprue. Ann Intern Med 1972;76(2):203–10.

131. Ghoshal UC, Srivastava D, Verma A, et al. Tropical sprue in 2014: the new face of an old disease. Curr Gastroenterol Rep 2014;16(6):391.

132. Korpe PS, Petri WA Jr. Environmental enteropathy: critical implications of a poorly understood condition. Trends Mol Med 2012;18(6):328–36.

133. Kosek MN, Investigators M-EN. Causal Pathways from Enteropathogens to Environmental Enteropathy: Findings from the MAL-ED Birth Cohort Study. EBioMedicine 2017;18:109–17.

134. Baker SJ, Mathan VI. Tropical enteropathy and tropical sprue. Am J Clin Nutr 1972;25(10):1047–55.

135. Crane RJ, Jones KD, Berkley JA. Environmental enteric dysfunction: an overview. Food Nutr Bull 2015;36(1 Suppl):S76–87.

136. Rogawski ET, Guerrant RL. The Burden of Enteropathy and "Subclinical" Infections. Pediatr Clin North Am 2017;64(4):815–36.

137. Black RE, Brown KH, Becker S. Effects of diarrhea associated with specific enteropathogens on the growth of children in rural Bangladesh. Pediatrics 1984;73(6):799–805.

138. Platts-Mills JA, Taniuchi M, Uddin MJ, et al. Association between enteropathogens and malnutrition in children aged 6-23 mo in Bangladesh: a case-control study. Am J Clin Nutr 2017;105(5):1132–8.

139. George CM, Burrowes V, Perin J, et al. Enteric Infections in Young Children are Associated with Environmental Enteropathy and Impaired Growth. Trop Med Int Health 2018;23(1):26–33.

140. Cybulski RJ Jr, Bateman AC, Bourassa L, et al. Clinical impact of a multiplex gastrointestinal polymerase chain reaction panel in patients with acute gastroenteritis. Clin Infect Dis 2018;67(11):1688–96.

141. Shane AL, Mody RK, Crump JA, et al. 2017 Infectious Diseases Society of America clinical practice guidelines for the diagnosis and management of infectious diarrhea. Clin Infect Dis 2017;65(12):1963–73.

142. Tack DM, Marder EP, Griffin PM, et al. Preliminary incidence and trends of infections with pathogens transmitted commonly through food - foodborne diseases active surveillance network, 10 U.S. Sites, 2015-2018. MMWR Morb Mortal Wkly Rep 2019;68(16):369–73.

143. Riddle MS, DuPont HL, Connor BA. ACG clinical guideline: diagnosis, treatment, and prevention of acute diarrheal infections in adults. Am J Gastroenterol 2016;111(5):602–22.

144. Taylor DN, Hamer DH, Shlim DR. Medications for the prevention and treatment of travellers' diarrhea. J Trav Med 2017;24(suppl_1):S17–22.

145. Guiral E, Goncalves Quiles M, Munoz L, et al. Emergence of resistance to quinolones and beta-lactam antibiotics in enteroaggregative and enterotoxigenic Escherichia coli causing traveler's diarrhea. Antimicrob Agents Chemother 2019;63(2). e01745-18.

146. Smith KE, Besser JM, Hedberg CW, et al. Quinolone-resistant Campylobacter jejuni infections in Minnesota, 1992-1998. Investigation Team. N Engl J Med 1999;340(20):1525–32.

147. U.S. Department of Health and Human Services C. CDC. Antibiotic resistance threats in the United States, 2019. Atlanta (GA): CDC; 2019.

148. Murray K, Reddy V, Kornblum JS, et al. Increasing Antibiotic Resistance in Shigella spp. from Infected New York City Residents, New York, USA. Emerg Infect Dis 2017;23(2):332–5.

149. Thanh Duy P, Thi Nguyen TN, Vu Thuy D, et al. Commensal Escherichia coli are a reservoir for the transfer of XDR plasmids into epidemic fluoroquinolone-resistant Shigella sonnei. Nat Microbiol 2020;5(2):256–64.

150. Kantele A, Laaveri T, Mero S, et al. Antimicrobials increase travelers' risk of colonization by extended-spectrum betalactamase-producing Enterobacteriaceae. Clin Infect Dis 2015;60(6):837–46.

151. Keeney KM, Yurist-Doutsch S, Arrieta MC, et al. Effects of antibiotics on human microbiota and subsequent disease. Annu Rev Microbiol 2014;68:217–35.

152. McDonald LC. Effects of short- and long-course antibiotics on the lower intestinal microbiome as they relate to traveller's diarrhea. J Trav Med 2017; 24(suppl_1):S35–8.

153. Langdon A, Crook N, Dantas G. The effects of antibiotics on the microbiome throughout development and alternative approaches for therapeutic modulation. Genome Med 2016;8(1):39.

154. Schwartz DJ, Langdon AE, Dantas G. Understanding the impact of antibiotic perturbation on the human microbiome. Genome Med 2020;12(1):82.

155. Marchant J. When antibiotics turn toxic. Nature 2018;555(7697):431–3.

156. Osterholm MT, Norgan AP. The role of irradiation in food safety. N Engl J Med 2004;350(18):1898–901.

157. Thayer DW. Irradiation of food–helping to ensure food safety. N Engl J Med 2004;350(18):1811–2.

158. Lutter R. Policy forum: food safety. Food irradiation–the neglected solution to food-borne illness. Science 1999;286(5448):2275–6.

159. Voetsch AC, Van Gilder TJ, Angulo FJ, et al. FoodNet estimate of the burden of illness caused by nontyphoidal Salmonella infections in the United States. Clin Infect Dis 2004;38(Suppl 3):S127–34.

160. Montgomery MP, Robertson S, Koski L, et al. Multidrug-Resistant Campylobacter jejuni Outbreak Linked to Puppy Exposure - United States, 2016-2018. MMWR Morb Mortal Wkly Rep 2018;67(37):1032–5.

161. Centers for Disease Control and Prevention. Campylobacter jejuni infection associated with unpasteurized milk and cheese–Kansas, 2007. MMWR Morb Mortal Wkly Rep 2009;57(51):1377–9.

162. Centers for Disease Control and Prevention. Brief report: Gastroenteritis among attendees at a summer cAMP–Wyoming, June-July 2006. MMWR Morb Mortal Wkly Rep 2007;56(15):368–70.

163. Patrick ME, Gilbert MJ, Blaser MJ, et al. Human infections with new subspecies of *Campylobacter fetus*. Emerg Infect Dis 2013;19(10):1678–80.

164. Braden CR. *Salmonella enterica* serotype Enteritidis and eggs: a national epidemic in the United States. Clin Infect Dis 2006;43(4):512–7.

165. Heiman KE, Mody RK, Johnson SD, et al. *Escherichia coli* O157 Outbreaks in the United States, 2003-2012. Emerg Infect Dis 2015;21(8):1293–301.

166. Bowen A, Hurd J, Hoover C, et al. Importation and domestic transmission of *Shigella sonnei* resistant to ciprofloxacin - United States, May 2014-February 2015. MMWR Morb Mortal Wkly Rep 2015;64(12):318–20.

167. Gupta A, Polyak CS, Bishop RD, et al. Laboratory-confirmed shigellosis in the United States, 1989-2002: epidemiologic trends and patterns. Clin Infect Dis 2004;38(10):1372–7.

168. Hines JZ, Pinsent T, Rees K, et al. Notes from the field: shigellosis outbreak among men who have sex with men and homeless persons - Oregon, 2015-2016. MMWR Morb Mortal Wkly Rep 2016;65(31):812–3.

169. Black RE, Jackson RJ, Tsai T, et al. Epidemic *Yersinia enterocolitica* infection due to contaminated chocolate milk. N Engl J Med 1978;298(2):76–9.

170. Bottone EJ. *Yersinia enterocolitica*: the charisma continues. Clin Microbiol Rev 1997;10(2):257–76.

171. Newton AE, Garrett N, Stroika SG, et al. Increase in *Vibrio parahaemolyticus* infections associated with consumption of Atlantic Coast shellfish–2013. MMWR Morb Mortal Wkly Rep 2014;63(15):335–6.

172. Vugia DJ, Tabnak F, Newton AE, et al. Impact of 2003 state regulation on raw oyster-associated *Vibrio vulnificus* illnesses and deaths, California, USA. Emerg Infect Dis 2013;19(8):1276–80.

173. Daniels NA. *Vibrio vulnificus* oysters: pearls and perils. Clin Infect Dis 2011; 52(6):788–92.

174. Mayer HB, Wanke CA. Enteroaggregative *Escherichia coli* as a possible cause of diarrhea in an HIV-infected patient. N Engl J Med 1995;332(4):273–4.

175. Levine MM, Edelman R. Enteropathogenic *Escherichia coli* of classic serotypes associated with infant diarrhea: epidemiology and pathogenesis. Epidemiol Rev 1984;6:31–51.

176. Hebbelstrup Jensen B, Olsen KE, Struve C, et al. Epidemiology and clinical manifestations of enteroaggregative *Escherichia coli*. Clin Microbiol Rev 2014; 27(3):614–30.

177. Nayar DM, Vetrivel S, McElroy J, et al. Toxic megacolon complicating *Escherichia coli* O157 infection. J Infect 2006;52(4):e103–6.

178. Ajene AN, Fischer Walker CL, Black RE. Enteric pathogens and reactive arthritis: a systematic review of *Campylobacter, Salmonella and Shigella*-associated reactive arthritis. J Health Popul Nutr 2013;31(3):299–307.

179. Townes JM, Deodhar AA, Laine ES, et al. Reactive arthritis following culture-confirmed infections with bacterial enteric pathogens in Minnesota and Oregon: a population-based study. Ann Rheum Dis 2008;67(12):1689–96.

180. Porter CK, Choi D, Riddle MS. Pathogen-specific risk of reactive arthritis from bacterial causes of foodborne illness. J Rheumatol 2013;40(5):712–4.

181. Doorduyn Y, Van Pelt W, Siezen CL, et al. Novel insight in the association between salmonellosis or campylobacteriosis and chronic illness, and the role of

host genetics in susceptibility to these diseases. Epidemiol Infect 2008;136(9): 1225–34.

182. Townes JM. Reactive arthritis after enteric infections in the United States: the problem of definition. Clin Infect Dis 2010;50(2):247–54.

183. van Doorn PA, Ruts L, Jacobs BC. Clinical features, pathogenesis, and treatment of Guillain-Barre syndrome. Lancet Neurol 2008;7(10):939–50.

184. Morrison WM, Matheson JA, Hutchison RB, et al. *Salmonella* gastroenteritis associated with erythema nodosum. Br Med J (Clin Res Ed) 1983; 286(6367):765.

185. Debois J, Vandepitte J, Degreef H. *Yersinia enterocolitica* as a cause of erythema nodosum. Dermatologica 1978;156(2):65–78.

Viral Acute Gastroenteritis in Special Populations

Jeffery L. Meier, MD

KEYWORDS

- Acute gastroenteritis • Infectious diarrhea • Norovirus • Rotavirus
- Enteric adenovirus • Sapovirus • Astrovirus • And nitazoxanide

KEY POINTS

- Norovirus is the leading cause of sporadic cases and outbreaks of acute gastroenteritis (AGE) across all ages.
- Universal rotavirus vaccination of infants has reduced the frequency and severity of rotavirus AGE cases in young children and indirectly reduced cases in older adults.
- Other viral causes of AGE include sapoviruses, enteric adenoviruses 40 and 41, and astroviruses.
- Severe viral AGE episodes are more likely in persons at the age extremes or with underlying immunocompromising conditions.
- Viral AGE can result in protracted diarrheal illness in persons with immunocompromising conditions, that is distinguished from other causes of diarrhea through diagnostic testing.

ACUTE GASTROENTERITIS

The World Health Organization ranks acute diarrheal illness as the second leading cause of death among young children worldwide. These deaths largely occur in resource-limited regions of the world because of inadequacy or unavailability of countermeasures to mitigate diarrhea-related dehydration and malnutrition. The consensus definition of acute diarrhea entails having 3 or more loose or unformed stools per day. Acute gastroenteritis (AGE) generally represents the condition of acute watery diarrhea and/or vomiting. The US Centers for Disease Control and Prevention define AGE as acute diarrhea or vomiting.[1] Most AGE cases have diarrhea. AGE may be accompanied by abdominal cramps and low-grade fever. In most AGE cases, the diarrhea resolves in 2 days to 5 days. Diarrhea lasting 14 days to 29 days is classified as persistent diarrhea, whereas chronic diarrhea lasts greater than or equal to 30 days.[2,3] Although AGE incidence is highest among young children, sporadic and outbreak AGE cases commonly involve people of all ages.

Division of Infectious Diseases, Department of Internal Medicine, University of Iowa Carver College of Medicine, Iowa City Veterans Affairs Healthcare System, SW34 GH, 200 Hawkins Dr., Iowa City, IA 52242, USA
E-mail address: jeffery-meier@uiowa.edu

Gastroenterol Clin N Am 50 (2021) 305–322
https://doi.org/10.1016/j.gtc.2021.02.003
0889-8553/21/© 2021 Elsevier Inc. All rights reserved.

gastro.theclinics.com

NOROVIRUS AND ROTAVIRUS ACUTE GASTROENTERITIS

Noroviruses cause a majority of sporadic cases and outbreaks of AGE worldwide.[4] In recent years, norovirus has caused approximately 60% of AGE outbreaks in the United States in which an etiology was determined.[5] The median attack rate was 32% among residents or guests where the norovirus outbreaks took place. Direct person-to-person contact propagated most of these outbreaks. Environmental contamination and foodborne transmission, however, also contribute significantly to norovirus AGE outbreaks,[5,6] and waterborne transmission also is possible.[7] Norovirus outbreaks occur with greater frequency during the winter season and in congregate settings (eg, long-term care facility, health care, school, daycare, and military settings).[5,7] During 2009 to 2013, long-term care facilities accounted for 79% of reported norovirus outbreaks in the United States.[5] Outbreaks on cruise ships are infrequent but draw heightened media attention. Contaminated raspberries were the source of norovirus outbreaks aboard several ships operated by the same cruise line in 2019.[8]

The decline of rotavirus disease after rotavirus vaccination has resulted in norovirus becoming the lead cause of severe AGE in children in several countries.[9] Young children are more likely than older children to have severe AGE. An observational study of norovirus illness in children in Japan revealed that the mean duration of illness was 7 days in children less than 2 years of age compared with 3.5 days for ages 2 years to 4 years.[10] Necrotizing enterocolitis is a feared serious complication of norovirus infection in preterm and term neonates.[11–14] Adults greater than or equal to 65 years of age also are at higher risk of severe norovirus AGE and attributable hospitalization and mortality.[9,15–17] Norovirus caused 82% of the 459 deaths among the 340 AGE outbreaks in the United States during 2009 to 2013, in which an associated death was reported.[5] Most of these deaths involved residents of long-term care facilities. A prospective study of norovirus AGE outbreaks in health care settings in the United Kingdom revealed that the duration of illness was significantly longer in hospitalized patients (median duration 2 days; 75th percentile, 5 days) than in hospital staff (median duration of 2 days; 75th percentile, 4 days).[18] The genogroup 2, genotype 4 (GII.4) norovirus strain has been associated with increased severity of illness in the many AGE outbreaks it has produced across the globe, and the associated deaths were more likely to occur in outbreaks taking place in health care settings, which include long-term care faciliities.[19]

Immunity to norovirus disease after reinfection or re-exposure appears to be specific to the same norovirus strain causing the previous infection.[7] Antigen drift among common norovirus genotypes (ie, GII.4 genotype) has caused global epidemics of norovirus infections.[20,21] Inherited host traits affect susceptibility to norovirus disease. One such trait determines the amount of ABH histo-blood group antigens on the intestinal mucosal surface to which the norovirus attaches. Having antibody that blocks binding of the norovirus to the ABH histo-blood group antigen is associated with decreased risk of illness.[22]

Rotaviruses are a common cause of acute diarrheal illness in young children less than 5 years of age.[22,23] Since 2006, the implementation of rotavirus vaccination of young children in greater than 100 countries has produced a 36% decrease in cases of AGE mortality and a 60% decrease in rotavirus-associated hospitalizations, with larger reductions noted in countries with low childhood mortality and higher vaccine coverage.[24] Severe rotavirus disease occurs with higher frequency in children ages 4 months to 23 months who have not received the rotavirus vaccine.[22] Maternal-fetal transfer of maternal antibody likely accounts for infants younger than 4 months having milder rotavirus illness. Natural rotavirus infection induces sufficient immunity to dampen or prevent symptoms of subsequent reinfections but does not stop all re-infections.[25] The sporadic cases and rare outbreaks of rotavirus AGE that afflict immu-nocompetent adults usually produce mild illness.[25–31] Severe illness requiring hospitalization is more likely to occur in older adults.[25–31] Rates of rotavirus infections in adults have decreased as an indirect effect of rotavirus vaccination of children.[32,33]

OTHER CAUSES OF ACUTE GASTROENTERITIS

Other viral causes of AGE include sapoviruses, enteric adenoviruses 40 and 41, and astroviruses. Sapoviruses cause 3% to 17% of AGE cases in children,[34,35] which can be severe and necessitate hospitalization.[36] Persons ages 65 and older also commonly are affected.[37] Both sapoviruses and noroviruses are members of the Cal-icivirus family and their modes of transmission are similar. Although sapovirus AGE outbreaks increasingly are recognized, they accounted for less than 1% of AGE out-breaks in the United States during 2009 to 2013.[5] A recent study of moderate to severe diarrhea in young children in Africa and Asia versus matched asymptomatic controls found that enteric adenoviruses 40 or 41 ranked next behind rotavirus as most com-mon viral cause of diarrhea.[38] Enteric adenoviruses were not linked to any of the 10,756 AGE outbreaks reported in the United States during 2009 to 2013.[5] Astrovi-ruses are non-enveloped viruses that are transmitted by the fecal-oral route.[39] They cause sporadic cases of AGE in young children and occasionally cause AGE out-breaks.[34,40,41] Adults also may be affected.[40,42,43] Reports published during the se-vere acute respiratory syndrome coronavirus 2 (SARS-Cov-2) pandemic indicate that SARS-Cov-2 infection may present as AGE in infants, children, or adults.[44–46]

In the United States, shigella and salmonella have been the most common nonviral infectious causes of AGE outbreaks, followed in descending order by Shiga toxin-pro-ducing Escherichia coli, campylobacter, clostridium, cryptosporidium, giardia, yersi-nia, listeria, and Cyclospora.[5] Foodborne AGE outbreaks from ingestion of Bacillus cereus toxin or staphylococcal enterotoxin also occasionally were encountered. These nonviral etiologies also can cause sporadic cases of AGE.

IMMUNOCOMPROMISED HOST

Viral AGE in immunocompromised hosts is more likely to result in hospitalization and death. A growing number of reports underscore the propensity of immunocompro-mised persons to develop severe and persistent diarrheal illness caused by rotavi-ruses, noroviruses, enteric adenoviruses, and, less frequently, sapoviruses and astroviruses. Determining whether the virus is a bona fide pathogen or innocent bystander, however, requires attention to the clinicopathologic correlates, because stool of asymptomatic persons may contain the same virus.[25,30,38,47] Also, finding the virus together with another putative pathogen in the diarrheal stool of immunocom-promised persons is not rare.

The incubation period for acute norovirus illness is 24 hours to 48 hours.[48] In the immunocompetent healthy adult, the diarrhea usually resolves in 1 day to 3 days.[7] The diarrhea is more likely to be severe and persistent in immunocompromised pa-tients.[49–52] Chronic continuous or intermittent diarrhea (lasting ≥30 days) may occur in hematopoietic stem cell transplant (HSCT) and solid organ transplant (SOT) recipi-ents.[49,53,54] Chronic norovirus diarrhea also complicates common variable immuno-deficiency that can result in intestinal villous atrophy and malabsorption.[55] In contrast, human immunodeficiency virus (HIV)-infected adults and children with acquired immunodeficiency syndrome (AIDS) develop severe or protracted bouts of norovirus diarrhea infrequently.[56,57]

Severe and persistent rotavirus diarrheal illness affects pediatric and adult HSCT recipients, SOT recipients, patients receiving chemotherapy for cancer, and patients with common variable immunodeficiency.[49,58–60] Allogeneic HCST recipients with severe rotavirus infections often also have graft-versus-host disease (GVHD).[49,61] Children receiving a T-cell–replete haploidentical HSCT and developing GVHD are at higher risk of rotavirus infection, which may be complicated by post-transplantation hemophagocytic syndrome.[62] Rotavirus diarrhea generally is not a greater problem in HIV-infected children,[56,57] and the live attenuated rotavirus vaccines are considered relatively safe for use in most HIV-infected infants.[63]

Immunocompromised persons commonly develop diarrhea for which there are many potential causes. For example, diarrhea in transplant recipients could result from HSCT conditioning chemotherapy, medications (eg, mycophenolate, calcineurin inhibitors, antibiotics, and proton pump inhibitors), GVHD, small bowel overgrowth, or infection. Bacteria, viruses, and parasites are among the wide range of possible etiologies that cause diarrhea in these patients (**Table 1**). Epstein-Barr virus–associated post-transplant lymphoproliferative disorder (PTLD) also can present with diarrhea, and the gastrointestinal tract is the most common extranodal site for PTLD. The relative likelihood of the different etiologies is dependent on several epidemiologic, individual, and transplant population-level variables. Commonly encountered pathogens in SOT recipients are *Clostridioides difficile* (formerly, *Clostridium difficile*), norovirus, and cytomegalovirus (CMV).[64] The relative risk for opportunistic infections is proportional to the degree of immunosuppression imposed by the various types of antirejection treatments. Children and adults living with HIV/AIDS and having $CD4^+$ T-cell counts in blood below 200 cells/mm^3 are predisposed to opportunistic infections with many of the same pathogens encountered in transplant recipients. Diarrhea also may be part of the clinical presentation of AIDS-associated disseminated histoplasmosis, acid-fast bacillus infection (eg, *Mycobacterium avium* complex and tuberculosis), and gastrointestinal Kaposi sarcoma or lymphoma. AIDS-associated diarrhea also may result from idiopathic AIDS enteropathy and small bowel overgrowth.

Table 1
Infectious causes of diarrhea in immunocompromised hosts

Viruses	Bacteria	Protozoa	Mycobacteria	Fungi
Norovirus	Enterotoxigenic *E coli*	*Giardia*	*M avium* complex	Histoplasma
Rotavirus	Shiga-toxin–producing *E coli*	*Cryptosporidium*	*M tuberculosis*	
Enteric adenoviruses	*Salmonella* species	*Cyclospora*		
Sapovirus	*Campylobacter* species	*Cystoisospora*		
Astrovirus	*Shigella* species	*Entamoeba*		
CMV	*C difficile*	*Microsporidia*		
Other adenoviruses	*Yersinia enterocolitica*	*Blastocystis*		
	Listeria monocytogenes			
	Small bowel overgrowth			

CMV produces patchy ulcerative and necroinflammatory disease anywhere along the gastrointestinal tract, from esophagus to rectum, in patients with profound cellular immunodeficiency. In AIDS, CMV disease usually does not develop until the CD4$^+$ T-cell count drops below 50 cells/mm^3 and the anti-HIV therapy is lacking or inadequate. The range in anatomic locations of CMV disease yields a spectrum of symptoms and signs. Occasionally, gastrointestinal CMV disease manifests as acute-onset watery diarrhea.[65–67] Epigastric discomfort, nausea, and dyspepsia also may occur. CMV colitis typically presents as persistent or chronic diarrhea that may be accompanied by abdominal discomfort or cramps, fever, and anorexia. The stool may contain blood.

Adenovirus infection in allogenic HSCT and SOT recipients produces a range of illness, including diarrhea with or without concomitant disseminated adenovirus disease.[49,68–72] The adenovirus species linked most commonly to invasive infections include species A, B, and C. Adenovirus species F, which includes adenoviruses 40 and 41, rarely produces disseminated disease. In an outbreak of adenovirus 41 AGE in 6 pediatric HSCT recipients, however, 4 of the children had adenovirus DNAemia of 10^5 copies/mL in blood, but the severity of disease was less than that caused by adenovirus species C.[70] In another AGE outbreak involving adenovirus A31, 8 pediatric HSCT recipients had prolonged course of diarrhea and DNAemia.[73] Invasive adenovirus infections are more likely to occur in pediatric transplant recipients than in adult recipients.[74,75] In allogenic HSCT recipients, risk factors for adenovirus infection include transplantation with a haploidentical, unrelated, or T-cell–depleted donor graft, severe lymphopenia, severe GVHD, and treatment with alemtuzumab.[74] Adenovirus enteritis is common in intestinal transplants.[75]

TRAVELER'S DIARRHEA

Traveler's diarrhea is an acute diarrhea that affects people who are traveling in resource-limited regions of the world where the level of sanitation may be substandard.[76] This usually develops in the first 2 weeks of travel and is less likely to develop thereafter. The probability of developing traveler's diarrhea depends on travel destination and traveler characteristics. Traveler's diarrhea may be accompanied by fever, nausea, vomiting, abdominal cramps, and fecal urgency. Although the average duration of the untreated diarrhea is 4 days to 5 days, short-term disability as a consequence is a common and a few percent of such travelers have greater than 10 diarrheal stools per day or develop dysentery (eg, visible blood in stool).[76–78] Infants and toddlers often have more severe illness. Travel-related diarrhea accounts for a considerable number of medical visits in returned travelers. Bacteria cause most traveler's diarrhea cases, with enterotoxigenic *Escherichia coli*, enteroaggregative *Escherichia coli*, and diffusely adherent *Escherichia coli* leading the list. Invasive bacterial pathogens, such as salmonella species, *Campylobacter jejuni*, and shigella species, account for 10% to 20% of traveler's diarrhea cases.[79] Less common are vibrio species, *C difficile*, and miscellaneous bacteria types. Remarkably, noroviruses account for 15% to 25% of traveler's diarrhea cases originating in regions of Latin America/Caribbean, Africa, and South Asia.[76] Occasionally, giardia, cryptosporidium, and *Entamoeba histolytica* are the culpable pathogens. Postinfectious irritable bowel syndrome complicates approximately 5% of traveler's diarrhea cases.[78] This troubling sequela may improve gradually over time.

DIAGNOSIS OF INFECTIOUS ACUTE GASTROENTERITIS AND DIARRHEA

Clinical presentation alone often is insufficient to distinguish between viral and bacterial causes of AGE. Acute diarrhea is the predominant feature of most AGE cases.

Clinical information collected from AGE outbreaks in the United States indicates that vomiting does not accompany 33% and 61% of norovirus and salmonella AGE cases, respectively.[5] The 2016 American College of Gastroenterology clinical guideline[3] and 2017 Infectious Disease Society of America clinical practice guidelines[2] lay out approaches to evaluating acute diarrheal illness. This subject also has been addressed recently in published reviews on acute infectious diarrhea in immunocompetent adults[80] and traveler's diarrhea.[76] Guidelines also are available for the evaluation of diarrhea in SOT recipients,[54] traveler's diarrhea,[79] and pathogen-specific causes of diarrhea in AIDS.[63,81]

Most people who develop acute watery diarrhea have an uncomplicated course of self-limited illness. Diagnostic testing to determine etiology is not warranted in these cases unless this information is needed for an outbreak investigation or infection control. Conditions that warrant laboratory testing to determine etiology include the following: visible blood or mucus in stool, signs of sepsis or hemolytic uremic syndrome, severe abdominal pain or tenderness, persistent diarrhea, moderate–severe diarrhea greater than or equal to 3 days with fever greater than or equal to 38.3°C, or traveler's diarrhea lasting greater than 7 days. These conditions include those that increase the probability of involvement of an enteropathogen for which antimicrobial therapy is indicated. Testing for C difficile infection should be considered in people greater than 2 years of age who have a history of diarrhea following antibiotic use within the preceding 8 weeks to 12 weeks or have health care–associated diarrhea. Immunocompromising conditions lower the threshold for initiating diagnostic testing, especially when there is high pretest probability of C difficile–associated disease or clinicoepidemiologic factors raising concern for another enteropathogen.

DIAGNOSTIC TESTS

The nucleic acid amplification test (NAAT) largely is supplanting use of cultures and immunoassays to detect enteric pathogens in stool because the NAAT method (1) quickly provides accurate and highly sensitive test results that likely reduce antibiotic use and procedures[82,83] and (2) requires very little stool specimen that may be collected by rectal swab.[84] Several multiplex NAAT panels have been Food and Drug Administration (FDA) cleared for detection of enteric pathogens. The broad-range multiplex NAAT panel that targets many types of enteric pathogens is used widely. This broad approach to laboratory testing is facing scrutiny as to cost-benefit compared with a tiered approach that might entail use of minipanels and to the reliability of current guideline-based criteria for test utilization.[85] Although the practice of omitting bacterial cultures precludes the determination of the bacteria's antimicrobial susceptibilities to guide antibiotic selection, such susceptibility testing is not needed routinely for antibiotic selection. The lack of culture specimens has hindered public health efforts to detect, investigate, and control outbreaks of enteric bacterial illness using molecular subtyping of infecting bacterial strains and to trend antibiotic resistance in the community.

NAAT-based detection of enteric viruses has been a major advance in elucidating the role and extent of these viruses in diarrheal illness. The clinical interpretation of these results, however, requires an understanding that not all people with presence of enteric viral nucleic acid in stool have illness and that finding more than 1 possible pathogen in stool is not uncommon. Children and immunocompromised hosts are more likely to carry these viruses without symptoms. When more than a single infectious agent is present, the determination of the culpable enteropathogen sometimes can pose a conundrum. This is exemplified in a study of stool test findings in patients diagnosed with community-associated *C difficile* infection, in which approximately 12% of these patients had evidence of viral coinfections with norovirus (6.5% of patients), adenovirus, rotavirus, or sapovirus.[86] The patients with viral coinfection (94% of them were adults) were more likely to have nausea or vomiting, a negative *C difficile* toxin enzyme immunoassay, and negative *C difficile* stool culture. This suggests that *C difficile* may have been an innocent bystander and the virus was the actual pathogen, although other explanations are possible. Routine testing for *C difficile* infection in infants and young children experiencing diarrhea is not recommended because of high prevalence of asymptomatic carriage of toxigenic *C difficile* in the pediatric population.[87]

NAATs focusing only on norovirus detection are commercially available and more sensitive than is the enzyme immunoassay. Multiplex NAATs targeting many different pathogens are designed to reliably detect rotavirus A and norovirus genogroups GI and GII, which are the viral strains causing most cases of rotavirus and norovirus diarrhea, respectively.[82,88] The BioFire FilmArray GI Panel (BioFire Diagnositics, Salt Lake City, UT, USA) additionally detects enteric adenoviruses 40 and 41, sapoviruses, and astrovirus, whereas the Verigene Enteric Pathogen (Luminex Corporation) and Luminex xTAG Gastrointestinal Pathogen Panels (Luminex Corporation) detect enteric adenoviruses 40 and 41. Testing for presence of viral antigen in diarrheal stool using FDA-cleared assays is another way of detecting rotavirus, norovirus, or adenoviruses 40/41. There is no clinical role for a viral culture of stool or viral serologies.

Both BioFire FilmArray GI Panel and Luminex xTAG Gastrointestinal Pathogen Panel additionally detect *Salmonella* species, *Campylobacter* species, Shiga-like toxin-producing *E coli* (*stx1* and *stx2*), enterotoxigenic *E coli*, *Shigella*, *Vibrio* species, *C difficile* toxin A/B, and *Yersinia enterocolitica* as well as the parasites *Giardia lamblia* and *Cryptosporidium*. The BioFire FilmArray GI Panel also detects enteroaggregative *E coli*, enteropathogenic *E coli*, enteroinvasive *E coli*, *E histolytica*, and *Cyclospora cayetanensis*. The Nanosphere Verigene Enteric Panel is designed to detect *Salmonella* species, *Campylobacter* species, *Shigella* species, Shiga toxin-producing *E coli* (*stx1 and stx2*), and *Yersinia enterocolitica* as well as rotavirus A and norovirus GI/GII. Although the broadest range multiplex NAAT commonly is used to evaluate prolonged diarrhea illness in returned travelers, it does not cover the entire gamut of possible infectious etiologies. Stool analysis for ova and parasites (eg, *Balantidium coli*, *Dientamoeba fragilis*, *Cystoisospora*, and *Cyclospora*) is recommended in cases of persistent diarrhea. Blood cultures are recommended for travelers who had consumed food in areas where *Salmonella enterica* serovar Typhi or Paratyphi is endemic or are suspected of having enteric fever. Blood cultures also are indicated for infants less than 3 years of age and in persons with signs of septicemia, regardless of travel history.

DIAGNOSIS IN THE IMMUNOCOMPROMISED HOST

Diarrhea frequently is encountered in immunocompromised populations. Although a wide array of infectious etiologies is possible, *C difficile* and norovirus often are the commonest bacterial and viral causes of diarrhea in this population.[50,51,53,89,90] The SOT guidelines recommend a tiered approach to testing by beginning with a dedicated *C difficile* toxin test and enteric bacterial pathogens culture or NAAT panel applied to stool as well as a quantitative NAAT for CMV DNA detection in plasma/serum or whole blood.[54] The guidelines leave open the option of performing broad range multiplex NAAT for enteric pathogens, if available. Evidence of CMV DNAemia is an indication for anti-CMV treatment. The second tier of testing should include NAAT for norovirus and analyses of parasites, especially *Giardia* and *Cryptosporidium*. The BioFire FilmArray GI Panel reliably provides NAAT-based detection of *Giardia*,

Cryptosporidium, and *Cyclospora.*[91,92] If adenovirus is suspected, a dedicated NAAT for adenovirus DNA should be performed on the relevant clinical specimens (eg, blood and tissue), because this detects all adenovirus types and is more sensitive than the multiplex NAAT.[75] Breath test for bacterial overgrowth also should be considered given the frequency of this problem in the SOT population. If these tests are negative, colonoscopy with or without esophagogastroduodenoscopy should be considered to evaluate possibilities of PTLD, GVHD, CMV, mycobacterial infection, microsporidiosis, and inflammatory bowel disease. Not all CMV disease of the gut is accompanied by CMV DNAemia in blood. Unlike SOT and HSCT, the finding of CMV DNAemia in AIDS is a poor marker of CMV end-organ disease and is not an indication for anti-CMV treatment in the absence of documented end-organ disease.[81] In AIDS, disseminated histoplasmosis may present with diarrhea, fever, abdominal pain, and weight loss.[93,94] Histoplasma antigen usually is detectable in urine and serum of these patients. The same symptoms also can be a manifestation of AIDS-associated disseminated *M avium* complex.[95] The *M avium* complex organism usually is recovered by acid-fast bacteria culture of blood or bone marrow of these patients.[81] Evidence of the opportunistic pathogen in biopsy specimens of gastrointestinal tissues cinches the diagnosis.

POSTINFECTIOUS IRRITABLE BOWEL SYNDROME

AGE is a risk factor for postinfectious irritable bowel syndrome. This syndrome follows approximately 5% to 15% of infectious diarrhea cases caused by bacterial pathogens.[96] Viral diarrhea is viewed as less likely to cause this syndrome. A massive norovirus AGE outbreak arising from a contaminated municipal water supply was subjected to a prospective population-based study with a control group to assess the incidence of postinfectious irritable bowel syndrome in adults.[97] This study found that norovirus AGE led to the development of postinfectious irritable bowel syndrome in 13% of the patients. Thus, the most common cause of sporadic cases and outbreaks of AGE has the potential to produce postinfectious irritable bowel syndrome.

MANAGEMENT OF VIRAL ACUTE GASTROENTERITIS

The management of AGE-like illness and specific treatments of the different pathogens causing diarrhea are detailed in clinical practice guidelines,[2,3] including guidelines specifically focusing on travelers,[79] SOT recipients,[54] persons with AIDS,[63,81] and persons having *C difficile* infection.[87] Attention to hydration and salt replacement is essential. Use of oral rehydration solutions (consisting of glucose, sodium, potassium, chloride, and sodium citrate) is the cornerstone of prevention or treatment of dehydration in children having diarrhea and/or vomiting. In low-income regions, underlying malnutrition and zinc deficiency are common and contribute to worse outcomes in children with acute diarrhea. Maintaining adequate protein-calorie intake during the diarrhea is especially important in this setting. The World Health Organization also recommends daily zinc supplementation for 10 days to 14 days in infants and young children living in low-income regions.

Most AGE episodes are short lived and uncomplicated. For an AGE producing watery diarrhea, age-appropriate use of an antimotility drug (eg, loperamide) can be considered in an immunocompetent host if fever is absent or low grade. Empiric antibiotic therapy should not be given in this situation. Travel-related watery diarrhea with moderate to severe illness is an exception in which empiric antibiotic therapy may be warranted. Dysenteric diarrheal stools (visible blood in stool) should be tested for presence of bacterial pathogens and antimicrobial treatment directed at the specific pathogen if not a Shiga-toxin-producing *E coli*. Empiric antibiotic therapy is considered for bloody diarrhea in infants less than 3 months old, immunocompromised persons with severe illness, or febrile travelers having visited areas in which the pathogens causing dysentery are endemic. *C difficile* infection usually does not produce visible blood in stool. The specific antimicrobial drugs used to treat the various nonviral enteric pathogens fall outside the scope of this report.

ANTIVIRAL TREATMENT

In immunocompromised hosts, the reduction in immunosuppressive therapy, if feasible, is a key step in ameliorating gastrointestinal illness caused by viruses. There are no clinically proved effective antiviral treatments for infections with rotavirus, norovirus, sapovirus, or astrovirus. Passive immunization with oral or parenteral immunoglobulin has been used but efficacy has not been established clearly. Case series and a small case-control study have produced mixed results as to benefit of oral immunoglobulin use for treatment of norovirus diarrhea in transplant recipients and other immunocompromised patients.[98–101] Anecdotal reports citing improvement of rotavirus diarrhea in association with use of enteral immunoglobulin in transplant recipients and other immunocompromise patients have not been tested in a randomized controlled trial.[61,101–103] A meta-analysis of clinical studies evaluating oral immunoglobulin Y, which is derived from the yolk of eggs of chickens vaccinated with rotavirus, suggests efficacy of this investigational treatment of infantile rotavirus enteritis.[104]

Nitazoxanide has antiviral activity against rotavirus, norovirus, and astrovirus.[105–107] Nitazoxanide is FDA approved for treatment of diarrhea caused by *Giardia lamblia* or *Cryptosporidium parvum* in people ages greater than or equal to 1 year and is administered orally as a tablet or oral suspension. Several case reports and small case series speak to the variable success of using nitazoxanide to treat norovirus diarrhea in immunocompromised patients.[108–112] An ongoing phase 2, randomized, double-blind, placebo-controlled study (NCT03395405) will determine efficacy and safety of nitazoxanide for treatment of norovirus diarrhea in HSCT and SOT recipients. Nitazoxanide also has been used for treatment of rotavirus diarrhea. A small, randomized, double-blind, placebo-controlled trial of nitazoxanide for treatment of rotavirus diarrhea in young children found nitazoxanide to decrease duration of severe diarrheal illness.[113] Nitazoxanide also decreased duration of acute rotavirus diarrhea in Bolivian children, based on results of a randomized single-blind controlled trial.[114] Ribavirin also has been used for treatment of norovirus diarrhea in immunocompromised patients,[55,112,115] with case reports of treatment success and failure.

Severe adenovirus infections in immunocompromised patients may require treatment with intravenous cidofovir, although dose-limiting nephrotoxicity is common. Guidelines have been issued on the treatment of adenovirus infections in SOT[75] and HSCT[74,116] recipients. Invasive CMV infection of the gastrointestinal tract usually is treated initially with intravenous ganciclovir until a patient's condition allows the use of oral valganciclovir for a total treatment duration of 2 weeks to 3 weeks. Guidelines for treatment of gastrointestinal CMV disease are available for the clinical settings of AIDS,[81] SOT,[117] HSCT,[118] and inflammatory bowel disease.[119]

PREVENTION OF VIRAL ACUTE GASTROENTERITIS

Rotavirus AGE is preventable by vaccination. Oral live-attenuated rotavirus vaccines, for example, RotaTeq (Merck and CO., INC., Whitehouse Station, NJ, USA) and ROTARIX (GlaxoSmithKline Biologicals, Rixesart, Belgium), have been licensed for use in many countries, including the United States. The first dose of the vaccine is administered to the child at 6 weeks of age and not later than 15 weeks.[120] The vaccine is contraindicated in children with severe immunodeficiency because of risk for severe, protracted illness. Although it is recommended that rotavirus vaccine is delayed until after 6 months of age if an infant was exposed in utero to an anti–tumor necrosis factor (TNF)-α monoclonal antibody that can cross the placenta, residual anti–TNF-α antibody does not appear to affect response to the vaccine.[121] It is advisable to vaccinate infants living in households with a person with immunodeficiency as well as non-immunocompromised infants with preexisting chronic gastrointestinal disease. Mild temporary diarrhea and vomiting are known possible side effects. Reports of vaccine-associated intussusception are rare.[122] Norovirus vaccine candidates are in various stages of preclinical and clinical development.[123,124] The immunologic correlates of protection from norovirus infection are poorly understood.[124] Norovirus human challenge studies reveal that norovirus immunity is strain-specific and only lasts for a few years.[123] Challenge studies also suggest that vomiting may be an underappreciated source of viral spread, because approximately half of AGE cases did not have diarrhea and the emesis contained 10^4 to 10^5 viral genome equivalents/mL.[125] Public health control measures that limit the spread of norovirus to others include hand hygiene, environmental disinfection, and activity or work restrictions for ill staff members.[7] The Healthcare Infection Control Practices Advisory Committee has provided national guidelines for the prevention and control of norovirus AGE outbreaks in health care settings,[126] although state-level guidelines may vary somewhat from these guidelines.[127] The same prevention measures are applied to other AGE-causing viruses that are transmitted predominately by the fecal-oral route. They do not apply to CMV because this virus is horizontally transmitted by close mucosal contact with infectious body fluids, such as saliva, urine, breast milk, semen, and cervical secretions. CMV vaccine candidates are in clinical development. Probiotic use for prevention and management of infectious diarrhea have been addressed in recent guidelines.[2,3] Although there are differing recommendations, probiotic preparations may be considered for the purpose of decreasing symptom severity and duration of diarrhea in immunocompetent adults and children.

CLINICS CARE POINTS

- Individual and special population-level characteristics guide decision and approach to the diagnostic evaluation of AGE-related diarrhea illness.

- Nonviral causes of AGE-like illness are more common in the setting of traveler's diarrhea.

- Gastrointestinal pathogen nucleic acid detection panels are advantageous in the rapid diagnosis of viral and non-viral causes of AGE-related diarrheal illness, subject to diagnostic test stewardship.

- Cytomegalovirus and other opportunistic pathogens that cause diarrhea in immunocompromised persons require additional diagnostic strategies to identify the etiology and treat accordingly.

- The efficacy of oral and parenteral immunoglobulins and nitazoxanide treatment of persistent norovirus or rotavirus diarrhea in immunocompromised persons has not been clearly established.

DISCLOSURE

The author has nothing to disclose.

FUNDING SOURCES

United States Department of Veterans Affairs Merit award I01 BX004434.

REFERENCES

1. Hall AJ, Wikswo ME, Manikonda K, et al. Acute gastroenteritis surveillance through the national outbreak reporting system, United States. Emerg Infect Dis 2013;19(8):1305–9.
2. Shane AL, Mody RK, Crump JA, et al. 2017 Infectious diseases society of america clinical practice guidelines for the diagnosis and management of infectious diarrhea. Clin Infect Dis 2017;65(12):e45–80.
3. Riddle MS, DuPont HL, Connor BA. ACG clinical guideline: diagnosis, treatment, and prevention of acute diarrheal infections in adults. Am J Gastroenterol 2016;111(5):602–22.
4. Ahmed SM, Hall AJ, Robinson AE, et al. Global prevalence of norovirus in cases of gastroenteritis: a systematic review and meta-analysis. Lancet Infect Dis 2014;14(8):725–30.
5. Wikswo ME, Kambhampati A, Shioda K, et al. Outbreaks of acute gastroenteritis transmitted by person-to-person contact, environmental contamination, and unknown modes of transmission–United States, 2009-2013. MMWR Surveill Summ 2015;64(12):1–16.
6. Hall AJ, Eisenbart VG, Etingue AL, et al. Epidemiology of foodborne norovirus outbreaks, United States, 2001-2008. Emerg Infect Dis 2012;18(10):1566–73.
7. Robilotti E, Deresinski S, Pinsky BA. Norovirus. Clin Microbiol Rev 2015;28(1): 134–64.
8. Rispens JR, Freeland A, Wittry B, et al. Notes from the field: multiple cruise ship outbreaks of norovirus associated with frozen fruits and berries - United States, 2019. MMWR Morb Mortal Wkly Rep 2020;69(16):501–2.
9. Kowalzik F, Binder H, Zoller D, et al. Norovirus gastroenteritis among hospitalized patients, Germany, 2007-2012. Emerg Infect Dis 2018;24(11):2021–8.
10. Murata T, Katsushima N, Mizuta K, et al. Prolonged norovirus shedding in infants <or=6 months of age with gastroenteritis. Pediatr Infect Dis J 2007;26(1):46–9.
11. Bagci S, Eis-Hubinger AM, Yassin AF, et al. Clinical characteristics of viral intestinal infection in preterm and term neonates. Eur J Clin Microbiol Infect Dis 2010; 29(9):1079–84.
12. Pelizzo G, Nakib G, Goruppi I, et al. Isolated colon ischemia with norovirus infection in preterm babies: a case series. J Med Case Rep 2013;7:108.
13. Turcios-Ruiz RM, Axelrod P, St John K, et al. Outbreak of necrotizing enterocolitis caused by norovirus in a neonatal intensive care unit. J Pediatr 2008;153(3): 339–44.
14. Stuart RL, Tan K, Mahar JE, et al. An outbreak of necrotizing enterocolitis associated with norovirus genotype GII.3. Pediatr Infect Dis J 2010;29(7):644–7.
15. Lindsay L, Wolter J, De Coster I, et al. A decade of norovirus disease risk among older adults in upper-middle and high income countries: a systematic review. BMC Infect Dis 2015;15:425.
16. Hall AJ, Lopman BA, Payne DC, et al. Norovirus disease in the United States. Emerg Infect Dis 2013;19(8):1198–205.

17. Harris JP, Edmunds WJ, Pebody R, et al. Deaths from norovirus among the elderly, England and Wales. Emerg Infect Dis 2008;14(10):1546–52.

18. Lopman BA, Reacher MH, Vipond IB, et al. Clinical manifestation of norovirus gastroenteritis in health care settings. Clin Infect Dis 2004;39(3):318–24.

19. Desai R, Hembree CD, Handel A, et al. Severe outcomes are associated with genogroup 2 genotype 4 norovirus outbreaks: a systematic literature review. Clin Infect Dis 2012;55(2):189–93.

20. Siebenga JJ, Vennema H, Zheng DP, et al. Norovirus illness is a global problem: emergence and spread of norovirus GII.4 variants, 2001-2007. J Infect Dis 2009;200(5):802–12.

21. de Graaf M, van Beek J, Koopmans MP. Human norovirus transmission and evolution in a changing world. Nat Rev Microbiol 2016;14(7):421–33.

22. Banyai K, Estes MK, Martella V, et al. Viral gastroenteritis. Lancet 2018; 392(10142):175–86.

23. Crawford SE, Ramani S, Tate JE, et al. Rotavirus infection. Nat Rev Dis Primers 2017;3:17083.

24. Burnett E, Parashar UD, Tate JE. Global impact of rotavirus vaccination on diarrhea hospitalizations and deaths among children <5 years old: 2006-2019. J Infect Dis 2020. https://doi.org/10.1093/infdis/jiaa081.

25. Anderson EJ, Weber SG. Rotavirus infection in adults. Lancet Infect Dis 2004; 4(2):91–9.

26. Anderson EJ, Katz BZ, Polin JA, et al. Rotavirus in adults requiring hospitalization. J Infect 2012;64(1):89–95.

27. Anderson EJ, Shippee DB, Tate JE, et al. Clinical characteristics and genotypes of rotavirus in adults. J Infect 2015;70(6):683–7.

28. Friesema IH, De Boer RF, Duizer E, et al. Aetiology of acute gastroenteritis in adults requiring hospitalization in The Netherlands. Epidemiol Infect 2012; 140(10):1780–6.

29. Cardemil CV, Cortese MM, Medina-Marino A, et al. Two rotavirus outbreaks caused by genotype G2P[4] at large retirement communities: cohort studies. Ann Intern Med 2012;157(9):621–31.

30. Quee FA, de Hoog MLA, Schuurman R, et al. Community burden and transmission of acute gastroenteritis caused by norovirus and rotavirus in the Netherlands (RotaFam): a prospective household-based cohort study. Lancet Infect Dis 2020;20(5):598–606.

31. Beck-Friis T, Andersson M, Gustavsson L, et al. Burden of rotavirus infection in hospitalized elderly individuals prior to the introduction of rotavirus vaccination in Sweden. J Clin Virol 2019;119:1–5.

32. Gastanaduy PA, Curns AT, Parashar UD, et al. Gastroenteritis hospitalizations in older children and adults in the United States before and after implementation of infant rotavirus vaccination. JAMA 2013;310(8):851–3.

33. Baker JM, Tate JE, Steiner CA, et al. Longer-term Direct and indirect effects of infant rotavirus vaccination across all ages in the united states in 2000-2013: analysis of a large hospital discharge data set. Clin Infect Dis 2019;68(6): 976–83.

34. Hassan F, Kanwar N, Harrison CJ, et al. Viral etiology of acute gastroenteritis in <2-year-old us children in the post-rotavirus vaccine era. J Pediatric Infect Dis Soc 2019;8(5):414–21.

35. Becker-Dreps S, Bucardo F, Vinje J. Sapovirus: an important cause of acute gastroenteritis in children. Lancet Child Adolesc Health 2019;3(11):758–9.

36. Becker-Dreps S, Gonzalez F, Bucardo F. Sapovirus: an emerging cause of childhood diarrhea. Curr Opin Infect Dis 2020;33(5):388–97.

37. Pang XL, Lee BE, Tyrrell GJ, et al. Epidemiology and genotype analysis of sapovirus associated with gastroenteritis outbreaks in Alberta, Canada: 2004-2007. J Infect Dis 2009;199(4):547–51.

38. Liu J, Platts-Mills JA, Juma J, et al. Use of quantitative molecular diagnostic methods to identify causes of diarrhoea in children: a reanalysis of the GEMS case-control study. Lancet 2016;388(10051):1291–301.

39. Bosch A, Pinto RM, Guix S. Human astroviruses. Clin Microbiol Rev 2014;27(4): 1048–74.

40. Vu DL, Bosch A, Pinto RM, et al. Epidemiology of classic and novel human astrovirus: gastroenteritis and beyond. Viruses 2017;9(2):33.

41. Dennehy PH, Nelson SM, Spangenberger S, et al. A prospective case-control study of the role of astrovirus in acute diarrhea among hospitalized young children. J Infect Dis 2001;184(1):10–5.

42. Jarchow-Macdonald AA, Halley S, Chandler D, et al. First report of an astrovirus type 5 gastroenteritis outbreak in a residential elderly care home identified by sequencing. J Clin Virol 2015;73:115–9.

43. Belliot G, Laveran H, Monroe SS. Outbreak of gastroenteritis in military recruits associated with serotype 3 astrovirus infection. J Med Virol 1997;51(2):101–6.

44. Tariq R, Saha S, Furqan F, et al. Prevalence and mortality of COVID-19 patients with gastrointestinal symptoms: a systematic review and meta-analysis. Mayo Clin Proc 2020;95(8):1632–48.

45. Pan L, Mu M, Yang P, et al. Clinical characteristics of COVID-19 patients with digestive symptoms in hubei, china: a descriptive, cross-sectional, multicenter study. Am J Gastroenterol 2020;115(5):766–73.

46. Liu Q, Zhang Y, Long Y. A child infected with severe acute respiratory syndrome coronavirus 2 presenting with diarrhea without fever and cough: a case report. Medicine (Baltimore) 2020;99(33):e21427.

47. Phillips G, Lopman B, Rodrigues LC, et al. Asymptomatic rotavirus infections in England: prevalence, characteristics, and risk factors. Am J Epidemiol 2010; 171(9):1023–30.

48. Lee RM, Lessler J, Lee RA, et al. Incubation periods of viral gastroenteritis: a systematic review. BMC Infect Dis 2013;13:446.

49. Ghosh N, Malik FA, Daver RG, et al. Viral associated diarrhea in immunocompromised and cancer patients at a large comprehensive cancer center: a 10-year retrospective study. Infect Dis (Lond) 2017;49(2):113–9.

50. Munir N, Liu P, Gastanaduy P, et al. Norovirus infection in immunocompromised children and children with hospital-acquired acute gastroenteritis. J Med Virol 2014;86(7):1203–9.

51. Bok K, Green KY. Norovirus gastroenteritis in immunocompromised patients. N Engl J Med 2012;367(22):2126–32.

52. Swartling L, Ljungman P, Remberger M, et al. Norovirus causing severe gastrointestinal disease following allogeneic hematopoietic stem cell transplantation: A retrospective analysis. Transpl Infect Dis 2018;20(2):e12847.

53. Brown JR, Shah D, Breuer J. Viral gastrointestinal infections and norovirus genotypes in a paediatric UK hospital, 2014-2015. J Clin Virol 2016;84:1–6.

54. Angarone M, Snydman DR, Practice AICo. Diagnosis and management of diarrhea in solid-organ transplant recipients: Guidelines from the American society of transplantation infectious diseases community of practice. Clin Transplant 2019;33(9):e13550.

55. Woodward J, Gkrania-Klotsas E, Kumararatne D. Chronic norovirus infection and common variable immunodeficiency. Clin Exp Immunol 2017;188(3):363–70.
56. Grohmann GS, Glass RI, Pereira HG, et al. Enteric viruses and diarrhea in HIV-infected patients. Enteric opportunistic infections working group. N Engl J Med 1993;329(1):14–20.
57. Weber R, Ledergerber B, Zbinden R, et al. Enteric infections and diarrhea in human immunodeficiency virus-infected persons: prospective community-based cohort study. Swiss HIV Cohort Study. Arch Intern Med 1999;159(13):1473–80.
58. Bruijning-Verhagen P, Nipshagen MD, de Graaf H, et al. Rotavirus disease course among immunocompromised patients; 5-year observations from a tertiary care medical centre. J Infect 2017;75(5):448–54.
59. Rayani A, Bode U, Habas E, et al. Rotavirus infections in paediatric oncology patients: a matched-pairs analysis. Scand J Gastroenterol 2007;42(1):81–7.
60. Yin Y, Metselaar HJ, Sprengers D, et al. Rotavirus in organ transplantation: drug-virus-host interactions. Am J Transplant 2015;15(3):585–93.
61. Flerlage T, Hayden R, Cross SJ, et al. Rotavirus infection in pediatric allogeneic hematopoietic cell transplant recipients: clinical course and experience using nitazoxanide and enterally administered immunoglobulins. Pediatr Infect Dis J 2018;37(2):176–81.
62. Jaiswal SR, Bhakuni P, Chakrabarti A, et al. Rotavirus infection following post-transplantation cyclophosphamide based haploidentical hematopoietic cell transplantation in children is associated with hemophagocytic syndrome and high mortality. Transpl Infect Dis 2019;21(5):e13136.
63. Panel on opportunistic infections in HIV-exposed and HIV-infected children. guidelines for the prevention and treatment of opportunistic infections in hiv-exposed and hiv-infected children. Department of health and human services. Available at: https://clinicalinfo.hiv.gov/sites/default/files/guidelines/documents/OI_Guidelines_Pediatrics.pdf. Accessed March 16, 2021.
64. Echenique IA, Penugonda S, Stosor V, et al. Diagnostic yields in solid organ transplant recipients admitted with diarrhea. Clin Infect Dis 2015;60(5):729–37.
65. Seminari E, Fronti E, Contardi G, et al. Colitis in an elderly immunocompetent patient. J Clin Virol 2012;55(3):187–90.
66. Einbinder Y, Wolf DG, Pappo O, et al. The clinical spectrum of cytomegalovirus colitis in adults. Aliment Pharmacol Ther 2008;27(7):578–87.
67. Alhyraba M, Grim SA, Benedetti E, et al. Unusual presentation of cytomegalovirus enteritis after liver and kidney transplantation. Transpl Infect Dis 2007;9(4):343–6.
68. Baldwin A, Kingman H, Darville M, et al. Outcome and clinical course of 100 patients with adenovirus infection following bone marrow transplantation. Bone Marrow Transplant 2000;26(12):1333–8.
69. Jalal H, Bibby DF, Tang JW, et al. First reported outbreak of diarrhea due to adenovirus infection in a hematology unit for adults. J Clin Microbiol 2005;43(6):2575–80.
70. Mattner F, Sykora KW, Meissner B, et al. An adenovirus type F41 outbreak in a pediatric bone marrow transplant unit: analysis of clinical impact and preventive strategies. Pediatr Infect Dis J 2008;27(5):419–24.
71. Kim NJ, Hyun TS, Pergam SA, et al. Disseminated adenovirus infection after autologous stem cell transplant. Transpl Infect Dis 2020;22(1):e13238.
72. Cox GJ, Matsui SM, Lo RS, et al. Etiology and outcome of diarrhea after marrow transplantation: a prospective study. Gastroenterology 1994;107(5):1398–407.

73. Swartling L, Allard A, Torlen J, et al. Prolonged outbreak of adenovirus A31 in allogeneic stem cell transplant recipients. Transpl Infect Dis 2015;17(6):785–94.

74. Matthes-Martin S, Feuchtinger T, Shaw PJ, et al. European guidelines for diagnosis and treatment of adenovirus infection in leukemia and stem cell transplantation: summary of ECIL-4 (2011). Transpl Infect Dis 2012;14(6):555–63.

75. Florescu DF, Schaenman JM, Practice ASTIDCo. Adenovirus in solid organ transplant recipients: guidelines from the American society of transplantation infectious diseases community of practice. Clin Transplant 2019;33(9):e13527.

76. Steffen R, Hill DR, DuPont HL. Traveler's diarrhea: a clinical review. JAMA 2015; 313(1):71–80.

77. Porter CK, Olson S, Hall A, et al. Travelers' Diarrhea: an update on the incidence, etiology, and risk in military deployments and similar travel populations. Mil Med 2017;182(S2):4–10.

78. Steffen R. Epidemiology of travellers' diarrhea. J Travel Med 2017; 24(suppl_1):S2–5.

79. Riddle MS, Connor BA, Beeching NJ, et al. Guidelines for the prevention and treatment of travelers' diarrhea: a graded expert panel report. J Travel Med 2017;24(suppl_1):S57–74.

80. DuPont HL. Acute infectious diarrhea in immunocompetent adults. N Engl J Med 2014;370(16):1532–40.

81. Panel on opportunistic infections in HIV-infected adults and adolescents. Guidelines for the prevention and treatment of opportunistic infections in HIV-infected adults and adolescents: recommendations from the centers for disease control and prevention, the national institutes of health, and the HIV Medicine association of the infectious diseases society of America. Available at: https://clinicalinfo.hiv.gov/sites/default/files/guidelines/documents/Adult_OI.pdf. Accessed March 16, 2021.

82. Ramanan P, Bryson AL, Binnicker MJ, et al. Syndromic panel-based testing in clinical microbiology. Clin Microbiol Rev 2018;31(1):e00024-17.

83. Axelrad JE, Freedberg DE, Whittier S, et al. Impact of gastrointestinal panel implementation on health care utilization and outcomes. J Clin Microbiol 2019; 57(3):e01775-18.

84. Walker CR, Lechiile K, Mokomane M, et al. Evaluation of anatomically designed flocked rectal swabs for use with the biofire filmarray gastrointestinal panel for detection of enteric pathogens in children admitted to hospital with severe gastroenteritis. J Clin Microbiol 2019;57(12):e00962-19.

85. Clark SD, Sidlak M, Mathers AJ, et al. Clinical yield of a molecular diagnostic panel for enteric pathogens in adult outpatients with diarrhea and validation of guidelines-based criteria for testing. Open Forum Infect Dis 2019;6(4):ofz162.

86. Korhonen L, Cohen J, Gregoricus N, et al. Evaluation of viral co-infections among patients with community-associated Clostridioides difficile infection. PLoS One 2020;15(10):e0240549.

87. McDonald LC, Gerding DN, Johnson S, et al. Clinical practice guidelines for clostridium difficile infection in adults and children: 2017 update by the infectious diseases society of America (IDSA) and society for healthcare epidemiology of America (SHEA). Clin Infect Dis 2018;66(7):e1–48.

88. Chhabra P, Gregoricus N, Weinberg GA, et al. Comparison of three multiplex gastrointestinal platforms for the detection of gastroenteritis viruses. J Clin Virol 2017;95:66–71.

89. Alejo-Cancho I, Fernandez Aviles F, Capon A, et al. Evaluation of a multiplex panel for the diagnosis of acute infectious diarrhea in immunocompromised hematologic patients. PLoS One 2017;12(11):e0187458.

90. Daniel-Wayman S, Fahle G, Palmore T, et al. Norovirus, astrovirus, and sapovirus among immunocompromised patients at a tertiary care research hospital. Diagn Microbiol Infect Dis 2018;92(2):143–6.

91. Hitchcock MM, Hogan CA, Budvytiene I, et al. Reproducibility of positive results for rare pathogens on the FilmArray GI Panel. Diagn Microbiol Infect Dis 2019; 95(1):10–4.

92. Buss SN, Leber A, Chapin K, et al. Multicenter evaluation of the BioFire FilmArray gastrointestinal panel for etiologic diagnosis of infectious gastroenteritis. J Clin Microbiol 2015;53(3):915–25.

93. Assi M, McKinsey DS, Driks MR, et al. Gastrointestinal histoplasmosis in the acquired immunodeficiency syndrome: report of 18 cases and literature review. Diagn Microbiol Infect Dis 2006;55(3):195–201.

94. Gutierrez ME, Canton A, Sosa N, et al. Disseminated histoplasmosis in patients with AIDS in Panama: a review of 104 cases. Clin Infect Dis 2005;40(8): 1199–202.

95. Gordin FM, Cohn DL, Sullam PM, et al. Early manifestations of disseminated Mycobacterium avium complex disease: a prospective evaluation. J Infect Dis 1997;176(1):126–32.

96. Svendsen AT, Bytzer P, Engsbro AL. Systematic review with meta-analyses: does the pathogen matter in post-infectious irritable bowel syndrome? Scand J Gastroenterol 2019;54(5):546–62.

97. Zanini B, Ricci C, Bandera F, et al. Incidence of post-infectious irritable bowel syndrome and functional intestinal disorders following a water-borne viral gastroenteritis outbreak. Am J Gastroenterol 2012;107(6):891–9.

98. Florescu DF, Hermsen ED, Kwon JY, et al. Is there a role for oral human immunoglobulin in the treatment for norovirus enteritis in immunocompromised patients? Pediatr Transplant 2011;15(7):718–21.

99. Chagla Z, Quirt J, Woodward K, et al. Chronic norovirus infection in a transplant patient successfully treated with enterally administered immune globulin. J Clin Virol 2013;58(1):306–8.

100. Gairard-Dory AC, Degot T, Hirschi S, et al. Clinical usefulness of oral immunoglobulins in lung transplant recipients with norovirus gastroenteritis: a case series. Transplant Proc 2014;46(10):3603–5.

101. Alexander E, Hommeida S, Stephens MC, et al. The role of oral administration of immunoglobulin in managing diarrheal illness in immunocompromised children. Paediatr Drugs 2020;22(3):331–4.

102. Williams D. Treatment of rotavirus-associated diarrhea using enteral immunoglobulins for pediatric stem cell transplant patients. J Oncol Pharm Pract 2015;21(3):238–40.

103. Kanfer EJ, Abrahamson G, Taylor J, et al. Severe rotavirus-associated diarrhoea following bone marrow transplantation: treatment with oral immunoglobulin. Bone Marrow Transplant 1994;14(4):651–2.

104. Wang X, Song L, Tan W, et al. Clinical efficacy of oral immunoglobulin Y in infant rotavirus enteritis: systematic review and meta-analysis. Medicine (Baltimore) 2019;98(27):e16100.

105. Rossignol JF. Nitazoxanide: a first-in-class broad-spectrum antiviral agent. Antiviral Res 2014;110:94–103.

106. Hargest V, Sharp B, Livingston B, et al. Astrovirus replication is inhibited by ni-
     tazoxanide in vitro and in vivo. J Virol 2020;94.
107. Dang W, Xu L, Ma B, et al. Nitazoxanide inhibits human norovirus replication and
     synergizes with ribavirin by activation of cellular antiviral response. Antimicrobial
     Agents Chemother 2018;62(11):e00707-18.
108. Avery RK, Lonze BE, Kraus ES, et al. Severe chronic norovirus diarrheal disease
     in transplant recipients: Clinical features of an under-recognized syndrome.
     Transpl Infect Dis 2017;19(2). https://doi.org/10.1111/tid.12674.
109. Ghusson N, Vasquez G. Successfully treated norovirus- and sapovirus-
     associated diarrhea in three renal transplant patients. Case Rep Infect Dis
     2018;2018:6846873.
110. Siddiq DM, Koo HL, Adachi JA, et al. Norovirus gastroenteritis successfully
     treated with nitazoxanide. J Infect 2011;63(5):394–7.
111. Haubrich K, Gantt S, Blydt-Hansen T. Successful treatment of chronic norovirus
     gastroenteritis with nitazoxanide in a pediatric kidney transplant recipient. Pe-
     diatr Transplant 2018;22(4):e13186.
112. Brown LK, Ruis C, Clark I, et al. A comprehensive characterization of chronic
     norovirus infection in immunodeficient hosts. J Allergy Clin Immunol 2019;
     144(5):1450–3.
113. Rossignol J, Abu-Zekry M, Hussein A, et al. Effect of nitazoxanide for treatment
     of severe rotavirus diarrhoea: randomised double-blind placebo-controlled trial.
     Lancet 2006;368:124–9.
114. Teran CG, Teran-Escalera CN, Villarroel P. Nitazoxanide vs. probiotics for the
     treatment of acute rotavirus diarrhea in children: a randomized, single-blind,
     controlled trial in Bolivian children. Int J Infect Dis 2009;13(4):518–23.
115. Brown LK, Clark I, Brown JR, et al. Norovirus infection in primary immune defi-
     ciency. Rev Med Virol 2017;27(3):e1926.
116. Hiwarkar P, Kosulin K, Cesaro S, et al. Management of adenovirus infection in
     patients after haematopoietic stem cell transplantation: state-of-the-art and
     real-life current approach: a position statement on behalf of the infectious dis-
     eases working party of the european society of blood and marrow transplanta-
     tion. Rev Med Virol 2018;28(3):e1980.
117. Kotton CN, Kumar D, Caliendo AM, et al. The third international consensus
     guidelines on the management of cytomegalovirus in solid-organ transplanta-
     tion. Transplantation 2018;102(6):900–31.
118. Ljungman P, de la Camara R, Robin C, et al. Guidelines for the management of
     cytomegalovirus infection in patients with haematological malignancies and af-
     ter stem cell transplantation from the 2017 European conference on infections in
     leukaemia (ECIL 7). Lancet Infect Dis 2019;19(8):e260–72.
119. Lamb CA, Kennedy NA, Raine T, et al. British Society of Gastroenterology
     consensus guidelines on the management of inflammatory bowel disease in
     adults. Gut 2019;68(Suppl 3):s1–106.
120. Cortese MM, Parashar UD, Centers for Disease C, Prevention. Prevention of
     rotavirus gastroenteritis among infants and children: recommendations of the
     Advisory Committee on Immunization Practices (ACIP). MMWR Recomm Rep
     2009;58(RR-2):1–25.
121. Beaulieu DB, Ananthakrishnan AN, Martin C, et al. Use of biologic therapy by
     pregnant women with inflammatory bowel disease does not affect infant
     response to vaccines. Clin Gastroenterol Hepatol 2018;16(1):99–105.
122. Burnett E, Parashar U, Tate J. Rotavirus vaccines: effectiveness, safety, and
     future directions. Paediatr Drugs 2018;20(3):223–33.

123. Mattison CP, Cardemil CV, Hall AJ. Progress on norovirus vaccine research: public health considerations and future directions. Expert Rev Vaccines 2018; 17(9):773–84.
124. Cortes-Penfield NW, Ramani S, Estes MK, et al. Prospects and challenges in the development of a norovirus vaccine. Clin Ther 2017;39(8):1537–49.
125. Kirby AE, Streby A, Moe CL. Vomiting as a symptom and transmission risk in norovirus illness: evidence from human challenge studies. PLoS One 2016; 11(4):e0143759.
126. MacCannell T, Umscheid CA, Agarwal RK, et al. Guideline for the prevention and control of norovirus gastroenteritis outbreaks in healthcare settings. Infect Control Hosp Epidemiol 2011;32(10):939–69.
127. Grafe CJ, Staes CJ, Kawamoto K, et al. State-level adoption of national guidelines for norovirus outbreaks in health care settings. Am J Infect Control 2018; 46(10):1084–91.

A Review of *Clostridioides difficile* Infection and Antibiotic-Associated Diarrhea

Cybéle Lara R. Abad, MD[a], Nasia Safdar, MD, PhD[b],*

KEYWORDS

- *C. difficile* infection • Antibiotic-associated diarrhea • Diagnosis • Treatment
- Prevention

KEY POINTS

- *Clostridioides difficile* is a common etiology of antibiotic-associated diarrhea, and continues to be the most common cause of health care–associated diarrhea.
- The most important risk factors for hospital-acquired *C difficile* infection (CDI), including advanced age, hospitalization, and exposure to antibiotics, may not be present in community-acquired CDI.
- CDI can range from mild to profuse diarrhea, severe colitis, and rarely, toxic megacolon.
- Diagnosis can be challenging and involves both clinical symptoms and laboratory tests.
- Therapy for CDI is evolving, and many new agents with different mechanisms of action are under investigation.

INTRODUCTION

Antibiotic-associated diarrhea (AAD) is defined as diarrhea associated with antibiotic exposure, either while on antibiotics, or for up to 8 weeks after antibiotic discontinuation.[1,2] Although the etiologies for AAD are varied and not all the pathogens are identifiable, nearly one-third of AAD cases in adults are due to *Clostridioides difficile.*

C difficile is an anaerobic, gram-positive, spore-forming, toxin-producing bacillus that colonizes the gut of up to 70% of neonates and infants,[3] can form part of the commensal intestinal flora of asymptomatic adults,[4] and is ubiquitous in the natural environment. It was renamed *Clostridioides difficile* and reclassified to the genus *Peptoclostridium* in 2016, when molecular methods revealed that the organism was more similar to the family Peptostreptococcaceae than the genus *Clostridium.*[5]

[a] Department of Medicine, Section of Infectious Diseases, University of the Philippines-Manila, UP-Philippine General Hospital, Philippines; [b] Department of Medicine, Division of Infectious Diseases, William S. Middleton Memorial Veterans Hospital, University of Wisconsin-Madison, Madison, WI, USA
* Corresponding author.
E-mail address: ns2@medicine.wisc.edu

Gastroenterol Clin N Am 50 (2021) 323–340
https://doi.org/10.1016/j.gtc.2021.02.010
0889-8553/21/© 2021 Elsevier Inc. All rights reserved.

gastro.theclinics.com

C difficile infection (CDI) remains the most common cause of health care–associated diarrhea. In the United States, CDI has an estimated incidence rate of 453,000 cases per year and 29,000 deaths, based on 2011 data.[6] In Europe, the estimated number of cases is 124,000 per year[7] and *C difficile* was the sixth most frequent microorganism responsible for health care–associated infections during the 2016 to 2017 European point prevalence study.[8]

The burden of *C difficile* also extends to the community, and it is estimated to cause 51.9 episodes of community-associated infection per 100,000 persons.[6] It remains underrecognized because of a lack of screening by community physicians.[9,10] Epidemiologic studies have shown that community-associated CDI affects groups not previously at risk, including younger patients, and those with no exposure to antibiotics in the 12 weeks before infection,[11] highlighting that CDI may occur out of hospital in patients without traditional risk factors.

This article reviews both AAD and CDI, but focuses specifically on CDI and provides updated recommendations regarding the pathogenesis, diagnosis, treatment, and prevention of incident and recurrent CDI.

PATHOGENESIS AND RISK FACTORS

The indiscriminate use of broad-spectrum antimicrobial drugs disrupts the equilibrium of the normal intestinal microbiota and results in AAD.[12–15] AAD is one of the most common complications of antibiotic therapy, occurring in approximately 5% to 25% of patients receiving antibiotics, depending on the specific type of antibiotic, host factors, underlying pathologies, and the presence of other risk factors.[16–18] Based on the results of a recent meta-analysis involving 5496 total patients, *C difficile* accounts for 20% (95% confidence interval [CI] 13.0–28.0) of all AAD cases among hospitalized patients.[19] A comparison of AAD and CDI is presented in **Table 1**.

The most important risk factors for CDI include advanced age, hospitalization, and exposure to antibiotics.[20–22] Although any antibiotic is a potential risk factor for CDI, the use of clindamycin, broad-spectrum penicillins, and more recently cephalosporins and fluoroquinolones have been reported to present the highest risk for *C difficile*.[23–25]

Most CDIs occur after or during antibiotic treatment because alteration of normal gut flora through antimicrobial exposure allows *C difficile* to proliferate in the gut. Once there is gut dysbiosis, an imbalance among the types of organisms present in a person's natural flora in the gut, *C difficile* from either endogenous or exogenous sources can proliferate (**Fig. 1**). *C difficile* produces 3 toxins: toxin A, toxin B, and binary toxin. Exotoxins A and B trigger a cytotoxic response in the colonic mucosa, which results in neutrophil infiltration and cytokine production.[26] The binary toxin is produced by a hypervirulent, epidemic strain of CDI, named NAP1/027, which emerged in 2014 and posed a global threat due to increased severity of CDI and resistance to fluoroquinolones.[27]

CLINICAL MANIFESTATION AND DIAGNOSIS
Clinical Manifestations

The clinical picture of CDI is heterogeneous, and ranges from an asymptomatic carrier state to a life-threatening colitis. The incubation period is not well defined and can range from as short as a few days to much longer, depending on individual risk factors and published evidence.[28–31] CDI can affect every part of the colon, but the distal segment is most commonly infiltrated. Most patients with CDI suffer from mild diarrhea and experience recovery spontaneously after 5 to 10 days of antibiotic therapy withdrawal.

Table 1
A comparison of antibiotic-associated diarrhea and *Clostridioides difficile* infection

Parameter	Antibiotic-Associated Diarrhea	*C difficile* Infection (CDI)
Definition	Diarrhea associated with antibiotic exposure, either while on antibiotics or for up to 8 weeks after antimicrobial treatment	Presence of *C difficile* in the stool and the presence of gastrointestinal symptoms without another etiology being present
Incidence	7–33/100 in adult inpatients 2.5/100000 person-years for adult outpatient	4.3–131/10,000 for adult inpatients 1–11/10,000 for outpatients
Risk factors	Older age, female gender, antibiotic use, antacid use[83,84]	Older age, antibiotic use, hospitalization, proton pump inhibitors, H2 blockers
Incubation time	3–18 d	Initial episode of adult CDI cases 6–12 d; Delayed-onset >21 or 31 d post-discharge[29,85,86]
Complications	Prolonged length of stay, higher mortality rates higher cost[84,87]	Increased mortality, higher rates of surgery (colectomies), higher health care costs, longer lengths of stay for inpatients and readmissions to health care systems

Data from McFarland LV, Ozen M, Dinleyici EC, et al. Comparison of pediatric and adult antibiotic-associated diarrhea and Clostridium difficile infections. World journal of gastroenterology 2016;22(11):3078-3104.

CDI should be suspected in individuals who present with acute diarrhea defined as ≥3 loose stools in a 24-hour period, particularly in the setting of recent antimicrobial exposure, prolonged hospitalization, and/or old age. CDI is the most common enteric pathogen among patients hospitalized for more than 3 days.[16]

The extent of CDI can range from mild to profuse diarrhea, severe colitis, and rarely, toxic megacolon. Associated signs and symptoms can include fever, abdominal pain, and tenesmus.[32] Nausea, vomiting, and fever may occur but are not always present. Physical findings vary depending on the length and severity of disease. There may be signs of dehydration, the abdomen may be tender, and in severe cases peritoneal signs may be present. A leukemoid reaction can be seen with peripheral white blood cell counts greater than 25,000/mm^3. Often, leukocytosis of more than 15,000/mm^3, and creatinine greater than 1.5 mg/dL along with hypoalbuminemia, are markers of disease severity.[33] Fecal occult blood test is often positive, although active bleeding is rare.[28] The most severe clinical presentation of CDI may include significant dehydration, abdominal distension, hypo-albuminemia with peripheral edema, and subsequent circulatory shock. Other severe complications of CDI include toxic megacolon, colon perforation, intestinal paralysis, kidney failure, systemic inflammatory response syndrome, septicemia, and death.[28] Extracolonic manifestations of CDI are rare, and most commonly involve small intestine infiltration, reactive arthritis, and bacteremia.[34]

Diagnosis

The diagnosis of CDI is made based on a combination of clinical symptoms (eg, loose watery stools >3/d) and diagnostic tests. Watery stools are defined as "stools taking the shape of the container." A stool specimen is sent to detect the presence of either toxigenic *C difficile* organism, its toxin or toxin-producing gene. In the absence of

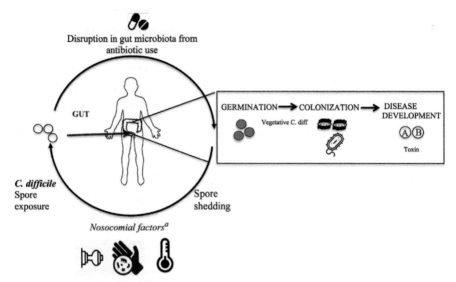

Fig. 1. Pathogenesis of *C difficile* in the hospital. [a] Hospital transmission via contaminated doorknobs, hands, thermometer. (*Modified from* Anna M. Seekatz, Vincent B. Young. Clostridium difficile and the microbiota. J Clin Invest. 2014;124(10):4182-4189. https://doi.org/10.1172/JCI72336; with permission.)

symptoms, sending stool for *C difficile* should be discouraged, because patients can carry the organism asymptomatically.[35] In addition, *C difficile* testing is not advised in patients who have received laxatives in the past 48 hours,[36] and stool samples should be also taken before initiating specific treatment for *C difficile* to avoid false negative results. Sunkesula and colleagues[37] showed that the cumulative number of patients converting from positive to negative polymerase chain reaction was 7 (14%) of 51, 18 (35%) of 51, and 23 (45%) of 51 after days 1, 2, and 3 of treatment, respectively.

Currently, methods used to diagnose CDI are imperfect. The gold standard references, toxigenic culture (TC) and cytotoxicity neutralization assay (CNNA), which detect *C difficile* toxin production, are rarely used because the procedures are cumbersome and the turnaround time impractical.[38] The most frequently used laboratory tests are enzyme immunoassays (EIAs) or nucleic acid amplification tests (NAATs, usually polymerase chain reaction [PCR] for toxin B). The EIAs may target glutamate dehydrogenase (GDH), an enzyme present in toxigenic and nontoxigenic CD isolates. GDH EIAs are highly sensitive for presence of *C difficile*, but not specific, predominantly due to detection of nontoxigenic strains. As a result, GDH is combined with a toxigenic *C difficile* specific test, either PCR detecting the presence of at least the toxin B gene (tcdB), which proves presence of toxigenic *C difficile* but not toxin production, or toxin EIA to at least toxin B, which proves production of toxin. As independent tests, toxin EIAs are suboptimal, as sensitivities range from 67% to 92%, risking missed cases, although proving toxin production.[39] In contrast, NAAT (PCR) for toxin B (tcdB) is highly sensitive and moderately specific with higher risk for detection of asymptomatic colonization[39] **(Table 2)**.

Different algorithms have been proposed for diagnosis of CDI. Both the Infectious Diseases Society of America (IDSA) and The European Society for Clinical Microbiology and Infectious Diseases (ESCMID) recommend a 2-step algorithm based on a

Table 2
Diagnostic tests for *Clostridioides. difficile*

Test	Percent Sensitivity	Percent Specificity	Comment
Colonoscopy	50	100	For detection of pseudomembranes and diagnostic sampling
Cell cytotoxicity	77–86	97–99	Considered a gold standard
EIA for toxins A and B	67–92 60–89	93–99 93–99	vs cell cytotoxicity vs toxigenic culture
EIA for GDH	71–100	67–99	Compared w/stool culture for C *difficile*
Toxigenic culture for C *difficile*	95–100	96–100	The more sensitive of 2 "gold standards"
Nucleic acid amplification test	88–100	88–97	Most sensitive rapid test, most expensive
GDH, 2 step[a] GDH, 3 step[b]	56–90 83–100	81–97 93–100	Discrepancy between GDH and toxin test is 13%–19%

Abbreviations: EIA, enzyme immuno assay; GDH, glutamate dehydrogenase.
[a] Two step: use of GDH enzyme immunoassay followed by a toxinA/B enzyme immunoassay.
[b] Three step: resolving discrepant GDH and toxin A/B enzyme immunoassay results with NAAT to reduce test costs.
Modified from Gerding DN, Young VB, Donseky CJ. Chapter 243: Clostriodioides difficile (Formerly Clostridium difficile) Infection. In: Bennett JE, Dolin R, Blaser MJ. Mandell, Douglas, and Bennett's Principles and Practice of Infectious Diseases. 9th ed. Elsevier; 2020: 2933-2947.e4.

sensitive screening method (nucleic acid amplification assay or GDH assay) followed, in the case of a positive result, by a more specific technique to detect free toxins in stools (EIA test for toxins or cytotoxicity neutralization assay)[28,40] (**Fig. 2**). Optional steps include performing a nucleic acid amplification assay for confirmation of GDH assay-positive, toxin enzyme immunoassay-negative samples or performing a combined test detecting GDH and toxins with an optional reflex nucleic acid amplification assay test in the case of GDH-positive, toxin-negative results. The IDSA also allows the use of nucleic acid amplification assay tests alone if appropriate stool selection is guaranteed.[28]

MANAGEMENT

The first consideration should always be potential discontinuation of antibiotic therapy in all patients with CDI, if doing so does not jeopardize recovery from other conditions. In a 10-year prospective study of 908 patients with documented C *difficile* diarrhea, 135 (15%) responded to cessation of antibiotic use alone.[41] Patients with mild infection, who are not at risk for severe disease, may be observed for a few days to determine whether discontinuation of antibiotic therapy is sufficient to resolve the condition.[42]

Anti-infectives

Classifying the severity of CDI is helpful for selecting initial appropriate antibiotic therapy. **Table 3** summarizes and compares CDI therapies from the American College of Gastroenterology,[43] the IDSA,[28] and the European Congress of Clinical Microbiology and Infectious Diseases[44] according to disease severity. Of these, the IDSA guideline is most recently updated.

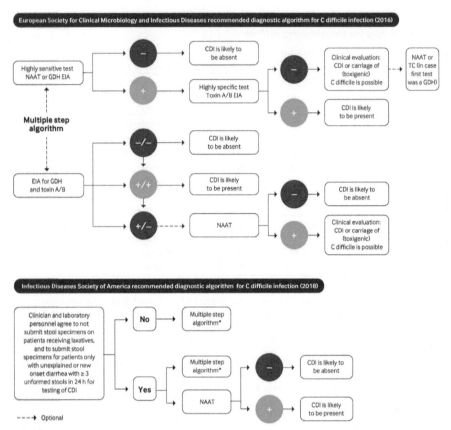

Fig. 2. European Society for Clinical Microbiology and Infectious Diseases recommended diagnostic algorithm for *C difficile* infection. *As recommended by the ESCMID. (*From* Guery B, Galperine T and Barbut F. Clostridioides difficile: Diagnosis and treatments. BMJ (Clinical research ed.) 2019;366:l4609.)

Metronidazole was once recommended as first-line therapy for mild to moderate CDI. However, recent data suggest that it is less effective than oral vancomycin: in one randomized trial, metronidazole had similar efficacy as vancomycin overall but was inferior in severe CDI.[45] Furthermore, metronidazole use may be associated with higher recurrence rates compared with vancomycin.[46,47] Given these concerns, in the updated 2018 IDSA guidelines, metronidazole is recommended for an initial episode of mild or moderate CDI only in the absence of vancomycin or fidaxomicin.[28] If metronidazole is used and symptoms do not improve within 5 to 7 days, or if clinical signs worsen at any point, a change to vancomycin or fidaxomicin should be considered. For fulminant CDI, defined as the need for colectomy or admission to the intensive care unit,[48] intravenous metronidazole is indicated along with vancomycin (see **Table 3**).

Vancomycin is now the standard therapy for mild or nonfulminant CDI at a dosage of 125 mg orally 4 times a day for 10 days. Oral vancomycin is poorly absorbed, resulting in limited systemic exposure and high concentrations in the stool. Higher doses are not recommended except for fulminant infection.

Table 3
Treatment of *Clostridioides difficile* infection

CDI Severity	ACG 2013[43]	ECCMID 2014[44]	IDSA 2017[28]
Initial Episode			
Mild to Moderate	• Metronidazole 500 mg TID for 10d • If unable to take metronidazole, vancomycin 125 mg QID × 10 d • If no improvement in 5–7 d, consider changing to vancomycin	• Metronidazole 500 mg TID × 10 d OR • Metronidazole 500 mg IV TID × 10 d if oral is not an option	• Vancomycin 125 mg orally QID for 10 d • Fidaxomicin 200 mg orally BID for 10 d • Metronidazole 500 mg orally TID for 10 d as alternative if neither are available
Severe	Vancomycin 125 mg QID × 10 d	Vancomycin 125 mg QID × 10 d OR If oral therapy is impossible, metronidazole 500 mg IV TID × 10 d, *and* intracolonic vancomycin (500 mg in 100 mL of normal saline) every 4–12 h with or without vancomycin 500 mg QID by NGT	• Vancomycin 125 mg orally QID for 10 d OR • Fidaxomicin 200 mg orally BID for 10 d
Fulminant	Vancomycin 500 mg QID *and* Metronidazole 500 mg IV every 8 h and Vancomycin per rectum (500 mg in 500 mL of normal saline) QID	NA	• Vancomycin 500 mg orally or via NGT QID *plus* • Vancomycin retention enema if ileus is present • Metronidazole 500 mg IV TID, particularly if ileus is present
Recurrent disease			
First	• Treat with same regimen used for initial episode; • If severe, use vancomycin	Vancomycin 125 mg QID × 10 d or Fidaxomicin 200 mg BID × 10 d	• Vancomycin 125 mg orally QID for 10 d then dose tapered over weeks OR • Fidaxomicin 200 mg orally BID for 10 d

(*continued on next page*)

Table 3 (continued)			
CDI Severity	ACG 2013[43]	ECCMID 2014[44]	IDSA 2017[28]
Second or subsequent	• Vancomycin 125 mg QID × 10 d *and* then 125 mg daily pulsed every 3 d for 10 doses • Consider FMT after third recurrence	• Vancomycin 125 mg QID × 10 d and then consider pulsed tapered strategy • Consider FMT after third recurrence	Vancomycin 125 mg orally QID for 10 d then dose tapered over weeks OR • Vancomycin 125 mg orally QID for 10 d followed by Rifaximin 400 mg orally TID for 20 d OR • Fidaxomicin 200 mg orally BID for 10 d if not previously used OR • FMT

Abbreviations: ACG, American College of Gastroenterology; BID, twice a day; CDI, *Clostridioides difficile* infection; d, day; ECCMID, European Congress of Clinical Microbiology; FMT, fecal microbiota transplant; IDSA, Infectious Diseases Society of America; IV, intravenously; NA, not applicable; NGT, nasogastric tube; QID, 4 times a day; TID, 3 times a day.

Fidaxomicin is an oral macrocyclic antibiotic with minimal systemic absorption, a narrow spectrum of activity against gram-positive aerobic and anaerobic bacteria, and less impact on the normal bowel flora.[49,50] Post hoc analyses from a randomized clinical trial comparing fidaxomicin and vancomycin demonstrated that fidaxomicin showed more microbiome preservation than the latter.[51] Fidaxomicin is also bactericidal against *C difficile,* whereas metronidazole and vancomycin are both bacteriostatic agents.[52] In 2 randomized, phase 3 clinical trials, fidaxomicin was noninferior to vancomycin for clinical cure (88.2% vs 85.8%; 91.7% vs 90.6%, respectively) and led to fewer recurrences (15.4% vs 25.3%; 12.7% vs 26.9%, respectively).[53,54] For treatment of patients with cancer, fidaxomicin was also superior to vancomycin, with higher cure rates and fewer recurrences.[55] The updated IDSA guidelines now recommend treatment with either vancomycin or fidaxomicin for an initial episode of nonfulminant CDI. Despite the evidence in favor of fidaxomicin, however, issues with cost[56,57] have made providers reluctant to use it, reserving it for cases of recurrent or refractory CDI.

High-dose vancomycin (500 mg orally 4 times a day) in combination with metronidazole (500 mg intravenously every 8 hours) is the preferred treatment for fulminant CDI (see **Table 3**). In a single-center, retrospective, observational study, mortality was lower among critically ill patients with CDI who received intravenous metronidazole in addition to vancomycin compared with patients who received vancomycin alone (15.9% vs 36.4%, $P = .03$).[58] In patients with severe ileus, rectal vancomycin (500 mg in 100 mL of normal saline) may be added,[43,59] and early surgical consultation for possible colectomy for fulminant disease should be considered.[43]

For those with recurrent CDI (rCDI), defined as recurrence of symptoms within 8 weeks of CDI, the IDSA guidelines[28] recommend treating a first recurrence with oral vancomycin as a tapered and pulsed regimen or a 10-day course of fidaxomicin, if vancomycin was used initially. If metronidazole was used for the initial infection, a

10-day course of vancomycin is recommended. Summary regimens for rCDI are detailed in **Table 3**.

Microbial Replacement Therapies

Because gut-induced dysbiosis is the pathology behind CDI, research into the development of microbial therapies has flourished. Fecal microbial replacement therapy (FMRT), such as fecal microbiota transplantation (FMT) has been the primary method for providing microbial replacement to treat rCDI.

In a recent systematic review, which included 7 randomized controlled trials and 30 case series, clinical resolution occurred in 92% of patients treated with FMT.[60] Ongoing clinical trials are assessing the use of FMT as primary treatment of moderate to severe CDI, the use of FMT or antibiotic therapy for initial treatment of rCDI, and the use of different modes of delivery for FMRT, such as by capsule. Current guidelines recommend FMT for prevention of further recurrences in patients who have had more than 2 episodes of CDI. Serious adverse events with FMT are rare and the most common adverse events are understandably gastrointestinal and include nausea, belching, or bloatedness, which are more frequently seen when FMT is given via the upper gastrointestinal route. Given the difficulties with endoscopic installation of FMT and increased cost, other routes such as enema or capsule-based microbiota replacements are also being developed and investigated.[61–65]

Immunologics

A robust immunologic response against *C difficile* toxins appears protective and seems to determine better outcomes. For example, higher serum concentrations of antibodies against toxin A have been associated with a decreased risk of CDI recurrence risk: patients with a single episode of *C difficile* diarrhea (n = 22) had higher concentrations of serum immunoglobulin (Ig)M against toxin A on day 3 of their first episode of diarrhea than those with recurrent diarrhea (n = 22, P = .004). The odds ratio for recurrence associated with a low concentration of serum IgG against toxin A, measured 12 days after onset of *C difficile* diarrhea, was 48.0 (95% CI 3.5–663).[66]

Bezlotoxumab is an intravenous monoclonal antibody that binds to *C difficile* toxin B and is approved by the Food and Drug Administration as an adjunctive therapy for preventing CDI in adults at high risk for recurrence. It was approved on the basis of 2 double-blind, randomized, placebo-controlled, phase 3 trials (MODIFY I and MODIFY II). In these trials, patients receiving bezlotoxumab in combination with standard oral antibiotic therapy had significantly lower rates of rCDI than patients treated with antibiotics alone (17% vs 28% in MODIFY I; 16% vs 26% in MODIFY II).[67] The benefit of bezlotoxumab was limited to patients who had risk factors for rCDI, including a prespecified age (ie, age >65), history of prior CDI, immunocompromised state, severe CDI, and infection with specific virulent epidemic strains of *C difficile*. Patients with any of these risk factors demonstrated significant reduction in recurrence with the exception of virulent epidemic *C difficile* strains, which showed benefit but did not reach statistical significance. The benefit of bezlotoxumab increased with the number of risk factors present, and there was no benefit if no risk factors for recurrence were present.

Probiotics

Probiotics are live microorganisms that provide a health benefit to the host.[68] These have been studied for the prevention and treatment of CDI with conflicting results.[69,70] In a more recent meta-analysis of 26 randomized controlled trials, *Lactobacillus*, *Saccharomyces*, and a mixture of probiotics reduced the risk of CDI in both adults and children treated with antibiotics in inpatient and outpatient settings (relative risk reduction: 63.7% with *Lactobacillus*, 58.5% with *Saccharomyces*, and 58.2% with a mixture of probiotics).[71] Overall, probiotic use reduced the risk by 60.5% (relative risk 0.395; 95% CI 0.294–0.531; P<.001). The absolute risk reduction was 2.3% and number needed to treat, 43 patients. However, more research is needed before robust recommendations can be made favoring the use of probiotics because of the heterogeneity among studies in the meta-analyses.

Investigational Therapies

There are many other novel and investigational therapies for the prevention of CDI. These include targeted-spectrum antimicrobials, antibiotic inhibition, vaccines, and biotherapeutics.

Ridinilazole (formerly known as SMT19969) is a new anti-infective that shows promise against CDI. In vitro studies have shown its high inhibitory activity against *C difficile* and minimal activity against both gram-positive and gram-negative aerobic and anaerobic intestinal microorganisms.[72–75] In a phase 2 randomized, double-blind, noninferiority study,[76] patients with confirmed *CDI* received oral ridinilazole (200 mg every 12 hour) or oral vancomycin (125 mg every 6 hours) for 10 days. The primary efficacy analysis included 69 patients (n = 36 in the ridinilazole group; n = 33 in the vancomycin group); 24 (66.7%) of 36 patients in the ridinilazole group versus 14 (42.4%) of 33 of those in the vancomycin group had a sustained clinical response (treatment difference 21.1%, 90% CI 3.1–39.1, P = .0004), establishing the noninferiority of ridinilazole and also showing statistical superiority at the 10% level. Ridinilazole was also well tolerated, with an adverse event profile similar to that of vancomycin.

Antibiotic inhibition neutralizes the effect of the antibiotic on the microbiota of the gastrointestinal (GI) tract, preserving "colonization resistance" of the microbiota against *C difficile*.[77] This is a challenging intervention, as the antibiotic inhibition cannot interfere with absorption of oral antibiotics in the upper GI tract, but must do so in the lower GI tract or colon to protect the microbiota. Two approaches are currently being evaluated in clinical trials. The first is to use an oral beta-lactamase to inactivate beta-lactam antibiotics (penicillins, cephalosporins, and carbapenems) in the lower GI tract, and the other is to use DAV132, an oral capsule formulation of activated charcoal designed for release in the distal ileum to adsorb antibiotics preventing disruption of the microbiome.[77]

Biotherapeutics, live bacterial products produced by in vitro fermentation for administration to patients to prevent or treat specific diseases, are also being studied for prevention of rCDI. Phase 2 and phase 3 vaccine trials for the primary prevention of CDI are also under way. A comprehensive review of these novel agents are beyond the scope of this article, but is available elsewhere.[77]

INFECTION CONTROL AND PREVENTION

Strategies for CDI prevention focus on 2 main components: antimicrobial stewardship and reduction of horizontal *C difficile* transmission within the health care setting. A summary of these measures is in **Table 4**.

Antibiotic Stewardship

Since the inciting event to developing CDI is gut dysbiosis, the primary means of preventing CDI is to limit the use of antibiotics, particularly those believed to carry high risk, these include clindamycin, higher generation cephalosporins, and fluoroquinolones.

Table 4
Infection prevention and control[28,88]

Preventive Measure	Comments
Isolation measures	• Patients with suspected CDI should be placed on preemptive contact precautions pending the *Clostridioides difficile* test results. • Patients with CDI should be admitted to a private room with a dedicated toilet to decrease transmission to other patients. • Continue contact precautions for at least 48 h after diarrhea has resolved. • Prolong contact precautions until discharge if CDI rates remain high despite implementation of standard infection control measures against CDI.
Patient cohorting	• If cohorting is desired, it is recommended to cohort patients infected or colonized with CDI.
Hand hygiene and PPE	• Health care personnel must use gown and gloves on entry to a room of a patient with CDI and while caring for patients with CDI. • In routine or endemic settings, perform hand hygiene before and after contact of a patient with CDI and after removing gloves with either soap and water or an alcohol-based hand hygiene product; if there is direct contact w/feces or areas w/fecal contamination, hand washing w/soap and water is preferred. • In CDI outbreaks or hyper endemic (sustained high rates) settings, perform hand hygiene with soap and water preferentially instead of alcohol-based hand hygiene products before and after caring for a patient with CDI given the increased efficacy of spore removal with soap and water. • Hand washing with soap and water is preferred if there is direct contact with feces or an area where fecal contamination is likely.
Disinfection/ cleaning	• Use disposable patient equipment when possible and ensure that reusable equipment is thoroughly cleaned and disinfected, preferentially with a sporicidal disinfectant that is equipment compatible. • Terminal room cleaning with a sporicidal agent should be considered in conjunction with other measures to prevent CDI during endemic high rates or outbreaks, or if there is evidence of repeated cases of CDI in the same room.
Stewardship	• Minimize the frequency and duration of high-risk antibiotic therapy and the number of antibiotic agents prescribed, to reduce CDI risk. • Implement an antibiotic stewardship program. • Antibiotics to be targeted should be based on the local epidemiology and the *C difficile* strains present. Restriction of fluoroquinolones, clindamycin, and cephalosporins (except for surgical antibiotic prophylaxis) should be considered.
PPIs	• Although there is an epidemiologic association between PPI use and CDI, and unnecessary PPIs should always be discontinued, there is insufficient evidence for discontinuation of PPIs as a measure for preventing CDI.
Probiotics	• There are insufficient data at this time to recommend administration of probiotics for primary prevention of CDI outside of clinical trials.

Abbreviations: CDI, *Clostridioides difficile* infection; PPE, personal protective equipment; PPI, proton pump inhibitor.

In the hospital setting, the implementation of an antimicrobial stewardship program or protocol is paramount and many strategies have been used, from restricting the use of high-risk drugs to routinely reviewing antibiotic therapy and giving feedback to the treating clinicians. Stewardship protocols can also focus on improving antibiotic use for specific syndromes or conditions, such as urinary tract infections and respiratory infections. A prospective controlled, interrupted time-series study of the geriatric service of a large teaching hospital evaluated the rates of CDI over 2 periods of 21 months, before and after institution of an antibiotic prescription protocol involving feedback on the appropriate use of narrow-spectrum antibiotics. After institution of the antibiotic policy, CDI decreased significantly (incidence rate ratio 0.35; $P = .009$).[78] Because of the increasing frequency of community-associated infection, antibiotic use among outpatients may also be an important contributor to CDI and monitoring such use may be a target for preventing these infections.

Infection Control

On the diagnosis of CDI, patients should be placed under contact precautions and ideally transferred to a private room.[28] It is recommended that contact precautions be continued until at least 48 hours after diarrhea has ceased, or maintained until duration of the hospital stay if CDI rates remain high despite standard infection control measures.[28]

Health care providers and visitors should also be educated about proper hand hygiene measures. Because alcohol-based hand rubs are not sporicidal and are less effective than soap and water at removing C difficile spores,[79] the use of soap and water is the preferred method of hand hygiene during outbreaks or in areas with high rates of CDI.[28,79] Handwashing with soap and water is also recommended if there is direct contact with stool or an area with fecal contamination or when hands are visibly soiled. Despite this recommendation, however, studies have failed to show a change in the rate of CDI when comparing alcohol-based hand products with soap and water across patient populations.[80,81] Because even soap and water against C difficile spores cannot achieve the usual 3-log to 4-log reductions commonly associated with alcohol against other bacteria,[82] the use of gloves are highly recommended and serve as a primary method of preventing C difficile transmission in the health care setting.

Disposable and dedicated medical equipment should be used when a patient with CDI is being treated. Reusable equipment should be thoroughly cleaned and disinfected after use with a sporicidal disinfectant registered by the U.S. Environmental Protection Agency.[28] Daily and terminal cleaning and disinfecting patient rooms, focusing on high-touch surfaces, should also be done.[28] During outbreak settings, terminal disinfection with a sporicidal agent in conjunction with other interventions to prevent CDI is recommended. However, this specific method of disinfection has not been associated with consistent reductions in CDI in non-outbreak settings. Therefore, sporicidal disinfection remains most appropriate as a supplemental intervention for outbreaks, hyperendemic settings, or evidence of several cases of CDI in the same room.[28]

SUMMARY/FUTURE DIRECTION

CDI continues to be a frequent cause of health care–associated diarrhea. Its diagnosis remains challenging despite the presence of more sensitive diagnostic tests. Treatment options continue to evolve, and metronidazole has fallen out of favor. More therapies that are directed to specifically address the underlying gut dysbiosis are now available, including FMT. Immunologics such as bezlotoxumab, new antimicrobials such as ridinilazole, and other investigational agents show promise. Diverse approaches to prevention are also under way, including vaccine development. Future research and approval of these additional effective modalities should make both the treatment and prevention of CDI and rCDI easier in the future.

CLINICS CARE POINTS

- CDI should be suspected among older, hospitalized patients given recent antimicrobial therapy, who develop more than 3 watery stools per day.
- Only unformed stool should be sent for *C difficile* testing, and laxatives should be avoided in the 48-hour window before stool submission.
- Vancomycin is now the drug of choice for mild to moderate CDI, but newer drugs show promise.
- Treatment of recurrent CDI usually involves pulse therapy with vancomycin, fidaxomicin, FMT, or bezlotoxumab.
- Many therapeutic agents targeting gut dysbiosis, or evaluating other mechanisms of treatment and prevention are under investigation.

DISCLOSURE

The authors have nothing to disclose.

REFERENCES

1. Alam S, Mushtaq M. Antibiotic associated diarrhea in children. Indian Pediatr 2009;46(6):491–6.
2. McFarland LV, Ozen M, Dinleyici EC, et al. Comparison of pediatric and adult antibiotic-associated diarrhea and *Clostridium difficile* infections. World J Gastroenterol 2016;22(11):3078–104.
3. Janezic S, Potocnik M, Zidaric V, et al. Highly divergent *Clostridium difficile* strains isolated from the environment. PLoS One 2016;11(11):e0167101.
4. Lees EA, Miyajima F, Pirmohamed M, et al. The role of *Clostridium difficile* in the paediatric and neonatal gut - a narrative review. Eur J Clin Microbiol Infect Dis 2016;35(7):1047–57.
5. The Lancet Infectious Diseases. *C difficile*-a rose by any other name. Lancet Infect Dis 2019;19(5):449.
6. Lessa FC, Gould CV, McDonald LC. Current status of *Clostridium difficile* infection epidemiology. Clin Infect Dis 2012;55(Suppl 2):S65–70.
7. Zarb P, Coignard B, Griskeviciene J, et al. The European Centre for Disease Prevention and Control (ECDC) pilot point prevalence survey of healthcare-associated infections and antimicrobial use. Euro Surveill 2012;17(46):20316.
8. Suetens C, Latour K, Kärki T, et al. Prevalence of healthcare-associated infections, estimated incidence and composite antimicrobial resistance index in acute care hospitals and long-term care facilities: results from two European point prevalence surveys, 2016 to 2017. Euro Surveill 2018;23(46):1800516.
9. Barbut F, Day N, Bouée S, et al. Toxigenic *Clostridium difficile* carriage in general practice: results of a laboratory-based cohort study. Clin Microbiol Infect 2019; 25(5):588–94.
10. Hensgens MP, Dekkers OM, Demeulemeester A, et al. Diarrhoea in general practice: when should a *Clostridium difficile* infection be considered? Results of a nested case-control study. Clin Microbiol Infect 2014;20(12):O1067–74.
11. Khanna S, Pardi DS, Aronson SL, et al. The epidemiology of community-acquired *Clostridium difficile* infection: a population-based study. Am J Gastroenterol 2012;107(1):89–95.

12. Bergogne-Bérézin E. Treatment and prevention of antibiotic associated diarrhea. Int J Antimicrob Agents 2000;16(4):521–6.

13. Legaria MC, Lumelsky G, Rosetti S. *Clostridium difficile*-associated diarrhea from a general hospital in Argentina. Anaerobe 2003;9(3):113–6.

14. Roldan GA, Cui AX, Pollock NR. Assessing the burden of *Clostridium difficile* infection in low- and middle-income countries. J Clin Microbiol 2018;56(3): e01747-17.

15. Ross CL, Spinler JK, Savidge TC. Structural and functional changes within the gut microbiota and susceptibility to *Clostridium difficile* infection. Anaerobe 2016;41: 37–43.

16. Bauer MP, Notermans DW, van Benthem BH, et al. *Clostridium difficile* infection in Europe: a hospital-based survey. Lancet 2011;377(9759):63–73.

17. Borren NZ, Ghadermarzi S, Hutfless S, et al. The emergence of *Clostridium difficile* infection in Asia: a systematic review and meta-analysis of incidence and impact. PLoS One 2017;12(5):e0176797.

18. Mavros MN, Alexiou VG, Vardakas KZ, et al. Underestimation of *Clostridium difficile* infection among clinicians: an international survey. Eur J Clin Microbiol Infect Dis 2012;31(9):2439–44.

19. Nasiri MJ, Goudarzi M, Hajikhani B, et al. *Clostridioides* (*Clostridium*) *difficile* infection in hospitalized patients with antibiotic-associated diarrhea: a systematic review and meta-analysis. Anaerobe 2018;50:32–7.

20. Loo VG, Bourgault AM, Poirier L, et al. Host and pathogen factors for *Clostridium difficile* infection and colonization. N Engl J Med 2011;365(18):1693–703.

21. McFarland LV. Antibiotic-associated diarrhea: epidemiology, trends and treatment. Future Microbiol 2008;3(5):563–78.

22. Pituch H, Obuch-Woszczatyński P, Luczak M, et al. *Clostridium difficile* and enterotoxigenic *Bacteroides fragilis* strains isolated from patients with antibiotic associated diarrhoea. Anaerobe 2003;9(4):161–3.

23. Goudarzi M, Goudarzi H, Alebouyeh M, et al. Antimicrobial susceptibility of clostridium difficile clinical isolates in Iran. Iran Red Crescent Med J 2013;15(8): 704–11.

24. Goudarzi M, Seyedjavadi SS, Goudarzi H, et al. *Clostridium difficile* infection: epidemiology, pathogenesis, risk factors, and therapeutic options. Scientifica 2014;2014:916826.

25. McFarland LV. Evidence-based review of probiotics for antibiotic-associated diarrhea and *Clostridium difficile* infections. Anaerobe 2009;15(6):274–80.

26. Lyon SA, Hutton ML, Rood JI, et al. CdtR regulates TcdA and TcdB production in *Clostridium difficile*. PLoS Pathog 2016;12(7):e1005758.

27. McDonald LC, Killgore GE, Thompson A, et al. An epidemic, toxin gene-variant strain of *Clostridium difficile*. N Engl J Med 2005;353(23):2433–41.

28. McDonald LC, Gerding DN, Johnson S, et al. Clinical practice guidelines for *Clostridium difficile* infection in adults and children: 2017 update by the Infectious Diseases Society of America (IDSA) and Society for Healthcare Epidemiology of America (SHEA). Clin Infect Dis 2018;66(7):987–94.

29. McFarland LV, Mulligan ME, Kwok RY, et al. Nosocomial acquisition of *Clostridium difficile* infection. N Engl J Med 1989;320(4):204–10.

30. Samore MH, DeGirolami PC, Tlucko A, et al. *Clostridium difficile* colonization and diarrhea at a tertiary care hospital. Clin Infect Dis 1994;18(2):181–7.

31. Toshniwal R, Silva J Jr, Fekety R, et al. Studies on the epidemiology of colitis due to *Clostridium difficile* in hamsters. J Infect Dis 1981;143(1):51–4.

32. Gebhard RL, Gerding DN, Olson MM, et al. Clinical and endoscopic findings in patients early in the course of *Clostridium difficile*-associated pseudomembranous colitis. Am J Med 1985;78(1):45–8.

33. Marinella MA, Burdette SD, Bedimo R, et al. Leukemoid reactions complicating colitis due to *Clostridium difficile*. South Med J 2004;97(10):959–63.

34. Vaishnavi C. Clinical spectrum & pathogenesis of *Clostridium difficile* associated diseases. Indian J Med Res 2010;131:487–99.

35. Riggs MM, Sethi AK, Zabarsky TF, et al. Asymptomatic carriers are a potential source for transmission of epidemic and nonepidemic *Clostridium difficile* strains among long-term care facility residents. Clin Infect Dis 2007;45(8):992–8.

36. Guery B, Galperine T, Barbut F. *Clostridioides difficile*: diagnosis and treatments. BMJ 2019;366:l4609.

37. Sunkesula VC, Kundrapu S, Muganda C, et al. Does empirical *Clostridium difficile* infection (CDI) therapy result in false-negative CDI diagnostic test results? Clin Infect Dis 2013;57(4):494–500.

38. Misch EA, Safdar N. *Clostridioides difficile* infection in the stem cell transplant and hematologic malignancy population. Infect Dis Clin North Am 2019;33(2): 447–66.

39. Tenover FC, Novak-Weekley S, Woods CW, et al. Impact of strain type on detection of toxigenic *Clostridium difficile*: comparison of molecular diagnostic and enzyme immunoassay approaches. J Clin Microbiol 2010;48(10):3719–24.

40. Crobach MJ, Dekkers OM, Wilcox MH, et al. European Society of Clinical Microbiology and Infectious Diseases (ESCMID): data review and recommendations for diagnosing *Clostridium difficile*-infection (CDI). Clin Microbiol Infect 2009; 15(12):1053–66.

41. Olson MM, Shanholtzer CJ, Lee JT Jr, et al. Ten years of prospective *Clostridium difficile*-associated disease surveillance and treatment at the Minneapolis VA Medical Center, 1982-1991. Infect Control Hosp Epidemiol 1994;15(6):371–81.

42. Guh AY, Kutty PK. *Clostridioides difficile* infection. Ann Intern Med 2018;169(7): ITC49–64.

43. Surawicz CM, Brandt LJ, Binion DG, et al. Guidelines for diagnosis, treatment, and prevention of *Clostridium difficile* infections. Am J Gastroenterol 2013; 108(4):478–98 [quiz: 499].

44. Debast SB, Bauer MP, Kuijper EJ. European Society of Clinical Microbiology and Infectious Diseases: update of the treatment guidance document for *Clostridium difficile* infection. Clin Microbiol Infect 2014;20(Suppl 2):1–26.

45. Zar FA, Bakkanagari SR, Moorthi KM, et al. A comparison of vancomycin and metronidazole for the treatment of *Clostridium difficile*-associated diarrhea, stratified by disease severity. Clin Infect Dis 2007;45(3):302–7.

46. Pepin J, Alary ME, Valiquette L, et al. Increasing risk of relapse after treatment of *Clostridium difficile* colitis in Quebec, Canada. Clin Infect Dis 2005;40(11): 1591–7.

47. Pépin J, Valiquette L, Alary ME, et al. *Clostridium difficile*-associated diarrhea in a region of Quebec from 1991 to 2003: a changing pattern of disease severity. CMAJ 2004;171(5):466–72.

48. Sailhamer EA, Carson K, Chang Y, et al. Fulminant *Clostridium difficile* colitis: patterns of care and predictors of mortality. Arch Surg 2009;144(5):433–9 [discussion: 439–40].

49. Gerber M, Ackermann G. OPT-80, a macrocyclic antimicrobial agent for the treatment of *Clostridium difficile* infections: a review. Expert Opin Investig Drugs 2008; 17(4):547–53.

50. Goldstein EJ, Babakhani F, Citron DM. Antimicrobial activities of fidaxomicin. Clin Infect Dis 2012;55(Suppl 2):S143–8.

51. Louie TJ, Cannon K, Byrne B, et al. Fidaxomicin preserves the intestinal microbiome during and after treatment of Clostridium difficile infection (CDI) and reduces both toxin reexpression and recurrence of CDI. Clin Infect Dis 2012; 55(Suppl 2):S132–42.

52. Venugopal AA, Johnson S. Fidaxomicin: a novel macrocyclic antibiotic approved for treatment of Clostridium difficile infection. Clin Infect Dis 2012;54(4):568–74.

53. Cornely OA, Crook DW, Esposito R, et al. Fidaxomicin versus vancomycin for infection with Clostridium difficile in Europe, Canada, and the USA: a double-blind, non-inferiority, randomised controlled trial. Lancet Infect Dis 2012;12(4):281–9.

54. Louie TJ, Miller MA, Mullane KM, et al. Fidaxomicin versus vancomycin for Clostridium difficile infection. N Engl J Med 2011;364(5):422–31.

55. Cornely OA, Miller MA, Fantin B, et al. Resolution of Clostridium difficile-associated diarrhea in patients with cancer treated with fidaxomicin or vancomycin. J Clin Oncol 2013;31(19):2493–9.

56. Ford DC, Schroeder MC, Ince D, et al. Cost-effectiveness analysis of initial treatment strategies for mild-to-moderate Clostridium difficile infection in hospitalized patients. Am J Health Syst Pharm 2018;75(15):1110–21.

57. Lam SW, Neuner EA, Fraser TG, et al. Cost-effectiveness of three different strategies for the treatment of first recurrent Clostridium difficile infection diagnosed in a community setting. Infect Control Hosp Epidemiol 2018;39(8):924–30.

58. Rokas KE, Johnson JW, Beardsley JR, et al. The addition of intravenous metronidazole to oral vancomycin is associated with improved mortality in critically ill patients with Clostridium difficile infection. Clin Infect Dis 2015;61(6):934–41.

59. Saffouri G, Khanna S, Estes L, et al. Outcomes from rectal vancomycin therapy in patients with Clostridium difficile infection. Am J Gastroenterol 2014;109(6):924–5.

60. Quraishi MN, Widlak M, Bhala N, et al. Systematic review with meta-analysis: the efficacy of faecal microbiota transplantation for the treatment of recurrent and refractory Clostridium difficile infection. Aliment Pharmacol Ther 2017;46(5):479–93.

61. Gerding DN, Meyer T, Lee C, et al. Administration of spores of nontoxigenic Clostridium difficile strain M3 for prevention of recurrent C. difficile infection: a randomized clinical trial. JAMA 2015;313(17):1719–27.

62. Hota SS, Sales V, Tomlinson G, et al. Oral vancomycin followed by fecal transplantation versus tapering oral vancomycin treatment for recurrent Clostridium difficile infection: an open-label, randomized controlled trial. Clin Infect Dis 2017;64(3):265–71.

63. Khanna S, Pardi DS, Kelly CR, et al. A novel microbiome therapeutic increases gut microbial diversity and prevents recurrent Clostridium difficile infection. J Infect Dis 2016;214(2):173–81.

64. Orenstein R, Dubberke E, Hardi R, et al. Safety and durability of RBX2660 (Microbiota Suspension) for recurrent Clostridium difficile infection: results of the PUNCH CD study. Clin Infect Dis 2016;62(5):596–602.

65. Youngster I, Mahabamunuge J, Systrom HK, et al. Oral, frozen fecal microbiota transplant (FMT) capsules for recurrent Clostridium difficile infection. BMC Med 2016;14(1):134.

66. Kyne L, Warny M, Qamar A, et al. Association between antibody response to toxin A and protection against recurrent *Clostridium difficile* diarrhoea. Lancet 2001; 357(9251):189–93.
67. Wilcox MH, Gerding DN, Poxton IR, et al. Bezlotoxumab for prevention of recurrent *Clostridium difficile* infection. N Engl J Med 2017;376(4):305–17.
68. Sanders ME. Probiotics: definition, sources, selection, and uses. Clin Infect Dis 2008;46(Suppl 2):S58–61 [discussion: S144–51].
69. McFarland LV. Meta-analysis of probiotics for the prevention of antibiotic associated diarrhea and the treatment of *Clostridium difficile* disease. Am J Gastroenterol 2006;101(4):812–22.
70. Pillai A, Nelson R. Probiotics for treatment of *Clostridium difficile*-associated colitis in adults. Cochrane Database Syst Rev 2008;(1):CD004611.
71. Lau CS, Chamberlain RS. Probiotics are effective at preventing *Clostridium difficile*-associated diarrhea: a systematic review and meta-analysis. Int J Gen Med 2016;9:27–37.
72. Baines SD, Crowther GS, Freeman J, et al. SMT19969 as a treatment for *Clostridium difficile* infection: an assessment of antimicrobial activity using conventional susceptibility testing and an in vitro gut model. J Antimicrob Chemother 2015;70(1):182–9.
73. Corbett D, Wise A, Birchall S, et al. In vitro susceptibility of *Clostridium difficile* to SMT19969 and comparators, as well as the killing kinetics and post-antibiotic effects of SMT19969 and comparators against *C. difficile*. J Antimicrob Chemother 2015;70(6):1751–6.
74. Goldstein EJ, Citron DM, Tyrrell KL. Comparative in vitro activities of SMT19969, a new antimicrobial agent, against 162 strains from 35 less frequently recovered intestinal *Clostridium* species: implications for *Clostridium difficile* recurrence. Antimicrob Agents Chemother 2014;58(2):1187–91.
75. Goldstein EJ, Citron DM, Tyrrell KL, et al. Comparative in vitro activities of SMT19969, a new antimicrobial agent, against *Clostridium difficile* and 350 gram-positive and gram-negative aerobic and anaerobic intestinal flora isolates. Antimicrob Agents Chemother 2013;57(10):4872–6.
76. Vickers RJ, Tillotson GS, Nathan R, et al. Efficacy and safety of ridinilazole compared with vancomycin for the treatment of *Clostridium difficile* infection: a phase 2, randomised, double-blind, active-controlled, non-inferiority study. Lancet Infect Dis 2017;17(7):735–44.
77. Khanna S, Gerding DN. Current and future trends in clostridioides (clostridium) difficile infection management. Anaerobe 2019;58:95–102.
78. Fowler S, Webber A, Cooper BS, et al. Successful use of feedback to improve antibiotic prescribing and reduce *Clostridium difficile* infection: a controlled interrupted time series. J Antimicrob Chemother 2007;59(5):990–5.
79. Dubberke ER, Burdette SD. *Clostridium difficile* infections in solid organ transplantation. Am J Transplant 2013;13(Suppl 4):42–9.
80. Rupp ME, Fitzgerald T, Puumala S, et al. Prospective, controlled, cross-over trial of alcohol-based hand gel in critical care units. Infect Control Hosp Epidemiol 2008;29(1):8–15.
81. Gordin FM, Schultz ME, Huber RA, et al. Reduction in nosocomial transmission of drug-resistant bacteria after introduction of an alcohol-based handrub. Infect Control Hosp Epidemiol 2005;26(7):650–3.
82. Edmonds SL, Zapka C, Kasper D, et al. Effectiveness of hand hygiene for removal of *Clostridium difficile* spores from hands. Infect Control Hosp Epidemiol 2013;34(3):302–5.

83. Asha NJ, Tompkins D, Wilcox MH. Comparative analysis of prevalence, risk factors, and molecular epidemiology of antibiotic-associated diarrhea due to *Clostridium difficile*, *Clostridium perfringens*, and *Staphylococcus aureus*. J Clin Microbiol 2006;44(8):2785–91.

84. Elseviers MM, Van Camp Y, Nayaert S, et al. Prevalence and management of antibiotic associated diarrhea in general hospitals. BMC Infect Dis 2015;15:129.

85. Chang HT, Krezolek D, Johnson S, et al. Onset of symptoms and time to diagnosis of *Clostridium difficile*-associated disease following discharge from an acute care hospital. Infect Control Hosp Epidemiol 2007;28(8):926–31.

86. Kutty PK, Benoit SR, Woods CW, et al. Assessment of *Clostridium difficile*-associated disease surveillance definitions, North Carolina, 2005. Infect Control Hosp Epidemiol 2008;29(3):197–202.

87. Selinger CP, Bell A, Cairns A, et al. Probiotic VSL#3 prevents antibiotic-associated diarrhoea in a double-blind, randomized, placebo-controlled clinical trial. J Hosp Infect 2013;84(2):159–65.

88. Mullane KM, Dubberke ER, Practice AICo. Management of *Clostridioides* (formerly *Clostridium*) *difficile* infection (CDI) in solid organ transplant recipients: guidelines from the American Society of Transplantation Community of Practice. Clin Transplant 2019;33(9):e13564.

Gastrointestinal and Abdominal Tuberculosis

Haluk Eraksoy, MD

KEYWORDS

- Extrapulmonary tuberculosis • Gastrointestinal tuberculosis
- Inflammatory bowel disease • Granulomatous hepatitis • Peritoneal tuberculosis
- Gastrointestinal *Mycobacterium avium* complex infection
- Tuberculosis-associated immune reconstitution inflammatory syndrome

KEY POINTS

- Gastrointestinal (GI) tuberculosis (TB) can present with involvement of any segment of the GI tract, associated viscera, and peritoneum. Diagnosis of GI TB is often delayed because of its nonspecific clinical presentation.
- Diagnosis in lesions of solid organs such as liver can be obtained by ultrasonography-guided aspiration. Suspected peritoneal TB is one of the few remaining indications for diagnostic laparoscopy.
- An important part of the differential diagnosis is Crohn disease for any patient in whom intestinal TB is a possible diagnosis.
- GI manifestations of TB-associated immune reconstitution inflammatory syndrome can occur as granulomatous hepatitis, intestinal lesions, peritonitis, ascites, or enlargement of intra-abdominal lymph nodes after initiation of antiretroviral therapy in advanced human immunodeficiency virus disease.
- Given the suboptimal accuracy of many of the diagnostic tests, it may be necessary to treat patients empirically with anti-TB drugs using strong clinical suspicion, especially in patients who come from areas where TB is endemic.

INTRODUCTION

Tuberculosis (TB) is an infectious disease that is one of the top 10 causes of death worldwide. About a quarter of the world's population is infected with bacteria belonging to the *Mycobacterium tuberculosis* complex and thus at risk of developing TB.[1] Gastrointestinal (GI) TB, as an extrapulmonary form, accounts for 1% to 3% of all TB cases worldwide.[2] It is now reemerging with the contributions of human immunodeficiency virus (HIV) infection and with multidrug-resistant (MDR) *M tuberculosis*.[3]

GI TB can occur as part of active pulmonary disease or as a primary infection without pulmonary involvement. It can present with involvement of any segment of the GI tract, associated viscera, and peritoneum.[4] Abdominal TB is an alternative

Department of Infectious Diseases and Clinical Microbiology, Istanbul Faculty of Medicine, Istanbul University, TR-34093 Istanbul, Turkey
E-mail address: haluk.eraksoy@gmail.com

Gastroenterol Clin N Am 50 (2021) 341–360
https://doi.org/10.1016/j.gtc.2021.02.004
0889-8553/21/© 2021 Elsevier Inc. All rights reserved.

term that describes a form of extrapulmonary TB that could involve the various organs of the abdominal cavity, including any part of the GI tract, singly or in combination.[5–9]

Diagnosis of GI TB is often delayed because of its nonspecific clinical presentation. Early initiation of anti-TB therapy is important in addition to a high index of suspicion for reducing morbidity and mortality. Standard anti-TB drugs are generally sufficient for GI TB.[4,7,10] Untreated GI TB has a 6% to 20% mortality.[7,11] Surgery is not required unless complications unresponsive to medical therapy, such as strictures or obstruction, have developed.[6,10,12,13]

This article summarizes the current information about cause, epidemiology, pathogenesis, pathophysiology, clinical evaluation, clinical forms, and treatment of GI TB.

CAUSE AND EPIDEMIOLOGY

GI TB is the result of infection with organisms of the *M tuberculosis* complex, which include *M tuberculosis*, *Mycobacterium bovis*, *Mycobacterium africanum*, *Mycobacterium microti*, and *Mycobacterium caprae*.[14] *Mycobacterium avium* complex (MAC) infection presents with disseminated disease in people living with HIV/acquired immunodeficiency syndrome (AIDS) (PLWHA), and typically occurs only after the cluster of differentiation (CD) 4 lymphocyte count decreases to less than 50 cells/μL. MAC may be responsible for involvement of any part of the GI tract or the liver in patients with AIDS.[15]

Extrapulmonary TB causes a significant morbidity and mortality in areas of Turkey accepting immigrants from lower socioeconomic populations.[16] The current percentage of extrapulmonary TB is around 40% of all TB cases throughout the country, and has been increasing over the last 10 years.[17] In contrast, extrapulmonary TB accounts for about 15% of all TB cases, globally.[1,9] As a fraction of extrapulmonary involvement, GI TB is seen less frequently than other forms of involvement, such as lymph nodes, genitourinary tract, bones and joints, or the central nervous system. GI TB accounts for 10% to 16% of cases.[9,18] Thus, it corresponds to 1% to 3% of all TB cases. In contrast, recent statistics in Turkey show that 5.4% of extrapulmonary TB cases have TB of the GI tract, including the peritoneum.[17]

GI TB shows no sex predisposition, and equal age distribution between 15 and 65 years.[5,11] People with lower socioeconomic status have a tendency to develop GI TB.[18] Major risk factors for the development of GI TB include HIV infection, underlying malignancies (such as lymphoma), cirrhosis, renal failure, diabetes mellitus, solid organ transplant, and treatment with glucocorticoids or anti–tumor necrosis factor (TNF) agents.[19,20] GI TB may be caused by ingestion of unpasteurized dairy products contaminated with *M bovis* in areas where bovine TB is uncontrolled.[21] Mycobacterial coinfections are the leading cause of death in PLWHA.[3,22] TB is a reportable disease; even if clinically suspected, public health authorities should be notified.

PATHOGENESIS AND PATHOPHYSIOLOGY

TB may occur via reactivation of latent *M tuberculosis* infection in any GI site.[4,9,10,23] TB can affect any of the following sites: peritoneum, oral cavity, esophagus, stomach, intestines, perianal area, liver, gallbladder, pancreas, and intra-abdominal lymph nodes. The most common forms of GI TB include involvement of the peritoneum and intestines.[2,4,10,20]

GI TB may be acquired from direct ingestion or biliary excretion of tubercle bacilli. Furthermore, infection can also result from hematogenous or lymphatic spread from distant sites as well as by means of direct extension from contiguous tissues. In the case of direct ingestion, the assumed route of infection is direct penetration of the mucosa by swallowed organisms, either in sputum or contaminated milk/food.[23]

CLINICAL EVALUATION
History and Physical Examination

Although some patients may be asymptomatic, common symptoms of GI TB are fever, anorexia, weight loss, nausea/vomiting, abdominal pain, diarrhea, and sometimes constipation. Hematemesis and melena are uncommon. On physical examination, signs such as pallor, abdominal distension, ascites, hepatomegaly, splenomegaly, rectal bleeding, and abdominal mass may be detected depending on the involved area of GI tract.[2,5–8,11,18,23,24]

A family history of TB is not obvious in all patients so GI TB must be kept in mind even in the absence of family history. Patients with GI TB do not necessarily have history of TB or concomitant active pulmonary TB.[4,8,9,25]

Laboratory Testing

General laboratory tests usually reveal mild anemia with a normal white blood cell (WBC) count, and increased levels of acute phase reactants (eg, C-reactive protein, erythrocyte sedimentation rate), although these are nonspecific. Fecal calprotectin may be useful in follow-up as a surrogate marker for healing in patients on anti-TB therapy.[6,18,24,26,27]

Sputum and gastric washings should be examined for tubercle bacilli if there is a suspicion of concomitant pulmonary disease. GI TB is a paucibacillary form of TB so acid-fast bacilli (AFB) may not be isolated from clinical specimens obtained by noninvasive or invasive techniques.[2,4,7,10] Although testing modalities for mycobacteria have high specificity in GI TB, poor sensitivities are reported for acid-fast staining, mycobacterial cultures, and polymerase chain reaction (PCR) tests.[28]

A direct smear of ascitic fluid is almost never positive because of the low concentration of mycobacteria in ascitic fluid in peritoneal TB.[2,4,16] Tubercle bacilli are detected with an acid-fast stain in around 20.5% of mucosal samples in intestinal TB, whereas sensitivity of PCR for this purpose is 64.1%.[19] A meta-analysis of studies showed that pooled sensitivity and specificity of PCR for AFB in endoscopic biopsies to distinguish intestinal TB from Crohn disease were 44% and 95%, respectively.[29] PCR testing in gastroscopic biopsy specimens may be also a promising method for early diagnosis of gastric TB.[30]

Multiplex PCR has been found to have higher sensitivity and specificity when assessed using a composite reference standard (CRS) comprising a combination of clinical characteristics and microbiological methods for diagnosis of TB.[31] Nevertheless, cultures are still required to determine susceptibility to antimicrobial agents.[9] A commercial nested PCR assay with automated amplification showed good sensitivity and specificity for detection of *M tuberculosis* and rifampin resistance gene in extrapulmonary TB compared with a CRS made up of smear and culture results and clinical, radiologic, and histopathologic findings.[32] It has been also reported that this test has a moderate sensitivity and excellent specificity, making it clinically useful on peritoneal tissue.[33] Meanwhile, detection of mycobacterial DNA in stool may potentially be practical as a rule-in test in patients with extrapulmonary TB, including intestinal TB.[34]

A positive tuberculin skin test (TST) or the interferon-γ release assay (IGRA), is not helpful because a positive test does not necessarily mean active disease. Bacille Calmette-Guérin (BCG) vaccination interferes with the result of TST in areas where it is given at birth. In addition, many patients, especially older people and PLWHA, have a negative TST if there is active GI TB.[4] The commercially available IGRA is reported to have better sensitivity and specificity than the traditional TST in differentiating intestinal TB from Crohn disease.[6,35] Specificity of IGRA could be increased by calculation of TB-specific antigen/phytohemagglutinin ratio, for distinguishing active TB from latent *M tuberculosis* infection.[36] False-negative IGRA results were found in 5.8% of patients with proven GI TB.[37] An enzyme-linked immunospot (ELISPOT) assay based on circulating and compartmentalized mononuclear cells for the diagnosis of active TB may be a useful adjunct in patients with suspected peritoneal TB.[38]

Measurement of adenosine deaminase (ADA) has been proposed as a useful test for detecting peritoneal TB.[39] Levels of ADA are typically increased in the ascitic fluid in peritoneal TB to differentiate peritoneal carcinomatosis.[40] However, in the United States, where greater than 50% of patients with peritoneal TB have underlying cirrhosis, the ADA level has been found to be too insensitive to be helpful.[41]

Imaging Studies

Computed tomography (CT) scan is the modality of choice for assessment of location and extension in GI TB.[6,23,28,42–44] MRI may be better than CT because of the absence of radiation, particularly for chronic cases in which repeated images might be needed.[20]

Radiologic appearance is diverse in intestinal TB.[23] CT can show asymmetric wall thickening of the terminal ileum, cecum, or ileocecal valves and massive lymphadenopathy with central necrosis. The cecum is contracted with disease on both sides of the valve, and the valve itself often is small and irregular because of fibrosis and stenosis. In the hypertrophic form, disease of colon can be diagnosed radiologically as cancer.[45,46] In contrast, multislice CT enterography and abdominal ultrasonography as cross-sectional imaging techniques have been found useful in evaluation of anti-TB therapy responses in patients with intestinal TB.[47]

Radiographic contrast studies of the gut show an array of changes, including mucosal ulceration, segmental narrowing, stricture, and fistula formation. The ileocecal region often reveals radiologic evidence of irritability and hypermotility, with hypersegmentation of the mucosal folds or poor filling of the region examined by barium enema.[43] TB lesions have shown positive uptake on [^{68}Ga-DOTA,1-Nal^3]-octreotide (^{68}Ga-DOTANOC) positron emission tomography/CT scan in a mesenteric mass resembling a carcinoid tumor, which resulted in the patient being operated erroneously.[48]

The presentation may mimic cancer, with an ulcerating mass lesion and paratracheal adenopathy on CT imaging in esophageal TB.[49] Radiographic studies reveal an enlarged stomach with a narrowed, deformed antrum and prepyloric ulcerations in gastric TB.[50]

CT imaging shows areas of high attenuation because of high protein and cellular content of ascitic fluid in peritoneal TB.[2] The diagnosis in the wet type of peritoneal TB (containing a large amount of viscous ascitic fluid in the peritoneal cavity) and abdominal lymphadenopathy can be approached by ultrasonography-guided aspiration followed by laparoscopy as needed.[9]

The diagnosis in lesions of solid organs such as liver can also be obtained by ultrasonography-guided aspiration.[9] The micronodular form of hepatic TB manifests as multiple small, low-attenuating nodules observed on the surface and throughout the parenchyma of liver on CT imaging.[42–44,51]

Although cross-sectional imaging with CT or MRI may show diffuse enlargement, the major challenge in imaging is to distinguish pancreatic TB from pancreatic adenocarcinoma.[4,52] Findings suggestive of TB include lack of vascular invasion or pancreatic duct dilatation, known as primary TB, and necrotic lymphadenopathy. On ultrasonography, pancreatic TB is seen as 1 or more solid hypoechoic masses in the parenchyma that may undergo central liquefaction.[23,46]

Gastroenterological Procedures

Endoscopy is often necessary to confirm active GI TB. When TB is suspected, use of N95 respirators is required to prevent inhalation of aerosolized tubercle bacilli by medical staff in the endoscopy suite.

Endoscopic findings of esophageal TB include shallow ulcers and conglomerated lesions mimicking neoplasia in addition to extrinsic compression of the esophagus.[53,54] Esophageal brush biopsies should be obtained, and specimens should be processed for acid-fast stain, mycobacterial culture, and PCR, in addition to routine studies.[55] Endoscopy may also be able to explore hypopharyngeal TB, a very rare location for TB.[56] Endoscopic findings in gastric TB include ulcers, thickened folds, nodules, and submucosal lesions.[57]

Although colonoscopy may detect asymptomatic cases when performed for other reasons, endoscopic findings in intestinal TB can be difficult to distinguish from other diseases of the colon.[58] Colonoscopic biopsies have been reported to reveal a 77.1% diagnostic accuracy, which is shown by a positive culture and/or histopathology. The yield of TB culture positivity may be improved when multiple tissue biopsies are obtained during colonoscopy.[59] It is difficult to differentiate Crohn disease from TB based on capsule endoscopic features alone.[6] Laparoscopy or laparotomy with histopathologic and mycobacteriologic examination of biopsies is the only means for diagnosis in some instances.[5]

Even though several noninvasive diagnostic tests are available to diagnose extrapulmonary TB, suspected peritoneal TB is one of the few remaining indications for diagnostic laparoscopy.[4,60] In contrast with a sensitivity of approximately 50% for ascitic fluid mycobacterial culture with optimal processing, laparoscopy with histopathology and culture of peritoneal biopsies has a sensitivity approaching 100% for detecting peritoneal TB.[4,9] The most common type of peritoneal TB is the wet type, which is characterized by a large amount of free or loculated viscous fluid. Fibrotic/fixed and dry/plastic types are less common. Several diseases, such as carcinomatosis, mesothelioma, and non-TB peritonitis, may have a similar appearance to peritoneal TB.[10,23,42,46]

Micronodular hepatic TB can be missed by CT scan and may be evident only on a liver biopsy.[9] Endoscopic retrograde cholangiopancreatography and stent placement have diagnostic and therapeutic roles, and are indicated in patients presenting with obstructive jaundice caused by hepatobiliary involvement.[4]

Endoscopic ultrasonography with diagnostic fine-needle aspiration has been shown to be effective as a means of obtaining a diagnosis in pancreatic TB.[61]

CLINICAL FORMS
Oral Tuberculosis

Oral TB is an uncommon form, and often presents as a painless ulceration with undermined edges on palate, lips, buccal mucosa, or tongue, and is usually associated with palpable cervical lymph nodes. The differential diagnosis includes traumatic ulcer, squamous cell carcinoma, aphthous ulcerations, syphilitic ulcer, actinomycosis, granulomatosis with polyangiitis, sarcoidosis, leishmaniasis, zygomycosis, and leprosy.[62]

Esophageal Tuberculosis

Esophageal involvement in TB occurs rarely, and most reports are from areas of endemic TB.[4] Usually, it has been seen to occur because of spread from adjacent mediastinal structures, which can compress or infiltrate the esophageal wall. There are well-documented cases of primary esophageal involvement as well.[63] It usually involves the middle one-third of the esophagus, at the level of the carina because of proximity to mediastinal lymph nodes.[6,43] Dysphagia and odynophagia are often accompanied by weight loss, cough, chest pain, and fever.[6,49,64]

Subsequent complications include bleeding, perforation, and fistula formation.[57,65] Choking on swallowing may indicate an underlying fistula between the esophagus and respiratory tract. Surgery is sometimes required to repair fistulas, perforations, and bleeding ulcers.[4,57]

Gastric Tuberculosis

Stomach is an uncommon location of TB even in endemic areas.[10,50] Protective factors against gastric TB are bactericidal acid environment, rapid transit of contents, and a relative absence of lymphoid tissue. Although gastroduodenal TB usually presents with gastric outlet obstruction, weight loss, and anorexia, it also may result in hematemesis and surgical obstructive jaundice.[6,12,50] Biopsies show necrotizing granulomas, but demonstration of AFB is uncommon.[66]

Intestinal Tuberculosis

Intestinal involvement secondary to pulmonary TB may result from swallowing of infected sputum or from biliary excretion of the organism from an infected liver. In the past, intestinal TB was associated with active pulmonary infection and especially with active laryngeal involvement, but, currently, fewer than half of patients have concomitant active pulmonary disease at the time of diagnosis of intestinal TB.[6] Acute miliary TB and direct extension from adjacent affected organs may also result in GI involvement.[25] Primary intestinal TB without pulmonary disease often results in hypertrophic mucosal changes and has been reported in the Asian countries.[67]

Ileocecal region and terminal ileum are areas of predilection for intestinal TB. Intestinal TB can occur because of a combination of factors, such as predominance of submucosal lymphatic tissue; areas of increased physiologic stasis; areas of increased rate of absorption; and areas where the intestinal contents are more completely digested, permitting freer contact of bacilli with the intestinal lining.[6,10] Other locations of involvement, in order of frequency, are ascending colon, jejunum, appendix, duodenum, stomach, esophagus, sigmoid colon, and rectum. Multiple areas of the intestines can be affected.[6]

Presentation of intestinal TB can be acute, acute on chronic, or chronic and insidious.[25] The symptoms of intestinal TB are nonspecific.[4,58] Colonic involvement is indistinguishable from small bowel involvement in terms of clinical presentation.[4] Hematochezia is the most common symptom in rectal involvement.[6] In addition to the classic constitutional symptoms of fever, night sweats, and weight loss, intestinal TB may manifest as distension caused by ascites when the abdominal cavity is involved.[20] Nonspecific chronic abdominal pain has been reported in 80% to 90% of patients.[68] Abdominal pain is often relieved by defecation or vomiting. Hemorrhage and presence of gross blood in the stool are distinctly uncommon in intestinal TB, perhaps because of the associated obliterative endarteritis.[67] A right lower quadrant mass is palpated in nearly 25% to 50% of patients.[25,68]

The gross appearance of intestinal TB is divided into the following 3 categories: ulcerative, hypertrophic or ulcerohypertrophic, and fibrous stricturing.[6,45] The ulcerative variety of TB commonly manifests with chronic diarrhea and malabsorption, whereas the hypertrophic variety more commonly causes abdominal pain and intestinal obstruction.[20,58]

TB is the great masquerader and can mimic almost any disease affecting the GI tract.[20,25] GI TB must be distinguished from Crohn disease, sarcoidosis, carcinoma, and infections including yersiniosis, histoplasmosis, actinomycosis, schistosomiasis, ameboma, syphilis, lymphogranuloma venereum, and periappendiceal abscess.[67]

Histopathologically, the distinguishing lesion is the granuloma, which is seen in more than half of patients with intestinal TB. A granuloma is an organized collection of activated macrophages, including epithelioid and multinucleated giant cells, surrounded by lymphocytes. Granulomas can either lead to localized elimination of *M tuberculosis* and mineralization or to caseation and necrosis that results in the release of the bacilli. However, histopathologic analysis may also reveal the presence of GI granulomas caused by many diseases other than TB. Granulomatous diseases may be either primary or secondary to environmental factors. Some causes of GI granulomas are shown in **Table 1**.

Demonstration of granulomas with caseous necrosis strongly suggests TB but it is not pathognomonic. Caseous necrosis is more frequently found in the mesenteric nodes than in intestinal tissue.[67] An important part of the differential diagnosis is Crohn disease for any patient in whom intestinal TB is a possible diagnosis. Crohn disease can manifest almost all of the alterations caused by intestinal TB except culture positivity for tubercle bacilli. Both sides of the ileocecal valve usually are involved in intestinal TB, leading to incompetence of the valve, a finding that can help to distinguish ileal TB from ileal Crohn disease. Clinical features distinguishing intestinal TB from Crohn disease are summarized in **Table 2**.[6,26,28,68–70] The diagnosis is made in

Table 1	
Infectious and noninfectious causes of gastrointestinal granulomas	
Categories	**Diseases**
Infectious disease	Systemic: tuberculosis, histoplasmosis, actinomycosis, Whipple disease Parasitic: enterobiasis, schistosomiasis Venereal: syphilis, lymphogranuloma venereum
Inflammatory bowel disease	Crohn disease
Vasculitis	Behçet disease Churg-Strauss syndrome Giant cell arteritis Granulomatosis with polyangiitis
Primary immunodeficiency disorder	Chronic granulomatous disease Common variable immunodeficiency
Foreign material	Barium Starch Suture Talc
Miscellaneous	Sarcoidosis Diverticular colitis Drugs (diclofenac, biologics) Eosinophilic granulomas Granulomatous gastritis and gastroenteritis

Table 2
Clinical features distinguishing intestinal tuberculosis from Crohn disease

Features	Intestinal Tuberculosis	Crohn Disease
Clinical manifestations	Fever, night sweats, concomitant pulmonary involvement, ascites, and positive interferon-γ release assay	Perianal disease, intestinal obstruction, extraintestinal manifestations, hematochezia, diarrhea
Endoscopic findings	Transverse or circumferential ulcers, thickening and incompetence of ileocecal valve	Linear ulcers, cobblestone appearance, mucosal bridge, rectal involvement, luminal stricture, aphthous ulcers, skip lesions, sigmoid involvement
Radiographic findings	Short segmental involvement, large and hypodense mesenteric lymph nodes, Stierlin sign	Asymmetric wall thickening, intestinal wall stratification, comb sign, fibrofatty proliferation
Pathologic findings	Caseating confluent granuloma, submucosal granuloma, lymphocyte cuffing around granuloma, ulcers lined by histiocytes	Chronic colitis with noncaseating granuloma

most cases by colonoscopy with a combination of biopsy for histopathology, culture (with drug sensitivities), and PCR tests, and posttreatment resolution of all abnormalities detected at initial investigation needs to be documented.

Complications of intestinal TB include perforation, peritonitis, and obstruction from hypertrophy, scarring, or tuberculoma.[6,67,71] Occasionally, surgical or percutaneous intervention may be required for obstructive disease and/or if intestinal perforation or hemorrhage occur.[4,12,13,68,71,72] Endoscopic balloon dilatation can be useful for the treatment of strictures caused by TB, instead of performing a surgical procedure.[4,6,73]

Anal Tuberculosis

Anal TB is rare, and represents only 1% of abdominal TB. Anorectal TB typically occurs in the setting of colonic involvement.[4] TB involving the rectal and anal areas may present as anal fissure, perirectal fistula, perirectal abscess, and nonhealing or recurrent perianal lesions. Initial diagnosis can be troublesome because of disease rareness, and such a presentation may mimic Crohn disease.[74] Complications such as massive rectal bleeding and rectal stricture have been reported. Severe disease may require surgical intervention in addition to standard anti-TB therapy.[4]

Peritoneal Tuberculosis

Peritoneal TB usually occurs with other TB forms of the abdominal cavity, and clinician suspicion is still the first step for the diagnosis.[4,7,11,20,75–77] Peritoneal involvement is secondary to necrotic mesenteric lymph node rupture.[10,76] Patients with HIV infection, cirrhosis, diabetes mellitus, and underlying malignancy are at increased risk.[4,43,78] The mortality of untreated peritoneal TB is 47% to 49%, but this can be reduced to less than 5% with anti-TB therapy.[60]

Ascites is the most frequent manifestation of peritoneal TB. Abdominal pain and abdominal distention are common symptoms in addition to fever, anorexia, and weight loss.[4,6,11,24,76–80] Classic doughy abdomen is uncommon.[6] Peritoneal TB rarely manifests as a clinical syndrome of acute abdomen.[81]

Patients nearly always have an increased ascitic fluid WBC count with a lymphocytic preponderance. Noncirrhotic patients with peritoneal TB often have ascitic fluid with a high protein content, low glucose concentration, and a low serum-to-ascitic-fluid albumin gradient (<1.1 g/dL).[4,11,75,79] The algorithm in the evaluation of patients with ascitic fluid that has a high lymphocyte count includes cytologic evaluation of the fluid and consideration of laparoscopy. If the clinical circumstances (eg, fever in an individual who comes from an area endemic for TB) and results of the initial ascitic fluid analysis suggest TB, an urgent laparoscopy should strongly be considered with histopathologic examination and mycobacterial culture of peritoneal biopsy specimens. In patients with cirrhosis, blind biopsy may be risky in the predictable presence of peritoneal collateral veins, and laparoscopically guided biopsy is preferable.[4,78]

Peritoneal TB may present as a pelvic mass on CT with increased serum levels of CA125 (cancer antigen 125), mimicking malignancies such as metastatic ovarian cancer. Therefore, it should be taken into consideration as a differential diagnosis in young women in order to avoid further complications or surgery that could lead to infertility.[20,82–84]

Patients with lymphocytic ascites and fever usually have TB, whereas afebrile patients usually have malignancy-related ascites. Cancer is the cause of lymphocytic ascites about 10 times more frequently than TB. If peritoneal carcinomatosis is present, the cytologic findings are positive more than 90% of the time, and the laparoscopy can be avoided. However, if the cytology is negative, laparoscopy is performed and is nearly 100% sensitive in detecting peritoneal TB.[60,78,85]

Peritoneal TB can easily be confused with spontaneous bacterial peritonitis, because both conditions are associated with abdominal pain and fever and half of the patients with peritoneal TB have cirrhosis. However, a negative bacterial culture and predominance of mononuclear cells in the differential count provide clues to the diagnosis of peritoneal TB. It should not be assumed that liver disease is the only cause of ascites in a febrile alcoholic patient if the ascitic fluid analysis is atypical. If the ascitic fluid lymphocyte count is unusually high, for example, peritoneal TB may be present.[86]

Hepatobiliary Tuberculosis

TB of the hepatobiliary tract is uncommon. Liver and bile ducts may be involved by hematogenous dissemination of tubercle bacilli from a pulmonary or extrapulmonary source, or direct intra-abdominal spread of mycobacteria.[4,10,43,76,87,88] Hepatobiliary or hepatic TB may manifest as pseudotumor, cholangitis, liver abscess, and hepatitis. Cases of obstructive jaundice secondary to TB, resulting from extrinsic compression of the biliary tree by enlarged lymph nodes, granulomas, or from direct involvement of biliary epithelium, are usually confused with pancreatic adenocarcinoma or cholangiocarcinoma.[4,23,87,88]

Symptoms of hepatic TB are nonspecific, and include upper abdominal pain, fever, and weight loss. Jaundice is uncommon; however, it can occur in the absence of biliary tract involvement.[4,23,87] Other clinical findings are hepatomegaly and splenomegaly. On palpation, the liver may be hard, rough, and tender.[4] Hepatic disease as part of miliary TB has been noted. Jaundice with increased serum alkaline phosphatase levels may occur in miliary TB. Massive miliary spread to the liver may cause acute liver failure as well as septic shock with multiorgan failure. Although levels of bilirubin and liver enzymes are often increased, laboratory testing is generally not diagnostic of hepatobiliary TB. Abnormalities in markers of synthetic liver functions, such as prolonged prothrombin time and decreased albumin, and decreased platelet count are less common.[4,88]

Hepatic TB can manifest as a micronodular or macronodular form. Micronodular hepatic TB corresponds to the miliary TB, resulting from hematogenous dissemination. The miliary pattern of disease is frequently associated with splenic involvement occurring as a diffuse hepatosplenomegaly. Macronodular liver involvement (tuberculoma) is rare, and nodules are fewer compared with the micronodular form.[42–44,46,51,76,87,88] The micronodular form can be mistaken for fungal abscesses, *Pneumocystis jirovecii* infection, or sarcoidosis, and correlation with clinical and biochemical findings is required. The macronodular pattern can be confused with pyogenic abscesses, metastases, and other tumors.[4,23,76]

Because the imaging findings are nonspecific, diagnosis of hepatic TB is made by isolating the organism or detecting caseating granulomas from liver tissue obtained by percutaneous or laparoscopic biopsy. The liver responds to *M tuberculosis* infection by granuloma formation. TNF is associated with granuloma formation in individuals with mycobacterial infections.[19] Granulomas are found in 2% to 15% of liver biopsies, most often near portal tracts. Although 10% to 30% of cases with hepatic granulomatous disease remain idiopathic, a lengthy list of underlying pathologic states should be taken into consideration in differential diagnosis when a granuloma is detected in histopathologic liver specimens, as shown in **Table 3**.[19,89–92] Primary biliary cirrhosis is the most common cause of hepatic granulomas in the developed world. Crohn disease commonly causes granulomatous inflammation in the luminal GI tract but only exceptionally in the liver. The most common causes of hepatic granulomas in the developing world are infectious diseases, especially TB. Both caseating and noncaseating granulomas are seen in hepatic TB.[19,51,88–90,92] Liver biopsy also helps the diagnosis of disseminated TB presenting with fever of unknown origin by revealing multiple hepatic granulomas (granulomatous hepatitis) in areas where TB is endemic.[11,93] AFB can be observed by appropriate staining of biopsy specimens. PCR may allow earlier diagnosis.[51,88,91] Mycobacteria other than *M tuberculosis* occasionally cause hepatic disease as well, including MAC, *Mycobacterium kansasii*, and BCG.[91]

Rarely, extrapulmonary TB may manifest within the gallbladder. Most frequently, TB involvement of the gallbladder presents with symptoms of biliary colic or cholecystitis. The diagnosis is only discovered after cholecystectomy and surgical pathology is reviewed.[4]

Pancreatic Tuberculosis

Pancreatic TB is a rare form, and may be isolated, associated with additional intestinal involvement, or occur in the setting of miliary TB.[4,52] The pancreatic body, head, and tail are involved in descending order of frequency. Pancreatic TB can present with epigastric pain that mimics acute pancreatitis, pancreatic abscess, or carcinoma.[23,46] Symptoms and signs of pancreatic TB have been reported as abdominal pain, jaundice, weight loss, hepatomegaly, fever, anorexia, supraclavicular lymphadenopathy, palpable gallbladder, and abdominal mass in order of frequency.[87] The diagnosis is usually established at laparotomy. Pancreatic TB is sometimes only identified after surgical resection of the affected pancreas. Complications including GI bleeding and pancreatic abscess have been reported.[4]

Gastrointestinal Involvement in Advanced Human Immunodeficiency Virus Disease

Although extrapulmonary TB is characteristic of advanced HIV disease, luminal GI tract involvement remains infrequent but, when present, usually involves the ileocecal

Table 3
Some causes of hepatic granulomas

Infections	Systemic Disorders	Hepatobiliary Disorders	Neoplastic Disorders	Drug-Induced Liver Injuries	Miscellaneous Causes
Mycobacterial:	CGD	Autoimmune hepatitis	Gastrointestinal adenocarcinoma	Allopurinol	*Chemicals:*
BCG disease	Churg-Strauss syndrome	Biliary obstruction	Hepatocellular carcinoma/adenoma	Amiodarone	Beryllium
Lepromatous leprosy	Crohn disease	Jejunoileal bypass	Hodgkin lymphoma	Acetylsalicylic acid	Copper sulfate
MAC infection	CVID	Metastases	Leukemias	Carbamazepine	Mineral oil
Tuberculosis	Erythema nodosum	PBC	Non-Hodgkin lymphoma	Cephalexin	*Dietary products:*
Bacterial:	Granulomatosis with polyangiitis	PSC	RCC	Chinidine	Green juice
Actinomycosis	Idiopathic eosinophilic enteritis	Steatosis		Chlorpromazine	Green-lipped mussel extract
Cat scratch disease	Polyarteritis nodosa Polymyalgia rheumatica			Chlorpropamide	*Parenteral foreign material reaction:*
Brucellosis	Sarcoidosis			Clofibrate	Silicone
LGV	Sjögren syndrome			Dapsone	Starch
Listeriosis	SLE			Diazepam	Talc
Lyme disease	Temporal arteritis			Dimethicone	
Melioidosis	Ulcerative colitis			Diltiazem	
Nocardiosis				Disopyramide	
Rhodococcus infection				Etanercept	
Syphilis				Feprazone	
Tularemia				Glyburide	
Typhoid fever				Gold	
Whipple disease				Halothane	
Yersiniosis				Hydralazine	
Rickettsial:				Hydrochlorothiazide	
African tick bite fever				Ipilimumab	
MSF				Isoniazid	
Q fever				Mesalamine	
Viral:				Metolazone	
Coxsackievirus infection				Methyldopa	
CMV disease				Nitrofurantoin	
EBV infection				Nivolumab	
Hepatitis B				Oral contraceptives	

(continued on next page)

Table 3
(continued)

Infections	Systemic Disorders	Hepatobiliary Disorders	Neoplastic Disorders	Drug-Induced Liver Injuries	Miscellaneous Causes
Hepatitis C				Oxacillin	
Fungal:				Papaverine	
Aspergillosis				Peginterferon	
Blastomycosis				Penicillins	
Candidiasis				Phenazone	
Coccidioidomycosis				Phenprocoumon	
Cryptococcosis				Phenylbutazone	
Histoplasmosis				Phenytoin	
Paracoccidioidomycosis				Prajmalium	
Pneumocystosis				Procainamide	
Zygomycosis				Procarbazine	
Parasitic:				Propylthiouracil	
Amebiasis				Quinidine	
Ascariasis				Quinine	
Capillariasis				Ranitidine	
Clonorchiasis				Rosiglitazone	
Enterobiasis				Sulfasalazine	
Fascioliasis				Sulfonamides	
Giardiasis				Tocainide	
Schistosomiasis				Tolbutamide	
Strongyloidiasis				Trichlormethiazide	
Toxoplasmosis					
Visceral larva migrans					
Visceral leishmaniasis					

Abbreviations: BCG, bacille Calmette-Guérin; CGD, chronic granulomatous disease; CMV, cytomegalovirus; CVID, common variable immunodeficiency; EBV, Epstein-Barr virus; LGV, lymphogranuloma venereum; MAC, *Mycobacterium avium* complex; MSF, Mediterranean spotted fever; PBC, primary biliary cirrhosis; PSC, primary sclerosing cholangitis; RCC, renal cell carcinoma; SLE, systemic lupus erythematosus.

region or colon.[94] The diagnostic criteria for patients with HIV infection differ from those who are not HIV infected. The common features of PLWHA have been reported as ascites, enlarged paraaortic lymph nodes, hepatosplenomegaly, and a mesenteric mass.[20] In contrast, MAC infection most commonly presents as disseminated disease with nonspecific symptoms in PLWHA.[15] GI MAC infection may present with fever, weight loss, and malabsorption in association with presence of yellow mucosal nodules in duodenal endoscopy. AFB are readily seen on endoscopic biopsy specimens, and the number of organisms is usually striking. Histopathology reveals blunting of villi and suffusion of macrophages with mycobacteria. As is typical of MAC infection, in advanced HIV disease, there is a poorly formed inflammatory response, and granulomas are rarely present.[95] Fecal acid-fast staining is much less sensitive than culture. Blood culture positivity confirms the diagnosis.[15]

Institution of antiretroviral therapy (ART) in PLWHA may improve immune function, hasten clinical resolution of mycobacterial infection, prevent relapse such that long-term anti-TB therapy becomes unnecessary, and enhance survival.[3,96] However, ART initiation in advanced HIV disease may cause immune reconstitution inflammatory syndrome (IRIS), typically occurring within 6 months after starting therapy in two forms. Firstly, IRIS can lead to a worse outcome compared with the clinical result achieved after treatment of opportunistic infections without the initiation of ART (ie, paradoxical form). Secondly, IRIS can also lead to appear the new clinical presentation of a previously quiescent or incubating pathogen (ie, unmasking form). TB-associated IRIS (TB-IRIS) has been reported in both paradoxical and unmasking forms among PLWHA. GI manifestations of TB-IRIS can occur as granulomatous hepatitis, intestinal lesions, peritonitis, ascites, or enlargement of intra-abdominal lymph nodes.[3,97,98] Lower baseline CD4 count and rapid increase in CD4 count are the major risk factors associated with the occurrence of paradoxical TB-IRIS.[99] Prednisone prophylaxis and early treatment can be effective in reducing the incidence of TB-IRIS and the severity of symptoms in selected patients.[100]

ART may also cause symptoms of MAC infection to flare up as IRIS until 90 days after its initiation. Although patients with MAC-IRIS are symptomatic for a longer period of time than MAC patients without IRIS, there is no difference in mortality between these groups.[101]

MAC infection is steadily responsible for the most common specific hepatic finding in advanced HIV disease. Distinctive feature of this infection is the presence of poorly formed granulomas containing AFB within foamy histiocytes. Organisms may be observed in the absence of granulomas and can be cultured from liver biopsy in the absence of infected histiocytes.[102] In contrast, TB is the most common opportunistic infection involving the liver in developing countries in particular, and may occur before PLWHA are severely immunocompromised, in contrast with MAC infection.[103] Patients with advanced HIV disease are also prone to hepatic granulomatous diseases other than mycobacterial infections, such as cytomegalovirus disease, histoplasmosis, cryptococcosis, and coccidioidomycosis.[89]

ANTITUBERCULOSIS THERAPY

Anti-TB therapy for extrapulmonary TB, including GI TB, is not different than that for pulmonary TB. A high index of suspicion ensures empiric anti-TB therapy pending the results of the culture and drug sensitivity testing.[2,4,10,16,25] A 6-month treatment course consisting of isoniazid, rifampin, pyrazinamide, and ethambutol for the first 8 weeks, followed by isoniazid and rifampin for the next 4 months, is considered adequate.[4,6–8,10,11,20,22,75,78,88,104] However, when there is a concern for disseminated TB with or without a miliary pattern, prolonged therapy may be needed.[10,24,78,88,104,105] Thus, each patient should be evaluated on an individual basis. Consultation with a specialist in infectious diseases and clinical microbiology is recommended. More anti-TB drugs may be necessary, depending on local susceptibility testing and the emergence of MDR strains. Patient compliance with the prescribed regimen is the most important predictor of a successful outcome. It should be kept in mind that erratic treatment leads to emergence of resistant strains.[2,5,11,106]

Given the suboptimal accuracy of many of the diagnostic tests, it may be necessary to treat the patient empirically with anti-TB drugs on the basis of a strong clinical suspicion, especially in areas where TB is endemic. A rapid clinical improvement, such as evidence of a healing ulcer or regressing ascites after anti-TB therapy, which often occurs within 2 weeks, may be accepted as a criterion for a correct diagnosis of GI TB, although the marked hyperplasia, masses, and stenosis of GI TB respond more slowly. When a definitive diagnosis remains in doubt after an extensive work-up in distinguishing intestinal TB from Crohn disease, it is logical to start an empiric anti-TB therapy before initiating immunosuppressive medications.[4–6,25,27,28,70,71,107]

The recommended standard therapy for infections caused by MAC consists of combination therapy with 1 macrolide such as azithromycin or clarithromycin in combination with ethambutol and rifabutin. Aminoglycosides such as streptomycin and amikacin are also used as second-line antimicrobials. Patients should be treated until culture negative on therapy for at least 1 year. Response to multidrug antibiotic therapy is variable and depends in part on the extent of immunocompromised state. However, eradication remains difficult.[5] In contrast with MAC, M tuberculosis infections in advanced HIV disease generally respond to multidrug therapy with clinical and microbiological cure.[3,22] Drug interactions can be avoided if rifampin is replaced by rifabutin, or protease inhibitors are not used in patients receiving concurrent ART with anti-TB therapy.[20]

The most common reason for discontinuation of anti-TB therapy is development of drug-induced liver injury (DILI).[6,88,104] Once a patient develops DILI, anti-TB therapy should continue with streptomycin, levofloxacin, and ethambutol, and then be switched to conventional therapy on resolution of DILI.[6,11,19,87] Half of the patients with peritoneal TB may have underlying cirrhosis (ie, mixed ascites). Therefore, they tolerate drug toxicity less well than do patients with a normal liver. The hepatotoxicity of the first-line drugs in cirrhotic patients may necessitate a modification in therapy.[75,78,108] Careful monitoring is required to assess for DILI in patients with hepatic TB as well, given that they already have some degree of liver injury. This monitoring should be done with frequent checks of liver enzymes, monthly at a minimum.[4,88,109]

Adjunctive corticosteroids may be useful by diminishing the inflammation and preventing the postinflammatory fibrosis. However, the role of corticosteroid therapy in GI TB is still controversial. Prospective studies are needed to better understand the contribution of corticosteroids.[20,75,78]

SUMMARY

GI TB remains a significant problem worldwide, and may involve the luminal GI tract from oral cavity to perianal area in addition to associated viscera and peritoneum. Although GI TB more commonly affects immunocompromised hosts, it can also occur in immunocompetent people. Diagnosis is difficult because it usually mimics a malignancy or inflammatory bowel disease. A high index of clinical suspicion and appropriate use of combined investigative methods help in early diagnosis, and reduce morbidity and mortality. Anti-TB therapy is the same as for pulmonary disease, and invasive and specialized interventions are reserved for selected complications.

CLINICS CARE POINTS

- GI TB is reemerging with the contributions of HIV infection and with MDR M tuberculosis.
- Major risk factors for the development of GI TB include HIV infection, underlying malignancies, cirrhosis, renal failure, diabetes mellitus, solid organ transplant and treatment with glucocorticoids or anti-TNF agents.
- GI TB is a paucibacillary form of TB so that AFB may not be isolated from clinical specimens obtained by noninvasive or invasive techniques.
- MRI may be better than CT for assessment of the location and extension in GI TB because of the absence of radiation, particularly for chronic cases in which repeated images might be needed.
- Crohn disease can manifest almost all of the alterations due to intestinal TB except culture positivity for tubercle bacilli.

DISCLOSURE

The author has nothing to disclose.

REFERENCES

1. World Health Organization. Global tuberculosis report 2019. Geneva (Switzerland): WHO; 2019.
2. Sheer TA, Coyle WJ. Gastrointestinal tuberculosis. Curr Gastroenterol Rep 2003; 5(4):273–8.
3. Kwan CK, Ernst JD. HIV and tuberculosis: A deadly human syndemic. Clin Microbiol Rev 2011;24(2):351–76.
4. Malikowski T, Mahmood M, Smyrk T, et al. Tuberculosis of the gastrointestinal tract and associated viscera. J Clin Tuberc Other Mycobact Dis 2018;12:1–8.
5. Uygur-Bayramiçli O, Dabak G, Dabak R. A clinical dilemma: Abdominal tuberculosis. World J Gastroenterol 2003;9(5):1098–101.
6. Rathi P, Gambhire P. Abdominal tuberculosis. J Assoc Physicians India 2016; 64(2):38–47.
7. Shreshtha S, Ghuliani D. Abdominal tuberculosis: A retrospective analysis of 45 cases. Indian J Tuberc 2016;63(4):219–24.
8. Chaudhary P, Kumar R, Ahirwar N, et al. A retrospective cohort study of 756 cases of abdominal tuberculosis: Two decades single centre experience. Indian J Tuberc 2016;63(4):245–50.
9. Abu-Zidan FM, Sheek-Hussein M. Diagnosis of abdominal tuberculosis: Lessons learned over 30 years: pectoral assay. World J Emerg Surg 2019;14:33.
10. Debi U, Ravisankar V, Prasad KK, et al. Abdominal tuberculosis of the gastrointestinal tract: Revisited. World J Gastroenterol 2014;20(40): 14831–40.
11. Singh A, Sahu MK, Panigrahi M, et al. Abdominal tuberculosis in Indians: Still very pertinent. J Clin Tuberc Other Mycobact Dis 2019;15:100097.
12. Manzelli A, Stolfi VM, Spina C, et al. Surgical treatment of gastric outlet obstruction due to gastroduodenal tuberculosis. J Infect Chemother 2008;14:371–3.
13. Lee CW, Chang WH, Shih SC, et al. Gastrointestinal tract pseudo-obstruction or obstruction due to Mycobacterium tuberculosis breakthrough. Int J Infect Dis 2009;13(4):e185–7.

14. Bayraktar B, Bulut E, Barış AB, et al. Species distribution of the Mycobacterium tuberculosis complex in clinical isolates from 2007 to 2010 in Turkey: A prospective study. J Clin Microbiol 2011;49(11):3837–41.

15. Marochi-Telles JP, Muniz R Jr, Sztajnbok J, et al. Disseminated Mycobacterium avium on HIV/AIDS: Historical and current literature review. AIDS Rev 2020; 22(1):9–15.

16. Sevgi DY, Derin O, Alpay AS, et al. Extrapulmonary tuberculosis: 7-year experience of a tertiary center in Istanbul. Eur J Intern Med 2013;24(8):864–7.

17. General Dictorate of Public Health. Tuberculosis in Turkey: 2019 report. Ankara (Turkey): Republic of Turkey Ministry of Health; 2020.

18. Udgirkar S, Jain S, Pawar S, et al. Clinical profile, drug resistance pattern and treatment outcomes of abdominal tuberculosis patients in Western India. Arq Gastroenterol 2019;56(2):178–83.

19. Almadi MA, Aljebreen AM, Sanai FM, et al. New insights into gastrointestinal and hepatic granulomatous disorders. Nat Rev Gastroenterol Hepatol 2011;8(8): 455–66.

20. Donoghue HD, Holton J. Intestinal tuberculosis. Curr Opin Infect Dis 2009;22(5): 490–6.

21. Deffontaines G, Vayr F, Rigaud E, et al. Guidelines for monitoring workers after occupational exposure to bovine tuberculosis. Med Mal Infect 2019;49(8): 563–73.

22. Crabtree-Ramírez B, Jenkins C, Jayathilake K, et al. HIV-related tuberculosis: Mortality risk in persons without vs. with culture-confirmed disease. Int J Tuberc Lung Dis 2019;23(3):306–14.

23. Lee WK, Van Tonder F, Tartaglia CJ, et al. CT appearances of abdominal tuberculosis. Clin Radiol 2012;67(6):596–604.

24. Muneef MA, Memish Z, Mahmoud SA, et al. Tuberculosis in the belly: A review of forty-six cases involving the gastrointestinal tract and peritoneum. Scand J Gastroenterol 2001;36(5):528–32.

25. Horvath KD, Whelan RL. Intestinal tuberculosis: Return of an old disease. Am J Gastroenterol 1998;93(5):692–6.

26. Watermeyer G, Thomson S. Differentiating Crohn's disease from intestinal tuberculosis at presentation in patients with tissue granulomas. S Afr Med J 2018; 108(5):399–402.

27. Sharma V, Mandavdhare HS, Lamoria S, et al. Serial C-reactive protein measurements in patients treated for suspected abdominal tuberculosis. Dig Liver Dis 2018;50(6):559–62.

28. Kedia S, Das P, Madhusudhan KS, et al. Differentiating Crohn's disease from intestinal tuberculosis. World J Gastroenterol 2019;25(4):418–32.

29. Jin T, Fei B, Zhang Y, et al. The diagnostic value of polymerase chain reaction for Mycobacterium tuberculosis to distinguish intestinal tuberculosis from Crohn's disease: A meta-analysis. Saudi J Gastroenterol 2017;23(1):3–10.

30. Ma J, Yin H, Xie H. Critical role of molecular test in early diagnosis of gastric tuberculosis: A rare case report and review of literature. BMC Infect Dis 2019; 19:589.

31. Malik S, Sharma K, Vaiphei K, et al. Multiplex polymerase chain reaction for diagnosis of gastrointestinal tuberculosis. JGH Open 2019;3(1):32–7.

32. Vadwai V, Boehme C, Nabeta P, et al. Xpert MTB/RIF: A new pillar in diagnosis of extrapulmonary tuberculosis? J Clin Microbiol 2011;49(7):2540–5.

33. Dahale AS, Puri AS, Kumar A, et al. Tissue Xpert® MTB/RIF assay in peritoneal tuberculosis: To be (done) or not to be (done). Cureus 2019;11(6):e5009.

34. Gaur M, Singh A, Sharma V, et al. Diagnostic performance of non-invasive, stool-based molecular assays in patients with paucibacillary tuberculosis. Sci Rep 2020;10(1):7102.

35. Li Y, Zhang LF, Liu XQ, et al. The role of in vitro interferon γ-release assay in differentiating intestinal tuberculosis from Crohn's disease in China. J Crohns Colitis 2012;6(3):317–23.

36. Bosco MJ, Hou H, Mao L, et al. The performance of the TBAg/PHA ratio in the diagnosis of active TB disease in immunocompromised patients. Int J Infect Dis 2017;59:55–60.

37. Kim YJ, Kang JY, Kim SI, et al. Predictors for false-negative QuantiFERON-TB Gold assay results in patients with extrapulmonary tuberculosis. BMC Infect Dis 2018;18(1):457.

38. Cho OH, Park KH, Park SJ, et al. Rapid diagnosis of tuberculous peritonitis by T cell–based assays on peripheral blood and peritoneal fluid mononuclear cells. J Infect 2011;62(6):462–71.

39. Riquelme A, Calvo M, Salech F, et al. Value of adenosine deaminase (ADA) in ascitic fluid for the diagnosis of tuberculous peritonitis: A meta-analysis. J Clin Gastroenterol 2006;40(8):705–10.

40. Kang SJ, Kim JW, Baek JH, et al. Role of ascites adenosine deaminase in differentiating between tuberculous peritonitis and peritoneal carcinomatosis. World J Gastroenterol 2012;18(22):2837–43.

41. Hillebrand DJ, Runyon BA, Yasmineh WG, et al. Ascitic fluid adenosine deaminase insensitivity in detecting tuberculous peritonitis in the United States. Hepatology 1996;24(6):1408–12.

42. Engin G, Acunaş B, Acunaş G, et al. Imaging of extrapulmonary tuberculosis. Radiographics 2000;20(2):471–88.

43. Raut AA, Naphade PS, Ramakantan R. Imaging spectrum of extrathoracic tuberculosis. Radiol Clin North Am 2016;54(3):475–501.

44. Gambhir S, Ravina M, Rangan K, et al. Imaging in extrapulmonary tuberculosis. Int J Infect Dis 2017;56:237–47.

45. Engin G, Balık E. Imaging findings of intestinal tuberculosis. J Comput Assist Tomogr 2005;29(1):37–41.

46. Prapruttam D, Hedgire SS, Mani SE, et al. Tuberculosis: The great mimicker. Semin Ultrasound CT MRI 2014;35(3):195–214.

47. Ma L, Zhu Q, Li Y, et al. The potential role of CT enterography and gastrointestinal ultrasound in the evaluation of anti-tubercular therapy response of intestinal tuberculosis: A retrospective study. BMC Gastroenterol 2019;19(1):106.

48. Razik A, Singh AN, Roy SG, et al. Mesenteric tuberculosis masquerading as carcinoid tumor on conventional imaging and DOTANOC positron emission tomography/computed tomography: Uncommon presentation of a common disease. Indian J Nucl Med 2019;34(3):216–9.

49. Faibis F, Demachy M-C, Abtahi M, et al. Esophageal tuberculosis in a patient on maintenance dialysis: Advantages of interferon-gamma release assay. Ren Fail 2009;31(3):248–50.

50. Chaudhary P, Khan AQ, Lal R, et al. Gastric tuberculosis. Indian J Tuberc 2019; 66(3):411–7.

51. Bächler P, Baladron MJ, Menias C, et al. Multimodality imaging of liver infections: Differential diagnosis and potential pitfalls. Radiographics 2016;36(4): 1001–23.

52. Cuadradoa NM, Berroa de la Rosa E, Jiménez BV, et al. Tuberculosis, one more consideration in the differential diagnosis of a pancreatic mass. Gastroenterol Hepatol 2017;40(9):619–21.

53. Kochhar R, Sriram PV, Rajwanshi A, et al. Transesophageal endoscopic fine-needle aspiration cytology in mediastinal tuberculosis. Gastrointest Endosc 1999;50(2):271–4.

54. Khanna V, Kumar A, Alexander N, et al. A case report on esophageal tuberculosis: A rare entity. Int J Surg Case Rep 2017;35:41–3.

55. Li YX, Nianb WD, Wang HH. A case of esophageal tuberculosis with unusual endoscopic feature. Clin Res Hepatol Gastroenterol 2018;42(1):e5–6.

56. Mayorga-Garcés A, Hernandez S, Otero-Regino W. Diagnostic reach of gastrointestinal endoscopy: Hypopharyngeal tuberculosis. Rev Gastroenterol Mex 2020;85(3):356–7.

57. Sharma V, Rana SS, Singh P. A case of upper gastrointestinal bleeding caused by gastric tuberculosis. Clin Gastroenterol Hepatol 2017;15:e107–8.

58. Lu S, Fu J, Guo Y, et al. Clinical diagnosis and endoscopic analysis of 10 cases of intestinal tuberculosis. Medicine (Baltimore) 2020;99(28):e21175.

59. Mehta V, Desai D, Abraham P, et al. Do additional colonoscopic biopsies increase the yield of Mycobacterium tuberculosis culture in suspected ileocolonic tuberculosis? Indian J Gastroenterol 2018;37(3):226–30.

60. Islam J, Clarke D, Thomson SR, et al. A prospective audit of the use of diagnostic laparoscopy to establish the diagnosis of abdominal tuberculosis. Surg Endosc 2014;28(6):1895–901.

61. Gupta P, Guleria S, Agarwal S. Role of endoscopic ultrasound guided FNAC in diagnosis of pancreatic TB presenting as mass lesion: A case report and review of literature. Indian J Tuberc 2011;58(3):120–4.

62. Santosh ABR, Reddy BVR. Oral mucosal infections: Insights into specimen collection and medication management. Dent Clin North Am 2017;61(2): 283–304.

63. González AE, Mendizábal EM, Dueñas CS, et al. Esophageal tuberculosis: a cause of dysphagia we should be aware of. Gastrointest Endosc 2018;88(6): 964–5.

64. Xu Q, Lv M, Xia Y, et al. Esophageal tuberculosis mimicking malignancy on 18F-FDG PET/CT. Rev Esp Med Nucl Imagen Mol 2020;39(3):182–3.

65. Fang HY, Lin TS, Cheng CY, et al. Esophageal tuberculosis: A rare presentation with massive hematemesis. Ann Thorac Surg 1999;68(6):2344–6.

66. Arabi NA, Musaad AM, Ahmed EE, et al. Primary gastric tuberculosis presenting as gastric outlet obstruction: a case report and review of the literature. J Med Case Rep 2015;9:265.

67. Lima AAM, Warren CA, Guerrant RL. Acute dysentery syndromes (diarrhea with fever). In: Bennett JE, Dolin R, Blaser MJ, editors. Mandell, Douglas, and Bennett's Principles and Practice of infectious diseases. 9th edition. Philadelphia, PA: Elsevier; 2020. p. 1357–64.

68. González-Puga C, Palomeque-Jiménez A, García-Saura PL, et al. Colonic tuberculosis mimicking Crohn's disease: An exceptional cause of massive surgical rectal bleeding. Med Mal Infect 2015;45(1–2):44–6.

69. Pulimood AB, Amarapurkar DN, Ghoshal U, et al. Differentiation of Crohn's disease from intestinal tuberculosis in India in 2010. World J Gastroenterol 2011; 17(4):433–43.

70. Limsrivilai J, Shreiner AB, Pongpaibul A, et al. Meta-analytic Bayesian model for differentiating intestinal tuberculosis from Crohn's disease. Am J Gastroenterol 2017;112(3):415–27.
71. Masood I, Majid Z, Rafiq A, et al. Multiple, pan-enteric perforation secondary to intestinal tuberculosis. Case Rep Surg 2015;2015:318678.
72. Bavunoglu I, Ayan F, Karabicak I, et al. Selective jejunal artery pseudoaneurysm embolization in a patient with massive gastrointestinal bleeding due to intestinal tuberculosis. J Emerg Med 2006;31(4):391–4.
73. Akarsu M, Akpinar H. Endoscopic balloon dilatation applied for the treatment of ileocecal valve stricture caused by tuberculosis. Dig Liver Dis 2007;39(6):597–8.
74. Tago S, Hirai Y, Ainoda Y, et al. Perianal tuberculosis: A case report and review of the literature. World J Clin Cases 2015;3(9):848–52.
75. Sanai FM, Bzeizi KI. Systematic review: Tuberculosis peritonitis. Presenting features, diagnostic strategies and treatment. Aliment Pharmacol Ther 2005;22(8):685–700.
76. Rodriguez-Takeuchi SY, Renjifo ME, Medina FJ. Extrapulmonary tuberculosis: Pathophysiology and imaging findings. Radiographics 2019;39(7):2023–37.
77. Tanrikulu AC, Aldemir M, Gurkan F, et al. Clinical review of tuberculous peritonitis in 39 patients in Diyarbakir, Turkey. J Gastroenterol Hepatol 2005;20(6):906–9.
78. Guirat A, Koubaa M, Mzali R, et al. Peritoneal tuberculosis. Clin Res Hepatol Gastroenterol 2011;35(1):60–9.
79. Poyrazoglu OK, Timurkaan M, Yalniz M, et al. Clinical review of 23 patients with tuberculous peritonitis: Presenting features and diagnosis. J Dig Dis 2008;9(3):170–4.
80. Jurado LF, Pinzon B, De La Rosa-Noriega ZR, et al. Peritoneal tuberculosis in a health-care worker, radio-pathological assessment and diagnosis, a case report. Radiol Infect Dis 2019;6(4):163–9.
81. Jacob JT, Mehta AK, Leonard MK. Acute forms of tuberculosis in adults. Am J Med 2009;122(1):12–7.
82. Ofluoglu R, Güler M, Unsal E, et al. Malignity-like peritoneal tuberculosis associated with abdominal mass, ascites and elevated serum Ca125 level. Acta Chir Belg 2009;109(1):71–4.
83. Abreu N, Serrado MA, Matos R, et al. Pelvic tuberculosis: A forgotten diagnosis – case report. Radiol Case Rep 2018;13(5):993–8.
84. Buinoiu NF, Enache SI, Chirculescu B, et al. Primary peritoneal tuberculosis, a forgotten localization. Case report. Indian J Tuberc 2018;65(3):257–9.
85. Hong KD, Lee SI, Moon HY. Comparison between laparoscopy and noninvasive tests for the diagnosis of tuberculous peritonitis. World J Surg 2011;35:2369–75.
86. Kim NJ, Choo EJ, Kwak YG, et al. Tuberculous peritonitis in cirrhotic patients: Comparison of spontaneous bacterial peritonitis caused by Escherichia coli with tuberculous peritonitis. Scand J Infect Dis 2009;41(11–12):852–6.
87. Saluja SS, Ray S, Pal S, et al. Hepatobiliary and pancreatic tuberculosis: A two decade experience. BMC Surg 2007;7:10.
88. Chaudhary P. Hepatobiliary tuberculosis. Ann Gastroenterol 2014;27(3):207–11.
89. Bhardwaj SS, Saxena R, Kwo PY. Granulomatous liver disease. Curr Gastroenterol Rep 2009;11(1):42–9.
90. Lagana SM, Moreira RK, Lefkowitch JH. Hepatic granulomas: Pathogenesis and differential diagnosis. Clin Liver Dis 2010;14(4):605–17.
91. Lamps LW. Hepatic granulomas: A review with emphasis on infectious causes. Arch Pathol Lab Med 2015;139(7):867–75.

92. Choi EK, Lamps LW. Granulomas in the liver, with a focus on infectious causes. Surg Pathol Clin 2018;11(2):231–50.
93. Kucukardali Y, Oncul O, Cavuslu S, et al. The spectrum of diseases causing fever of unknown origin in Turkey: A multicenter study. Int J Infect Dis 2008; 12(1):71–9.
94. Smith M, Boyars M, Veasey S, et al. Generalized tuberculosis in the acquired immune deficiency syndrome. A clinicopathologic analysis based on autopsy findings. Arch Pathol Lab Med 2000;124(9):1267–74.
95. Khan AS, Latif SU, Weber FH. Mycobacterium avium complex enteritis. Clin Gastroenterol Hepatol 2011;9(2):e11–2.
96. Farel CE, Dennis AM. Why everyone (almost) with HIV needs to be on treatment. Infect Dis Clin North Am 2019;33(3):663–79.
97. Lanzafame M, Vento S. Tuberculosis-immune reconstitution inflammatory syndrome. J Clin Tuberc Other Mycobact Dis 2016;3:6–9.
98. Meintjes G, Rabie H, Wilkinson RJ, et al. Tuberculosis-associated immune reconstitution inflammatory syndrome and unmasking of tuberculosis by antiretroviral therapy. Clin Chest Med 2009;30(4):797–810.
99. Xue M, Xie R, Pang Y, et al. Prevalence and risk factors of paradoxical tuberculosis associated immune reconstitution inflammatory syndrome among HIV-infected patients in Beijing, China. BMC Infect Dis 2020;20(1):554.
100. Meintjes G, Stek C, Blumenthal L, et al. Prednisone for the prevention of paradoxical tuberculosis-associated IRIS. N Engl J Med 2018;379(20):1915–25.
101. Smibert OC, Trubiano JA, Cross GB, et al. Mycobacterium avium complex infection and immune reconstitution inflammatory syndrome remain a challenge in the era of effective antiretroviral therapy. AIDS Res Hum Retroviruses 2017; 33(12):1202–4.
102. Amarapurkar A, Sangle N. Histological spectrum of liver in HIV. Autopsy study. Ann Hepatol 2005;4(1):47–51.
103. Aaron L, Saadoun D, Calatroni I, et al. Tuberculosis in HIV-infected patients: A comprehensive review. Clin Microbiol Infect 2004;10(5):388–98.
104. Zha BS, Nahid P. Treatment of drug susceptible tuberculosis. Clin Chest Med 2019;40(4):763–74.
105. Chien K, Seemangal J, Batt J, et al. Abdominal tuberculosis: A descriptive case series of the experience in a Canadian tuberculosis clinic. Int J Tuberc Lung Dis 2018;22(6):681–5.
106. Mase SR, Chorba T. Treatment of drug-resistant tuberculosis. Clin Chest Med 2019;40(4):775–95.
107. Manoria P, Gulwani HV. Gastric tuberculosis presenting as non healing ulcer: A case report. Indian J Tuberc 2019;66(4):502–4.
108. Wang NT, Huang YS, Lin MH, et al. Chronic hepatitis B infection and risk of antituberculosis drug-induced liver injury: Systematic review and meta-analysis. J Chin Med Assoc 2016;79(7):368–74.
109. Tostmann A, Boeree MJ, Aarnoutse RE, et al. Antituberculosis drug-induced hepatotoxicity: Concise up-to-date review. J Gastroenterol Hepatol 2008;23(2): 192–202.

Parasitic Infections of the Gastrointestinal Track and Liver

Annie L. Braseth, MD[a], David E. Elliott, MD, PhD[b],
M. Nedim Ince, MD[b],*

KEYWORDS

- Parasite • Protozoan • Helminth • Infectious gastroenteritis

KEY POINTS

- Protozoa or helminths are rare causes of gastroenteritis in industrialized countries, but in developing countries they cause significant morbidity.
- Certain exposures (eg. drinking shallow well water and eating raw or poorly cooked meats) or medical conditions (eg. immune suppression) can permit devastating parasitic infections in gastrointestinal tract.
- Helminths alter the composition of gut microbiota. In this context, helminth infection is investigated as a regulator of immune diseases.

INTRODUCTION

Parasites are unicellular or multicellular organisms, classified as protozoa, helminths, or arthropods. Colonization of human gut by certain protozoa (**Table 1**) or helminths (**Table 2**) can result in gastroenteritis. The frequency of parasitic gastroenteritis displays wide variation throughout the world, where the incidence and prevalence of disease parallel the frequency of parasites in endemic versus nonendemic geographies. Specific exposures, such as drinking river water and eating raw meats, predispose to parasitic gastroenteritis regardless of location in endemic landscapes. Moreover, patient populations, for example, organ transplant recipients, are at high risk of developing intense parasitic infections due to immunosuppression.

In the United States, infections by protozoa are the most frequent causes of parasitic gastroenteritis.[1] Illness due to helminthic infections, however, occur especially in people with previous travel to or residence in locations where these agents are

a Division of Gastroenterology and Hepatology, Department of Internal Medicine, University of Iowa, Carver College of Medicine, Iowa City, IA 52242, USA; b Division of Gastroenterology and Hepatology, Department of Internal Medicine, University of Iowa, Carver College of Medicine, 4546 JCP, 200 Hawkins Drive, Iowa City, IA 52242, USA
* Corresponding author.
E-mail address: m-nedim-ince@uiowa.edu

Gastroenterol Clin N Am 50 (2021) 361–381
https://doi.org/10.1016/j.gtc.2021.02.011
0889-8553/21/Published by Elsevier Inc.

gastro.theclinics.com

Table 1
Overview of protozoal infections causing gastroenteritis

Parasite	Geographic Region	At-risk Populations	Symptoms	Diagnosis	Treatment
Giardia	Worldwide, usually due to contaminated surface water	Affects both immunocompetent and immunocompromised	Bloating and diarrhea	Stool examination for trophozoites and cysts	Metronidazole, 500 mg, twice daily for 5–7 d
Cryptos-poridiosis	Worldwide	Affects both immunocompetent and immunocompromised but prolonged and more severe infection in immunosuppressed individuals (AIDS or organ transplant recipients)	Profuse diarrhea	ELISA for *Cryptosporidia* antigen	Supportive care for immunocompetent patients Can consider nitazoxanide or trimethroprim-sulfamethoxazole if immunocompromised
Cystoisospora	Tropical and subtropical climates	Immigrants and immunosuppressed patients (AIDS)	Nonbloody diarrhea	Direct visualization of oocysts in stool	Trimethroprim-sulfamethoxazole
Amebic dysentery	Tropical climate, more common in areas with poor sanitation	Men who have sex with men	Abdominal pain Bloody diarrhea	Identification of trophozoits and cysts in stool	Metronidazole, 500–750 mg, 3 times daily for 10 d + intraluminal agent

Table 2
Overview of helminth infections causing gastroenteritis

Parasite	Geographic Region	At-risk Populations	Symptoms	Diagnosis	Treatment
Ascaris lumbricoides	Worldwide, but more prevalent in less-developed countries	Poor sanitation Affects both immunocompetent and immunocompromised	Usually asymptomatic, but can present with obstructive symptoms	Direct visualization of eggs in stool	Albendazole, 400 mg, 1-time dose
S stercoralis	Tropical and semitropical regions	More severe infection in immunocompromised and alcoholic patients	Nausea, abdominal pain, or occult blood loss	ELISA for IgG against *S stercoralis*	Ivermectin, 200 µg/kg, 1-time dose
C philippinensis	Philippines Thailand Egypt	Affects both immunocompetent and immunocompromised	Protein-losing enteropathy, steatorrhea	Direct visualization of eggs or larvae in stool	Albendazole, 200 mg, twice daily for 10 d Mebendazole, 200 mg, twice daily for 20 d
Hookworm—*Necator americanus, Ancylostoma duodenale*	Americas, South Pacific, Indonesia, Southern Asia, and Central Africa	Affects both immunocompetent and immunocompromised	Iron deficiency anemia	Direct visualization of eggs or larvae in stool	Albendazole, 400 mg, once Mebendazole, 100, mg, twice daily for 3 d
Whipworm—*Trichuis trichiura*	Temperate and tropical countries, more prevalent in areas with poor sanitation	Children	Iron deficiency anemia Abdominal pain Rectal bleeding Rectal prolapse	Direct visualization of eggs or larvae in stool	Albendazole, 400 mg, and ivermectin, 200 µg /kg, 1 dose Mebendazole, 100 mg, twice daily for 3 e Albendazole, 400 mg, daily for 3 d

(continued on next page)

Table 2
(continued)

Parasite	Geographic Region	At-risk Populations	Symptoms	Diagnosis	Treatment
Pinworm—*Enterobius vermicularis*	No geographic constraints	Affects both immunocompetent and immunocompromised	Perianal pruritus	Cellophane tape test	Albendazole, 400 mg, once Mebendazole, 100 mg, once Administer second dose, 15 d after first to prevent reinfection
Hymenolepis species	Worldwide	Affects both immunocompetent and immunocompromised	Usually asymptomatic but heavy infections cause anorexia and diarrhea	Direct visualization of eggs in stool	Praziquantel, 25 mg/kg, once. Consider treating family members.
Diphyllobothrium species	Northern Europe, Russia, and Alaska	Most common in middle-aged men	Vitamin B_{12} deficiency, abdominal pain, diarrhea, constipation	Direct visualization of eggs or larvae in stool	Praziquantel, 10 mg/kg, as a single dose
Taenia species	Worldwide	Affects both immunocompetent and immunocompromised	Intestinal infection is largely asymptomatic but can cause abdominal pain and diarrhea	Direct visualization of eggs in stool	Praziquantel, 10 mg/kg, as a single dose Albendazole, 400 mg, daily for 3 d
Schistosoma species	Tropical	People living in tropical rural areas with frequent fresh water contact	Noncirrhotic portal hypertension, variceal bleeding	Direct visualization of eggs in stool	Praziquantel 40-60 mg/kg (one or two divided doses)

endemic. Diarrhea is a frequent symptom of protozoal gastroenteritis but not helminth infection. Parasites also can cause eosinophilic inflammation. Therefore, parasite and especially helminth infections should be included in differential diagnosis for patients who present with peripheral eosinophilia or in whom biopsies from the gastrointestinal tract show eosinophilic infiltrates.[2] Stool studies often are essential in diagnostic work-up.

Although well appreciated for causing morbidity and mortality, some parasites also may benefit human health by improving the diversity of intestinal microbiota and assisting in development of a homeostatic healthy immune system. In this context, parasites that enhance immunoregulation may help protect from allergy, autoimmunity, and other immune-mediated disorders.[3,4] This article focuses only on the diseases caused by parasites, but these complex eukaryotic organisms also may illuminate novel approaches of therapy for the chronic immune-mediated diseases now epidemic in highly industrialized locales.

PROTOZOAL GASTROENTERITIS

Four groups of protozoa, *Giardia*, *Cryptosporidia*, *Isosopora*, and *Amoeba or Entamoeba*, can cause gastroenteritis. Outbreaks of protozoal gastroenteritis usually are associated with poor sanitary conditions, and infection usually occurs after drinking contaminated water. A fifth protozoan, *Toxoplasma gondii*, utilizes the gastrointestinal tract of the cat as its definitive host for sexual reproduction. Humans serve as intermediary host but Toxoplasma sporozoites can invade the intestinal epithelium of humans and rarely cause intestinal symptoms.

GIARDIA GASTROENTERITIS

G intestinalis, also known as *G lamblia* or *G duodenalis*, is a microscopic protozoan, with adult trophozoites 10 μm to 20 μm in length. The source of infection usually is ingestion of contaminated water, such as lakes, ponds, or rivers. Although the *Giardia* trophozoites inhabit the human gut, they are shed in cyst form with the stool. *Giardia* cysts enable the parasite to survive outside the host and render the parasite resistant to chlorine-mediated disinfection. Therefore, swimming pools or public water supplies, if contaminated with human feces or agricultural overspills, can cause *Giardia* outbreaks. Although the infection usually is self-limited and responds to antibiotics, *Giardia* infection can create lasting gastrointestinal symptoms, such as gas, bloating, and diarrhea, which can be due to lactose or fructose intolerance, associated with disaccharides deficiency[5,6] on intestinal brush border. *Giardia* infection also constitutes a frequent cause of nonulcer dyspepsia.

In clinical practice, *Giardia* infestation usually is diagnosed with stool studies, including nucleic acid amplification tests (NAATs). Direct duodenal biopsy has poor sensitivity, although NAATs are under investigation to see whether they can increase the diagnostic yield from duodenal biopsies.[7] The disease is treated easily with metronidazole in most cases, although drug resistance has been reported in recent years.[3]

INTESTINAL CRYPTOSPORIDIOSIS

Cryptosporidium parvum causes a self-limited gastroenteritis in immunocompetent individuals, which presents with profuse diarrhea. It is transmitted easily because ingestion of as little as few hundred protozoa can cause diarrheal disease, and *Cryptosporidia* have constituted the leading cause waterborne outbreaks from pools or recreational water parks in recent years.[8] Furthermore, *Cryptosporidia* cause severe and long-lasting diarrhea in immunosuppressed individuals, such as those with acquired immunodeficiency syndrome (AIDS) or organ transplant recipients. Diagnosis of *Cryptosporidia* in stool is difficult. Therefore, patients with suspected cryptosporidiosis are asked to send several stool samples, for identification of the parasite by acid-fast staining or its antigens by immunofluorescence or ELISA.[9,10] Rarely, *Cryptosporidia* are diagnosed by careful examination of intestinal biopsies during histopathology and identification of basophilic, spherical structures, 3 μm to 8 μm in size, clustered along the epithelium.[9] Cryptosporidiosis in immunocompetent patients does not require treatment, except making sure that patients (especially young children) do not get dehydrated. Immune reconstitution in patients treated for human immunodeficiency virus (HIV)-AIDS reduces colonization and, likewise, reducing immunosuppression should be considered in transplant recipients with profuse diarrhea due to *C parvum*. Immunocompetent patients with cryptosporidiosis can be treated with nitazoxanide, although the benefit of this approach in immunosuppressed patients is questionable.[11]

CYSTOISOSPORA GASTROENTERITIS

Cystoisospora belli is a unicellular protozoan, which inhabits the human intestine in tropical and subtropical climates. The parasite causes gastroenteritis associated with nonbloody diarrhea. *Cystoisospora* gastroenteritis is rare in developed countries. The infection is seen mostly in patients with HIV-AIDS, especially in sub-Saharan Africa or in immigrants from this region.[12,13] Unlike cryptosporidiosis, gastroenteritis due to *Cystoisospora* rarely is seen in immunosuppressed patients and but can occur.[14] Diagnosis is established by showing the oocysts in stool. Repeat sampling often is needed to increase the yield. Rarely, microscopic examination of duodenal aspirates or histopathologic examination of intestinal biopsies may make a diagnosis. Trimethoprim/sulfamethoxazole is the treatment of choice.

AMEBIC DYSENTERY

The protozoon *Entamoeba histolytica* causes bloody diarrhea called amebic dysentery. The parasite is transmitted fecal-orally. Tropical climate and poor sanitary conditions facilitate the transmission of the parasite. It also can affect men involved in sexual relationship with other men. A majority of infections due to *E histolytica* have a mild course with abdominal pain and loose bowel movements. A minority of patients, however, present with systemic symptoms, fever, and amebic dysentery. These cases can require differentiation from inflammatory bowel disease (IBD), especially in patients whose presentation mimics ulcerative colitis but lack the clinical, colonoscopic, or histopathologic evidence for chronicity seen with IBD. The predilection of the pathogen for cecum and the ascending colon can help differentiate from ulcerative colitis, which uniformly affects the rectum and can involve more proximal segments of the colon in a contiguous fashion. The visualization of flask-shaped ulcers in colonic biopsies also can help with the differentiation of amebic dysentery from other causes of bloody diarrhea. Diagnosis rests on identification of organisms in freshly isolated stool specimens or colonic biopsies. *E dispar* is morphologically identical to *E histolytica* but rarely is pathogenic,[15] if pathogenic at all. The 2 species can be distinguished by NAATs or by detection of antigens unique to *E histolytica* using immunochemistry or ELISA tests.[16] Systemic treatment is with a 10-day course of metronidazole, which acts only on the trophozoite stage. Patients also should be treated with a luminally acting agent, such as paromomycin (a nonabsorbable aminoglycoside), to eradicate cysts and prevent reinfection.

HELMINTH INFECTIONS

Parasitic worms (helminths) now are encountered in nonendemic locales due to ease of travel and consumption of exotic cuisines. Helminths are grouped by phylum: nematodes (roundworms) and platyhelminthes (flatworms), the latter made up of cestodes (tapeworms) and trematodes (flukes). Although they all are called worms, they are evolutionarily vastly distant. Infection easily can be missed by health care providers, especially if a careful travel or emigration history is not obtained. Many helminths can survive for decades in a host. In areas where these infections are rare, they usually are diagnosed incidentally while testing for more common diseases. Helminth infection also can be hard to diagnose because it can cause little to no symptoms. Diagnosis may be made by stool studies, direct visualization, or serologic studies.[17]

NEMATODES (ROUNDWORMS)
Ascaris lumbricoides

Ascaris lumbricoides is a parasitic roundworm and a member of the group of soil-transmitted helminths (STHs). It is the largest nematode that can colonize humans. It infects as many as a quarter of the population of the world and is the most prevalent STH infection in humans.[18] It infects mainly children living in lower socioeconomic locales.[19] The adult parasites live in the human intestine. Infection occurs by ingesting eggs that are passed in the feces of infected individuals. This can occur through fecal-oral routes with handling contaminated detritus or through consumption of vegetables or fruits that have been exposed.[20,21] The eggs are relatively sticky and can adhere to the surface of many items that then are ngested.[22] Risk factors for developing infection include poverty, poor living conditions, and inadequate sewage disposal.[20] Unfortunately, sterilizing immunity does not develop after infection. Eggs are infective only once they are embryonated and contain third-stage larvae. The ingested eggs hatch in the small bowel (duodenum/jejunum). Larvae migrate to the lungs, exit through the alveoli, are coughed-up, and then are swallowed to re-reach the intestine. They become mature adults after 14 days to 20 days, with female adults releasing millions of eggs into feces by approximately 70 days after ingestion. The adult worms live for approximately 1 year. The worms are unable to multiply in the host because their eggs require incubation outside the host to reach infectivity.[20,23]

Often infection is asymptomatic and worms are found unexpectedly on endoscopy or seen in radiographic imaging. Clinical manifestation typically occurs in those only with heavy worm burden. Symptoms of heavy infection reflect effects of larval migration and adult worm behavior. Pulmonary symptoms can include cough, wheezing, and fever. As the larvae move into the lung alveoli, they can cause hemorrhage and consolidation. Gastrointestinal tract infection can lead to abdominal pain, nausea, vomiting, or diarrhea. A large number of adult worms can cause partial or complete small bowel obstruction. Worms also may invade the bile ducts, liver, or pancreatic ducts, leading to abscesses, ascending cholangitis, acalculous cholecystitis, or acute pancreatitis. Rare fatal infection occurs when obstruction leads to intestinal necrosis and bowel perforation.[20,21,23]

Infection usually is diagnosed after an adult worm is passed with defecation. Microscopic eggs are identifiable in stool but this requires direct visual identification by experienced personnel.[24] Furthermore, identification can be problematic with low worm burden. Even double-slide Kato-Katz (2 separate slides from the same sample) has a sensitivity of only 64.6% and can be as low as 55% in low parasitic burden.[25] A recent study looked at identifying helminth DNA in stool using NAATs showed higher sensitivity for *Ascaris* but more studies are needed to determine implications for clinical practice.[18,24] Adult worms can be identified during endoscopy or on imaging. They have characteristic appearance on ultrasound, appearing as long stripes that do not cast acoustic shadows. Serum antibody testing is not done routinely because it may not reflect active infection in patients from endemic areas. Chronic infection usually is not associated with peripheral eosinophilia because the adult worms reside in the intestinal lumen.[26]

Current drugs approved for treatment include albendazole, mebendazole, levamisole, and pyrantel pamoate, with a cure rate of more than 95% (93.2–97.3).[23,27] Asymptomatic colonization typically is treated with a single dose of albendazole at 400 mg. Albendazole has potential teratogenicity; so typically pregnant women are treated with pyrantel pamoate, although studies have shown no adverse events from albendazole compared with placebo.[28] A recent Cochrane review compared albendazole, mebendazole, and ivermectin. All drugs were highly effective for both parasitologic cure and reduced egg excretion. There was no clear difference in efficacy among the 3 drugs.[19] If pulmonary manifestations are present, a 400-mg dose of albendazole dose should be given twice, 1 month apart. Patients also should receive steroids to reduce the risk of developing pneumonitis. Intestinal obstruction should be treated conservatively with bowel rest, decompression, and a single dose of albendazole. If the worms migrate into the biliary system, treatment should be given for several days because the worms are susceptible to the drug only after they migrate out of the bile duct. Endoscopic retrograde cholangiopancreatography (ERCP) for worm extraction may be needed in cases of biliary obstruction and ascending cholangitis. Although the infection typically is easy to treat, in most endemic areas, patients become rapidly reinfected.[20,27] Health education and improved sanitation become inconsequential for long-term infection control.[20,23]

Strongyloides stercoralis

Strongyloides stercoralis is a roundworm whose larvae reside in soil in tropical and subtropical regions. Adults reside in the small intestine.[29] The parasite is estimated to infect upwards of 370 million people worldwide. Although infections most often are asymptomatic, mortality rates can reach as high as 85% in immunocompromised patients.

The life cycle of the nematode parasite occurs in 2 parts. Infection begins after filariform larvae residing in soil penetrate skin. The first stage of infection usually is asymptomatic, but when symptoms are present, they result from a local allergic reaction or urticarial serpiginous rash at the site of larva entry.[29,30] Larvae then migrate through the skin into the blood stream and to the lungs. Passage through the lungs can cause Loeffler syndrome, with symptoms of wheezing, cough, and shortness of breath. Pulmonary infiltrates also may be present on radiologic imaging. Entry into the gut is accomplished after larvae penetrate alveoli, migrate up the tracheobronchial tree, and subsequently are swallowed. Maturation is completed in the small intestine when adult worms lodge in submucosal tissue and molt. Gastrointestinal symptoms may occur beginning 2 weeks after exposure and usually are fairly nonspecific and can include pain, diarrhea, weight loss, and malabsorption.[30] Acute infection that goes undiagnosed can progress to chronic infection. Deposited parasite eggs hatch in the small intestinal lumen, releasing rhabditiform larvae that pass with the stool. Some of the rhabditiform larvae can develop into infective filariform larvae, penetrate the intestinal epithelium, and restart the life cycle. This ability to cause autoinfection allows the parasite to persist its host for decades.[30] Most patients with chronic infection have uncomplicated disease and remain asymptomatic. Others have intermittent attacks of gastrointestinal or pulmonary symptoms. Many patients also have peripheral eosinophilia. A small subset of patients with chronic infection can present with hyperinfection syndrome or disseminated strongyloidiasis. In hyperinfection, systemic sepsis and multiorgan failure can occur as a consequence of extensive larva-induced injury.[29] Disseminated disease occurs when parasites are present in organs outside of lungs, skin, and the gastrointestinal track. Disseminated strongyloidiasis occurs mainly in immunocompromised hosts or can occur when asymptomatic patients are treated with steroids or immunosuppression for an unrelated condition.[29] Studies have documented increased prevalence of chronic infection in alcoholic patients. The exact mechanism is unclear but may be related to altered hypothalamic-pituitary-adrenal axis or reduced gastrointestinal transit.[31]

Diagnosis can be challenging because many infected individuals remain asymptomatic. Diagnosis can be made by detecting live larvae in feces on agar plate culture. Larvae often are present in the stool intermittently or in such low numbers that detection is difficult.[30,32] Diagnostic sensitivity improves from 50% to almost 100%, when the number of stool specimens tested is increased from 3 to 7.[30,33] Other diagnostic tests include NAATs on stool samples. Even NAATs require testing multiple stool samples.[30,33] Low sensitivity is thought to be due to nucleases and reaction inhibitors present in feces. Blood testing for IgG antibodies against *Strongyloides* species is the preferred method for detection. IgG antibodies against *S stercoralis* are detectable 2 weeks after infection, peak at 6, and then can be present up to 20 weeks after clearance of the infection. Antibody titer is lower in patients with mild or asymptomatic infections. Detection of IgG4 anti-*Strongyloides* antibodies has improved specificity compared with other classes of anti-*Stronglyloides* IgG.[30,34,35]

The treatment goal should be complete eradication to prevent autoinfection and associated hyperinfection and dissemination syndromes. Standard treatment is with a single dose of ivermectin, which is sufficient to kill adult worms but does not affect larvae migrating through tissue. Repeat doses of ivermectin, given 2 weeks after the first dose, prevent recurrent autoinfection. Recently, a multicenter study showed that a single dose was as effective as repeated dosing[36] so this repeat treatment may not be required. Immunocompromised patients or patients with hyperinfection continue to require repeat dosing at day 3, day 16, and day 17 after the initial dose.[20]

Capillaria philippinensis

Parasitic infection *with Capillaria philippinensis* occurs after eating parasites infected raw freshwater fish. The infection is deadly if not promptly treated.[37] The first reported cases were in the Philippines. Capillariasis is a zoonosis; freshwater fish are the intermediate host, with the definitive reservoir hosts being other animals that eat these fish (such as birds).[38,39] Larvae mature into adults in the small intestine of the definitive hosts and deposit shelled eggs that drop back into the water, embryonate, and are ingested by fish completing the life cycle. Female adults also deposit eggs that lack a shell and embryonate in the host to cause autoinfection. Escalating infection in humans produces a sprue-like illness characterized by protein-losing enteropathy and steatorrhea. Diagnosis is made by identifying egg and larvae in feces. The eggs have a characteristic peanut shape that aids in their identification. Stool ELISA tests detecting *C philippinensis* coproantigen or NAATs detecting its DNA have increased sensitivity and specificity greatly compared with microscopic examination.[38] Treatment consists of an extended course of either albendazole or mebendazole.[20]

Hookworms (Necator americanus and Ancylostoma duodenale)

Hookworms (*Necator americanus* and *Ancylostoma duodenale*) infect more than 400 million people worldwide. Infection is most prevalent in tropical regions of South America, Africa, and Asia. Chronic infection can cause a wide array of nonspecific symptoms, including fatigue, abdominal pain, weight loss, anemia, and diarrhea. Infection in pregnant women can lead to poor fetal outcomes, including increased mortality and low birthweight.[40]

The life cycle begins when eggs are passed out of the body and hatch to release larvae that mature through several stages before they become infective. The infective larvae penetrate human skin, pass through the blood stream to the lungs, gain access to the airway, and eventually are swallowed. Adult worms can live in the small intestine for up to 10 years.[40]

Symptoms are based on disease burden. Patients with low parasite burden usually are asymptomatic. A high parasitic burden can cause iron deficiency anemia as adult worms feed on intestinal epithelial cells and blood. Reinfection can occur after treatment, because there is no sterilizing host immunity.[20,41]

Diagnosis is made by direct visualization of eggs under the microscope using the Kato-Katz technique. Low-level infections may be missed with this method due to decreased egg excretion in the stool.[42] Formol-ether concentration techniques and NAATs have increased the sensitivity.[42,43]

Infection is treated either with 3 days of mebendazole or a single dose of albendazole.[41] In endemic areas, it is important to improve sanitation with clean water supply and sewage treatment.[43]

Whipworm (Trichuris trichiura)

The whipworm *Trichuris trichiura* is a roundworm that infects humans. Heavy disease burden is seen in children in areas with poor sanitation.[44] The life cycle begins when eggs from human feces are deposited in soil. The eggs mature in 2 weeks to 3 weeks and become infective. Warm and humid climates are important for this maturation. Due to poor hygiene, infectious eggs are ingested and then hatch in the small intestine. Most larvae then migrate to the cecum, where they mature and anchor to the mucosa.[45]

Most infections are asymptomatic but, when symptomatic, symptoms typically include abdominal pain and rectal bleeding. Nighttime stooling with mucus discharge also can be reported by patients. Heavy worm infestation can lead to rectal prolapse. Children can develop abnormal growth and impaired cognitive development as a result of iron deficiency anemia and poor nutrition worsened by the worm burden. The worm can live upwards of 4 years.

Diagnosis usually is made by direct visualization of eggs using the Kato-Katz method. The eggs have a characteristic lemon shape.[46] Diagnosis can be challenging because ability to detect eggs in stool samples is low with low parasite burden and is dependent on the timing of stool collection in relation to release of eggs from the female worm. Stool NAATs demonstrated higher sensitivity (93.7%) than microscopic examination but still had only moderate sample to sample reproducibility, suggesting the need to test multiple stool samples.[42]

Options for treatment include albendazole or mebendazole, although efficacy is less than in treatment of other STHs. The lower efficacy of current antihelminthic medications has spurred studies evaluating combination therapy. A recent study showed better efficacy with combined therapy of ivermectin-albendazole compared with monotherapy.[42] A recent randomized control trial assessed efficacy of moxidectin coadministered with albendazole versus moxidectin monotherapy for treatment. Cure rates of 62% to 69% with moxidectin with 400 mg of albendazole were achieved.[47] Another double-blind, randomized controlled trial in children looked at combination of albendazole with pyrantel pamoate compared with albendazole monotherapy. Unfortunately, this study showed that combination therapy did not improve cure rates or reduce egg burden[48] compared with monotherapy.

Pinworm (Enterobius vermicularis)

Humans are the only natural host for *Enterobius vermicularis*, commonly called pinworm. Infection typically occurs in children by direct ingestion of eggs.[49] Risk factors for developing the infection include poor hygiene and eating after touching contaminated items.[50] The organism spreads easily in confined living situations.

Once ingested, the eggs hatch to release larvae that migrate to the ileum and cecum, develop into adult worms, and begin to deposit eggs in approximately 1 month. The infection usually is asymptomatic. At night, female pinworms migrate to and deposit eggs in the perianal area, which can cause significant pruritus. Itching can cause a continued cycle of infection by ingesting the eggs from the fingers and restarting the life cycle of the worm.[51]

Symptoms, if present, typically embody perianal pruritus. With excessive itching, perianal excoriation can occur. Abdominal pain, watery diarrhea, insomnia (from itching), and vaginitis[52] also have been reported. If the worms cause local inflammation around the appendiceal opening, appendicitis can occur.[50]

Diagnosis is made after isolating the organism on an adhesive surface and examining it under the microscope. This typically occurs by placing tape over the perianal area. Stool studies are not helpful because the egg deposition occurs outside the intestine.[51]

Treatment consists of albendazole, 400 mg, given twice with the second dose occurring 2 weeks after the initial dose. Mebendazole also can be given in a similar fashion but at a dose of 100 mg. Reinfection can occur especially within the same household, so the entire household should be treated regardless of symptoms once 1 member is diagnosed.

Anisakiasis

Anisakiasis is caused by transient infection with *Anisakis simplex, A pegreffii,* or *A decipiens* after consumption of raw fish. The worms cause a self-limited infestation in humans[53] **(Fig. 1)**, which can cause erosions, ulcers, or even perforation in the stomach, when they try to escape the lumen. The risk of bleeding gastric ulcers is approximately only 0.5%. Treatment includes albendazole or endoscopic removal of worms.[54,55]

CESTODES (TAPEWORMS)
Hymenolepis nana and Hymenolepis diminuta

Dwarf tapeworm (*Hymenolepis nana*) is the most common cestode that infects humans. Adults measure 1.5 cm to 4.0 cm in length. *H diminuta* can grow to nearly twice that length. Among cestodes, *H nana* is unique in that it can be transmitted directly from person to person. This direct pathway permits autoinfection with increasing symptoms. *H nana* also infects rodents but the strains that infect rodents appear to be different than the strains that infect people. The rodent tapeworm (*H diminuta*) normally infect rodents but humans also can harbor the parasite (zoonotic infection).[56] Hymenolepis eggs from either species are passed with stool and can be ingested by small arthropods like flour beetles or grain beetles. There they hatch to release an oncosphere and develop into cysticercoid larvae. Rodents or humans that ingest the infected arthropods acquire the helminth, which evaginates to form a scolex that attaches to the intestinal mucosa and matures to form a chain of

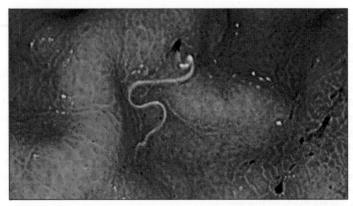

Fig. 1. Endoscopic appearance of *A simplex* in a patient seen for abdominal pain. (*From* Kondo T. DWoe sushi: gastric anisakiasis, The Lancet 2018;392(10155):1340; with permission.)

proglottids, each containing numerous eggs. *H nana* can dispense with the need for an arthropod intermediate host. Ingested eggs hatch in the human small intestine, each releasing an oncosphere that penetrates the mucosa and develops into a cysticercoid larva. The cysticercoid escapes from a ruptured villus, forms a scolex and completes the life cycle, as discussed previously. It even is possible for the *H nana* eggs to hatch directly without needing passage outside of the host (autoinfection). Direct infection permits spread to close associates (eg, household members) and autoinfection permits escalation of symptoms. Patients usually are asymptomatic but with heavy infections can have anorexia, bloating, cramps, and diarrhea. Diagnosis is by finding eggs in the stool or serendipitously by seeing the adult tapeworms on endoscopy.[57] Treatment of infection with either species is 1 dose of praziquantel, 25 mg/kg. Patients with *H nana* should have a second dose of 25 mg/kg, 1 week after the first. Household members also should be tested and treated for *H nana*.

Diphyllobothrium Species

Diphyllobothriasis (fish tapeworm) is a parasitic zoonosis caused by eating poorly cooked fish harboring infectious larvae. Infection can cause a wide array of symptoms and disease severity. There are a total of 18 described species of *Diphyllobothrium* that can infect humans but a majority are due to either *D latum* or *D nihonkaiense*. Infection is most common in middle-aged men. It is postulated that infection rates may increase with rising preference for eating raw fish and new methods for rapidly freezing fish.[58]

The complex life cycle begins with embryonation of eggs in water under favorable conditions. Transmission to humans occurs with ingestion of raw or undercooked fish infected with plerocercoid larvae. Once ingested, the mature tapeworm attaches to the host's small intestine and matures into a tapeworm. In the small intestine, these worms can cause changes in structure and neuroendocrine response and secretion.[58] The classic symptom of *D latum* infection is pernicious anemia due to vitamin B_{12} deficiency because the parasite competes with the host's absorption and use of the vitamin. Diagnosis is made by direct visualization of eggs or proglottids in stool with molecular testing to determine species.[16] Treatment consists of a single dose of praziquantel. Praziquantel can be given safely in pregnancy.[59]

Taenia Species

Zoonotic tapeworms that infect people include beef tapeworm (*Taenia saginata*) and pork tapeworms (*T solium* and *T asiatica*). In addition to cattle, intermediate hosts for *T saginata* include reindeer, and buffalo. *T saginata* is the most common tapeworm infection in humans. The prevalence is higher in the Pacific and Asia and in areas with poor sanitation where there is not routine enforcement of meat inspection.[60] Infection occurs after humans consume raw or undercooked meat that contains encysted parasitic larvae.[61,62]

The reproductive cycle begins when cattle or swine ingest water or a vegetation contaminated with stool containing parasitic eggs. Ingested eggs release oncospheres that break through the intestinal wall and disseminate through the body where the cysticerci encyst in striated muscle other tissues. After ingestion of raw or undercooked meat, the cysticerci evaginate in human body to create a scolex that attaches to the jejunum. Once attached, the parasite forms a tape-like chain of proglottids which mature, break from the distal end, and release eggs that pass with the stool. Worms can live in the human intestine for many years.

Symptoms can include abdominal pain and diarrhea although most people are asymptomatic. The eggs of *T saginata* are not infective to humans whereas the eggs of *T solium* are infective. Ingesting eggs of *T solium* leads to cysticercosis. Dissemination to the brain results in neurocysticercosis, which is a frequent cause of epilepsy in endemic regions.

Diagnosis usually is made by microscopic examination to find eggs or proglottids in the stool. Fecal examination often allows for diagnosis of the genus but not the species as the eggs are indistinguishable. If proglottids are seen, these can be distinguished by length and number of uterine branches. Species can be differentiated using NAATs[63] or through antibody detection for *T solium* excretory-secretory antigen. Cysticercosis can be tested for serologically[64] but neurocysticercosis requires imaging in addition to serodiagnosis.[65]

Common antihelmintic drugs typically provide good coverage for treatment. Historically, praziquantel and niclosamide are considered first-line treatment options although niclosamide is not available in the United States. Albendazole also is effective. Albendazole and praziquantel cross the blood-brain barrier and can cause neurologic symptoms in patients with latent neurocysticercosis. Neurocysticercosis is treated with albendazole and the addition of an antiepileptic along with glucocorticoids to limit neuroinflammation.[65]

Echinococcus Species

Cystic echinococcosis, also called hydatid cyst disease, results from a zoonotic infection by one of the tapeworms of the *Echinococcus* species, with *E granulosus* the most well-known.[66] Humans serve as intermediate hosts harboring the metacestode form. Ingested parasite eggs hatch in the intestinal lumen, each releasing an oncosphere that penetrates the mucosa and travels with the portal blood to the liver and mesenteric tissues. The parasite develops into a fluid-filled cyst harboring many (thousands) protoscolices. If the cyst ruptures, the released protoscolices can develop into disseminated secondary cysts. Rupture also result in anaphylaxis due to release of antigenic fluid contents. Most often, the infection is asymptomatic unless the cyst size affects organ function or erodes into a bile duct (cystobiliary fistula). Humans do not harbor adult worms, so no eggs are present in stool. Diagnosis is made by ultrasound or MRI of cysts.[67] Calcification is not a reliable sign of cyst nonviability. Treatment depends on cyst location, cyst complexity, and secondary complications.

Treatment options include surgery, sclerosis (puncture, aspiration, injection, or reaspiration) to kill the germinal layer of the cyst, and drug therapy with albendazole (2 doses of 5 mg/kg/d, for up to 6 months).[66]

TREMATODES (FLUKES)
Blood Flukes (Schistosoma Species)

Schistosomiasis is a parasitic disease caused by 1 of several species of the Schistosoma that reside in veins draining the hollow viscera. Infection occurs by contacting contaminated water.[68] In humans, infection in the intestinal and hepatic system is caused by S mansoni, S japonicum, S intercalatum, or S mekongi. The life cycle is complex, needing the use of a tropical aquatic snail as an intermediate host. After multiplying asexually in the snails, larvae (cercariae) escape into the water and enter the human body by penetrating through the host's intact skin. From the skin, they pass with blood to the lungs and eventually migrate to the mesenteric venules, where they mature and begin to deposit eggs intravascularly.[69] Acute symptoms may consist of abdominal pain, diarrhea, fever, or malaise. Chronic disease occurs from the local inflammation precipitated by eggs trapped in surrounding tissue. Disease burden and symptoms depend on the organ system involved. In intestinal involvement, eggs either are trapped in tissue or pass through the intestinal wall to cause granulomatous inflammation, bleeding, or even pseudopolyps. In the liver, eggs can be trapped in the presinusoidal vessels causing presinusoidal (pipestem) fibrosis, noncirrhotic portal hypertension, and esophageal varices.[70] Diagnosis typically is made by detection of eggs in feces. Nonetheless, diagnosis of a patient with schistosomiasis may require a high degree of suspicion guided by serology and classic radiologic findings. Rarely, investigation may find Schistosoma eggs and the granulomas in tissue biopsies[71] (**Fig. 2**), although this is very insensitive. Treatment typically consists of praziquantel, 40 mg/kg, as a single dose.[68,70]

Intestinal Flukes

There are many intestinal flukes that can infect humans, but the most common offenders are Fasciolopsis buski, Echinostoma species, and Heterophyes species.

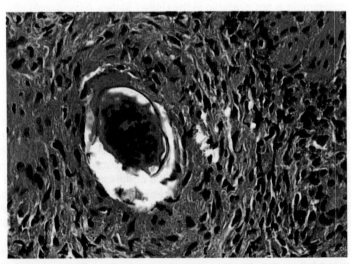

Fig. 2. Colonic biopsy from a patient with schistosomiasis with the egg embedded in lamina propria and surrounded by granulomatous reaction (hematoxylin-eosin, 400x original magnification). (*Courtesy of* Dr Sarag Boukhar, University of Iowa.)

They all have a complex life cycle: adult worms deposit eggs that pass in the stool, eggs hatch in water to release miracidia that infect snails, infected snails release cercariae, cercariae encyst on plants (*F buski*) or infect then encyst in fish and/or mollusks (*Echinostoma* spp and *Heterophyes* spp) as metacercariae. Once ingested, metacercariae excyst in the intestine, attach to the mucosa, and mature into adult worms. Intestinal flukes do not produce symptoms in most people but can cause abdominal discomfort and diarrhea if present in high numbers. Diagnosis is made by identifying flukes on endoscopy[72,73] or, more commonly, by identifying eggs passed with stool. Treatment is with 1 dose of praziquantel, 25 mg/kg.

Liver Flukes

Liver flukes reside in the bile ducts. They have a complex lifecycle employing freshwater snails as an intermediate host. People acquire these parasites by eating metacercariae encysted on freshwater plants (*Fasciola hepatica* and *F gigantica*) or in raw or undercooked fish (*Clonorchis sinensis*, *Opisthorchis viverrini*, and *O felineus*). *Fasciola* metacercariae excyst in the small intestine, burrow through the intestinal wall to the peritoneal cavity, migrate to the liver, and then journey through the hepatic parenchyma to the bile ducts. *C sinensis* and *Opisthorchis* spp excyst in the stomach and small bowel then migrate along the mucosa to the ampulla and then enter the bile duct. Once in the bile ducts, the organisms mature into adult worms that release eggs that pass with bile into the stool, and if deposited in fresh water, hatch to release miracidia that then infect snails. Liver flukes are long-lived (decades) and cause no symptoms in most people. When symptomatic, liver flukes cause recurrent cholangitis, biliary duct dilation/obstruction, and rarely pancreatitis or eosinophilic liver abscess.[74] The most worrisome complication from *C sinensis* and *O viverrine* is cholangiocarcinoma.[75,76] The longevity of the parasite and the risk for cholangiocarcinoma drive the recommendation to screen individuals from endemic areas for these liver flukes.

Diagnosis is made by finding eggs in the stool or by seeing curvilinear lucencies in the bile duct on ERCP.[77,78] Fascioliasis requires treatment with triclabendazole (10 mg/kg, single dose) whereas *C sinensis* and *Opisthorchis* spp can be treated with praziquantel (25 mg/kg, every 8 hours for 3 doses).

HELMINTHS AS IMMUNE MODULATORS

According to hygiene hypothesis, early childhood exposure to infectious agents, such as helminths, protect from immune-mediated diseases.[79] Helminth infections are common in developing countries, in which public hygiene is less advanced and immune-mediated diseases are less frequent, whereas immune-mediated diseases are on the rise in industrialized societies practicing high levels of sanitation.[80,81] The idea that helminths can regulate aberrant immune reactivity in these disorders was promoted by further experimental data demonstrating that helminths stimulate immune regulatory pathways and suppress inflammation in animal models.[82] Furthermore, some human trials have reported potential benefit in using helminths to regulate immunity in patients with celiac disease, IBD, or other immune-mediated disorders.[82–84] These observations gave rise to current research to determine the immunologic pathways exploited by helminths that protect from various immune-mediated pathologies.[85]

Helminths alter immune reactivity of mammalian host through the effect of their own products[85] or through altering the composition of intestinal microbiota.[86,87] In this context, intestinal microbiota has emerged as a factor contributing to the induction of or protection from immune-mediated diseases.[88] Further research on helminths and their interaction with microbiota is expected to lead to prevention and better management of immune-mediated disorders.

SUMMARY

Gastroenteritis and hepatobiliary disease due to various parasites continue to threaten public health despite advances in hygienic practices and sanitation. Parasites also can cause lethal and devastating gastroenteritis in immunosuppressed patient groups. Careful history and a thorough diagnostic work-up are essential for the diagnosis and management of parasitic infection. Basic research on helminthic parasites also can identify factors that may protect from developing immune-mediated disorders and improve clinical care of patients with these disorders.

CLINICS CARE POINTS

- In case of clinical suspicion, the healthcare provider should alert the laboratory for the possibility of a parasitic infection, because the laboratory may not routinely test for helminth eggs or check the specimen for the presence of protozoa.
- Parasitic infections and especially helminths should be included in the differential diagnosis for patients who present with peripheral eosinophilia.
- A careful history on travel or emigration is important in the diagnosis of parasitic diseases.
- Detection of a parasite can occasionally surprise the endoscopist during the diagnostic work-up.

DISCLOSURE

This work was supported by Merit Awards from the Department of Veterans Affairs BX002715 (D.E. Elliott) and BX002906 (M.N. Ince).

REFERENCES

1. La Via WV, B1P. Parasitic gastroenteritis. Pediatr Ann 1994;23(10):556–60.
2. Mehta P, Furuta GT. Eosinophils in gastrointestinal disorders: eosinophilic gastrointestinal diseases, celiac disease, inflammatory bowel diseases, and parasitic infections. Immunol Allergy Clin North Am 2015;35(3):413–37.
3. Leung AKC, Leung AAM, Wong AHC, et al. Giardiasis: an overview. Recent Pat Inflamm Allergy Drug Discov 2019;13(2):134–43.
4. Ayelign B, Akalu Y, Teferi B, et al. Helminth induced immunoregulation and novel therapeutic avenue of allergy. J Asthma Allergy 2020;13:439–51.
5. Trelis M, Taroncher-Ferrer S, Gozalbo M, et al. Giardia intestinalis and fructose malabsorption: a frequent association. Nutrients 2019;11(12):2973.
6. Rana SV, Bhasin DK, Vinayak VK. Lactose hydrogen breath test in Giardia lamblia-positive patients. Dig Dis Sci 2005;50(2):259–61.
7. Jangra M, Dutta U, Shah J, et al. Role of polymerase chain reaction in stool and duodenal biopsy for diagnosis of giardiasis in patients with persistent/chronic diarrhea. Dig Dis Sci 2020;65(8):2345–53.
8. Painter JE, Gargano JW, Collier SA, et al. Giardiasis surveillance – United States, 2011-2012. MMWR Suppl 2015;64(3):15–25.
9. Khurana S, Chaudhary P. Laboratory diagnosis of cryptosporidiosis. Trop Parasitol 2018;8(1):2–7.

10. Saha R, Saxena B, Jamir ST, et al. Prevalence of cryptosporidiosis in symptomatic immunocompetent children and comparative evaluation of its diagnosis by Ziehl-Neelsen staining and antigen detection techniques. Trop Parasitol 2019; 9(1):18–22.

11. La Hoz RM, Morris MI, Practice ASTIDCo. Intestinal parasites including cryptosporidium, cyclospora, giardia, and microsporidia, entamoeba histolytica, strongyloides, schistosomiasis, and echinococcus: guidelines from the American Society of Transplantation Infectious Diseases Community of Practice. Clin Transplant 2019;33(9):e13618.

12. Wang ZD, Liu Q, Liu HH, et al. Prevalence of Cryptosporidium, microsporidia and Isospora infection in HIV-infected people: a global systematic review and meta-analysis. Parasites & vectors 2018;11(1):28.

13. Lagrange-Xelot M, Porcher R, Sarfati C, et al. Isosporiasis in patients with HIV infection in the highly active antiretroviral therapy era in France. HIV Med 2008; 9(2):126–30.

14. Stein J, Tannich E, Hartmann F. An unusual complication in ulcerative colitis during treatment with azathioprine and infliximab: Isospora belli as 'Casus belli. BMJ Case Rep 2013;2013. bcr2013009837.

15. Oliveira FM, Neumann E, Gomes MA, et al. Entamoeba dispar: could it be pathogenic. Trop Parasitol 2015;5(1):9–14.

16. Gonin P, Trudel L. Detection and differentiation of Entamoeba histolytica and Entamoeba dispar isolates in clinical samples by PCR and enzyme-linked immunosorbent assay. J Clin Microbiol 2003;41(1):237–41.

17. Ince MN and Elliott DE. Intestinal worms. In: Feldman M, Friedman LS, Brandt L, editors. Schlesinger and Fortran's gastrointestinal and liver disease. 12th edition;-Philadelphia,USA:Elsevier.2020:114:1847-1867.e5.

18. Pilotte N, Maasch JRMA, Easton AV, et al. Targeting a highly repeated germline DNA sequence for improved real-time PCR-based detection of Ascaris infection in human stool. PLoS Negl Trop Dis. 2019;13(7):e0007593.

19. Conterno LO, Turchi MD, Corrêa I, et al. Anthelmintic drugs for treating ascariasis. Cochrane Database Syst Rev 2020;(4):CD010599.

20. Sleisenger, MH, Feldman M, Friedman LS, et al. Sleisenger & Fordtran's Gastrointestinal and Liver Disease: Pathophysiology, Diagnosis, Management. 8th edition.Philadelphia: Saunders, 2006.

21. Al-Tameemi K, Kabakli R. Ascaris lumbricoides: Epidemiology, diagnosis, treatment and control. Asian Journal of Pharmaceutical and Clinical Research 2020; 13(4):8–11.

22. Holland POLCV. The public health importance of Ascaris Lumbricoides Parasitology 2000.

23. Leung AK, Leung AA, Wong AH, et al. Human ascariasis: an updated review. Recent Pat Inflamm Allergy Drug Discov 2020;14(2):133–45.

24. Benjamin-Chung J, Pilotte N, Ercumen A, et al. Comparison of multi-parallel qPCR and double-slide Kato-Katz for detection of soil-transmitted helminth infection among children in rural Bangladesh. PLoS Negl Trop Dis 2020;14(4): e0008087.

25. Nikolay BBS, Pullan RL. Sensitivity of diagnostic tests for human soil-transmitted helminth infections: a meta-analysis in the absence of a true gold standard. Int J Parasitol 2014;44(11):765–74.

26. Weller PF. Eosinophilia in travelers. Med Clin North Am 1992;76(6):1413–32.

27. Chai JY, Sohn WM, Hong SJ, et al. Effect of mass drug administration with a single dose of albendazole on ascaris lumbricoides and trichuris trichiura infection

among school children in Yangon Region, Myanmar. Korean J Parasitol 2020; 58(2):195–200.

28. Ndibazza J, Muhangi L, Akishule D, et al. Effects of deworming during pregnancy on maternal and perinatal outcomes in Entebbe, Uganda: a randomized controlled trial. Clin Infect Dis 2010;50(4):531–40.

29. Karanam LS, Basavraj GK, Papireddy CKR. Strongyloides stercoralis Hyper infection Syndrome. Indian J Surg 2020, May 12;1–5.

30. Arifin N, Hanafiah KM, Ahmad H, et al. Serodiagnosis and early detection of Strongyloides stercoralis infection. J Microbiol Immunol Infect 2019;52(3):371–8.

31. de Souza JN, Oliveira CL, Araujo WAC, et al. Strongyloides stercoralis in alcoholic patients: implications of alcohol intake in the frequency of infection and parasite load. Pathogens 2020;9(6):422.

32. Kaewrat W, Sengthong C, Yingklang M, et al. Improved agar plate culture conditions for diagnosis of Strongyloides stercoralis. Acta Trop 2020;203:105291.

33. Dacal E, Saugar JM, Soler T, et al. Parasitological versus molecular diagnosis of strongyloidiasis in serial stool samples: how many? J Helminthol 2018;92(1):12–6.

34. Bisoffi Z, Buonfrate D, Sequi M, et al. Diagnostic accuracy of five serologic tests for Strongyloides stercoralis infection. PLoS Negl Trop Dis 2014;8(1):e2640.

35. Norsyahida A, Riazi M, Sadjjadi S, et al. Laboratory detection of strongyloidiasis: IgG-, IgG4-and IgE-ELISAs and cross-reactivity with lymphatic filariasis. Parasite Immunol 2013;35(5–6):174–9.

36. Buonfrate D, Salas-Coronas J, Munoz J, et al. Multiple-dose versus single-dose ivermectin for Strongyloides stercoralis infection (Strong Treat 1 to 4): a multicentre, open-label, phase 3, randomised controlled superiority trial. Lancet Infect Dis 2019;19(11):1181–90.

37. El-Dib N, Ali MI. Can thick-shelled eggs of Capillaria philippinensis embryonate within the host? J Parasit Dis 2020;44(3):666–9.

38. Khalifa MM, Abdel-Rahman SM, Bakir HY, et al. Comparison of the diagnostic performance of microscopic examination, Copro-ELISA, and Copro-PCR in the diagnosis of Capillaria philippinensis infections. PLoS One 2020;15(6):e0234746.

39. Attia RA, Tolba ME, Yones DA, et al. Capillaria philippinensis in Upper Egypt: has it become endemic? Am J Trop Med Hyg 2012;86(1):126–33.

40. Logan J, Pearson MS, Manda SS, et al. Comprehensive analysis of the secreted proteome of adult Necator americanus hookworms. PLoS Negl Trop Dis 2020; 14(5):e0008237.

41. Mourao Dias Magalhaes L, Silva Araujo Passos L, Toshio Fujiwara R, et al. Immunopathology and modulation induced by hookworms: from understanding to intervention. Parasite Immunol 2020;43(2):e12798.

42. Keller L, Patel C, Welsche S, et al. Performance of the Kato-Katz method and real time polymerase chain reaction for the diagnosis of soil-transmitted helminthiasis in the framework of a randomised controlled trial: treatment efficacy and day-to-day variation. Parasit Vectors 2020;13(1):517.

43. Riaz M, Aslam N, Zainab R, et al. Prevalence, risk factors, challenges, and the currently available diagnostic tools for the determination of helminth infections in humans. Eur J Inflamm 2020;18:1–15.

44. Bundy DA, Cooper ES. Trichuris and trichuriasis in humans. Adv Parasitol 1989; 28:107–73.

45. Chen CC, Liu KW, Tai CM. An unexpected worm hanging over the cecum. Gastroenterology 2014;146(7):e7–8.

46. Nejsum P, Andersen KL, Andersen SD, et al. Mebendazole treatment persistently alters the size profile and morphology of Trichuris trichiura eggs. Acta Trop 2020; 204:105347.
47. Keller L, Palmeirim MS, Ame SM, et al. Efficacy and safety of ascending dosages of moxidectin and moxidectin-albendazole against trichuris trichiura in adolescents: a randomized controlled trial. Clin Infect Dis 2020;70(6):1193–201.
48. Sapulete EJJ, de Dwi Lingga Utama IMG, Sanjaya Putra IGN, et al. Efficacy of albendazole-pyrantel pamoate compared to albendazole alone for trichuris trichiura infection in children: a double blind randomised controlled trial. Malays J Med Sci 2020;27(3):67–74.
49. Akinci O, Kepil N, Erzin YZ, et al. Enterobius vermicularis infestation mimicking rectal malignancy. Turkiye Parazitol Derg 2020;44(1):58–60.
50. Taghipour A, Olfatifar M, Javanmard E, et al. The neglected role of Enterobius vermicularis in appendicitis: a systematic review and meta-analysis. PLoS One 2020; 15(4):e0232143.
51. Wendt S, Trawinski H, Schubert S, et al. The diagnosis and treatment of pinworm infection. Dtsch Arztebl Int 2019;116(13):213–9.
52. Tsai CY, Junod R, Jacot-Guillarmod M, et al. Vaginal Enterobius vermicularis diagnosed on liquid-based cytology during Papanicolaou test cervical cancer screening: a report of two cases and a review of the literature. Diagn Cytopathol 2018;46(2):179–86.
53. Kondo T. Woe sushi: gastric anisakiasis. Lancet 2018;392(10155):1340.
54. Bernardo S, Castro-Pocas F. Gastric anisakiasis. Gastrointest Endosc 2018;88(4): 766–7.
55. Hamada K, Uedo N, Tomita Y, et al. A bleeding gastric ulcer caused by anisakiasis. Ann Gastroenterol 2016;29(3):378.
56. Panti-May JA, Rodriguez-Vivas RI, Garcia-Prieto L, et al. Worldwide overview of human infections with Hymenolepis diminuta. Parasitol Res 2020;119(7): 1997–2004.
57. Tanaka K, Hamada Y, Nakamura M, et al. Hymenolepis nana infection detected by magnifying colonoscopy with narrow-band imaging (with video). Gastrointest Endosc 2017;86(5):923–4.
58. Scholz T, Garcia HH, Kuchta R, et al. Update on the human broad tapeworm (genus diphyllobothrium), including clinical relevance. Clin Microbiol Rev 2009; 22(1):146–60. Table of Contents.
59. Friedman JF, Olveda RM, Mirochnick MH, et al. Praziquantel for the treatment of schistosomiasis during human pregnancy. Bull World Health Organ 2018;96(1): 59–65.
60. Braae UC, Thomas LF, Robertson LJ, et al. Epidemiology of Taenia saginata taeniosis/cysticercosis: a systematic review of the distribution in the Americas. Parasit Vectors 2018;11(1):518.
61. Eichenberger RM, Thomas LF, Gabriel S, et al. Epidemiology of Taenia saginata taeniosis/cysticercosis: a systematic review of the distribution in East, Southeast and South Asia. Parasit Vectors 2020;13(1):234.
62. Eom KS, Rim HJ, Jeon HK. Taenia asiatica: historical overview of taeniasis and cysticercosis with molecular characterization. Adv Parasitol 2020;108:133–73.
63. Nkouawa A, Sako Y, Okamoto M, et al. Simple identification of human taenia species by multiplex loop-mediated isothermal amplification in combination with dot enzyme-linked immunosorbent assay. Am J Trop Med Hyg 2016;94(6):1318–23.
64. Rodriguez S, Wilkins P, Dorny P. Immunological and molecular diagnosis of cysticercosis. Pathog Glob Health 2012;106(5):286–98.

65. White AC Jr, Coyle CM, Rajshekhar V, et al. Diagnosis and treatment of neurocysticercosis: 2017 clinical practice Guidelines by the Infectious Diseases Society of America (IDSA) and the American Society of Tropical Medicine and Hygiene (ASTMH). Am J Trop Med Hyg 2018;98(4):945–66.

66. Agudelo Higuita NI, Brunetti E, McCloskey C. Cystic echinococcosis. J Clin Microbiol 2016;54(3):518–23.

67. Brunetti E, Kern P, Vuitton DA, et al. Expert consensus for the diagnosis and treatment of cystic and alveolar echinococcosis in humans. Acta Trop 2010; 114(1):1–16.

68. Siqueira LDP, Fontes DAF, Aguilera CSB, et al. Schistosomiasis: drugs used and treatment strategies. Acta Trop 2017;176:179–87.

69. Di Bella S, Riccardi N, Giacobbe DR, et al. History of schistosomiasis (bilharziasis) in humans: from Egyptian medical papyri to molecular biology on mummies. Pathog Glob Health 2018;112(5):268–73.

70. McManus DP, Dunne DW, Sacko M, et al. Schistosomiasis. Nat Rev Dis Primers 2018;4(1):13.

71. Gray DJ, Ross AG, Li YS, et al. Diagnosis and management of schistosomiasis. BMJ 2011;342:d2651.

72. Lee TH, Huang CT, Chung CS. Education and imaging. Gastrointestinal: fasciolopsis buski infestation diagnosed by upper gastrointestinal endoscopy. J Gastroenterol Hepatol 2011;26(9):1464.

73. Sah R, Khadka S, Hamal R, et al. Human echinostomiasis: a case report. BMC Res Notes 2018;11(1):17.

74. Behzad C, Lahmi F, Iranshahi M, et al. Finding of biliary fascioliasis by endoscopic ultrasonography in a patient with eosinophilic liver abscess. Case Rep Gastroenterol 2014;8(2):310–8.

75. Hong ST, Fang Y. Clonorchis sinensis and clonorchiasis, an update. Parasitol Int 2012;61(1):17–24.

76. Sripa B, Brindley PJ, Mulvenna J, et al. The tumorigenic liver fluke Opisthorchis viverrini–multiple pathways to cancer. Trends Parasitol 2012;28(10):395–407.

77. Uskudar O, Parlak E. A swimmer in the bile duct. Diagnosis: Fasciola hepatica. Gastroenterology 2011;140(7):e3–4.

78. Choi BI, Han JK, Hong ST, et al. Clonorchiasis and cholangiocarcinoma: etiologic relationship and imaging diagnosis. Clin Microbiol Rev 2004;17(3):540–52, table of contents.

79. Varyani F, Fleming JO, Maizels RM. Helminths in the gastrointestinal tract as modulators of immunity and pathology. Am J Physiol Gastrointest Liver Physiol 2017; 312(6):G537–49.

80. Bach JF. The effect of infections on susceptibility to autoimmune and allergic diseases. N Engl J Med 2002;347(12):911–20.

81. Yazdanbakhsh M, Kremsner PG, van RR. Allergy, parasites, and the hygiene hypothesis. Science 2002;296(5567):490–4.

82. Elliott DE, Weinstock JV. Nematodes and human therapeutic trials for inflammatory disease. Parasite Immunol 2017;39(5).

83. Fleming JO, Weinstock JV. Clinical trials of helminth therapy in autoimmune diseases: rationale and findings. Parasite Immunol 2015;37(6):277–92.

84. Croese J, Giacomin P, Navarro S, et al. Experimental hookworm infection and gluten microchallenge promote tolerance in celiac disease. J Allergy Clin Immunol 2015;135(2):508–16.

85. Maizels RM, Smits HH, McSorley HJ. Modulation of host immunity by helminths: the expanding repertoire of parasite effector molecules. Immunity 2018;49(5): 801–18.
86. Lee SC, Tang MS, Easton AV, et al. Linking the effects of helminth infection, diet and the gut microbiota with human whole-blood signatures. PLoS Pathog 2019; 15(12):e1008066.
87. Martin I, Kaisar MMM, Wiria AE, et al. The effect of gut microbiome composition on human immune responses: an exploration of interference by helminth infections. Front Genet 2019;10:1028.
88. Wu WH, Zegarra-Ruiz DF, Diehl GE. Intestinal microbes in autoimmune and inflammatory disease. Front Immunol 2020;11:597966.

Hepatic Manifestations of Nonhepatotropic Infectious Agents Including Severe Acute Respiratory Syndrome Coronavirus-2, Adenovirus, Herpes Simplex Virus, and *Coxiella burnetii*

Saeed Ali, MBBS[a], Sameer Prakash, DO[a], Arvind R. Murali, MD[b],*

KEYWORDS

- Hepatitis • COVID-19 • Adenovirus hepatitis • HSV hepatitis • *Coxiella burnetii*

KEY POINTS

- Hepatic dysfunction is commonly encountered in patients with severe acute respiratory syndrome coronavirus-2 (SARS-CoV-2) infection. Presence of preexisting chronic liver disease and/or cirrhosis has been associated with poorer outcomes in patients infected with SARS-CoV-2.
- Adenovirus typically causes a self-limited viral illness. In immunocompromised individuals, it can cause severe infections involving the respiratory tract, gastrointestinal tract, heart, pancreas, liver, conjunctiva, meninges, and brain.
- Herpes simplex virus (HSV) hepatitis occurs as a part of disseminated HSV infection usually seen in immunocompromised patients and pregnant women. It is associated with high mortality if not identified and treated early, especially in pregnant women.
- Patient with acute Q fever from *Coxiella burnetii* may develop acute hepatitis, which is typically granulomatous hepatitis, ranging in severity from mild to severe.
- Flaviviruses such as dengue, Zika, and yellow fever, and Filoviruses such as Ebola virus and Marburg virus, can cause significant liver injury mimicking acute hepatitis.

[a] Department of Internal Medicine, University of Iowa Healthcare, 200 Hawkins Drive, SE 636 GH, Iowa City, IA 52242, USA; [b] Division of Gastroenterology-Hepatology, Department of Internal Medicine, University of Iowa Carver College of Medicine, University of Iowa, 200 Hawkins Drive, 4553 JCP, Iowa City, IA 52242, USA
* Corresponding author.
E-mail address: arvind-murali@uiowa.edu

Gastroenterol Clin N Am 50 (2021) 383–402
https://doi.org/10.1016/j.gtc.2021.02.012
0889-8553/21/© 2021 Elsevier Inc. All rights reserved.

INTRODUCTION

Hepatotropic viruses (A–E) are the most common causes of infectious hepatitis. Less commonly, nonhepatotropic viruses such as coronavirus, adenovirus, and herpes simplex virus (HSV), and bacteria such as *Coxiella burnetii*, may cause acute hepatitis. Hepatic injury may range from mild increase in aminotransferase level to severe acute hepatitis, or even acute liver failure. Clinical presentation of a patient with hepatitis from nonhepatotropic viruses may not be easily distinguishable from those with hepatotropic viral hepatitis. A high index of suspicion and knowledge of the clinicopathologic manifestations of important nonhepatotropic viruses and bacteria that can cause acute hepatitis is crucial in early diagnosis and appropriate management. This article discusses the hepatic manifestations of coronavirus, with a focus on severe acute respiratory syndrome coronavirus-2 (SARS-CoV-2) (coronavirus disease 2019 [COVID-19]), adenovirus, HSV, and *C burnetii*.

COVID-19 HEPATITIS
Virology and Transmission

Coronaviruses are single-stranded, positive-sense, single-stranded, enveloped RNA viruses that belong to the family Coronaviridae and the subfamily Orthocoronaviridae. They infect both humans and animals.[1] Coronaviruses are likely transmitted through respiratory droplets, either through direct contact or indirectly through fomites.[2,3] The COVID-19 virus is highly resilient and may remain viable for 2 hours to 14 days depending on environmental factors.[3,4]

Epidemiology

In December 2019, a series of patients developed severe and unexplained pneumonia, which was subsequently diagnosed as caused by a novel coronavirus named SARS-CoV2 or COVID-19. The infection spread rapidly throughout the world and, in March 2019, the World Health Organization (WHO) declared COVID-19 as a pandemic. As of September 16, 2020, the WHO has reported a worldwide number of 29.4 million cases and 931,000 deaths.[5] The mortality is approximately 3.8% and rapid viral transmission is attributed to a high asymptomatic carrier rate.[1]

Mechanism of Infection

The angiotensin-converting enzyme-2 (ACE-2) receptor plays a pivotal role in acquiring infection from the COVID-19 virus. SARS-CoV-2 binds to the susceptible ACE-2 receptor to enter the host tissue. ACE-2 receptors are abundantly expressed in type 2 alveolar cells of the lung. ACE-2 receptors are also highly expressed in the gastrointestinal tract, especially in the enterocytes of the small intestine and smooth muscles of the gastric and colonic mucosa. In the liver, ACE-2 receptors are predominantly expressed in cholangiocytes ($\sim$60%) but much less so in hepatocytes (2%–3%).[6] In addition, ACE-2 receptors are not expressed in sinusoidal endothelium but are expressed in the endothelium of small vessels in the liver.

Clinical Features

COVID-19 is typically a self-limiting viral disease in immunocompetent patients with mild symptoms such as fever, cough, fatigue, myalgia, and sore throat; however, severe infections, especially in immunocompromised patients, can quickly progress to bilateral pneumonia, severe multiorgan failure, and death.[2] The most common gastrointestinal symptoms in patients with COVID-19 are nausea, vomiting, and diarrhea. In a study by Han and colleagues,[6] patients presenting with gastrointestinal symptoms experienced a longer time interval between symptom onset and viral clearance and were more likely to be viral positive (73.3% vs 14.3%, P = .03) than those who had predominantly respiratory symptoms.

Hepatic Manifestations in COVID-19

Increased liver enzyme levels have been noted in patients infected with SARS-CoV-2, with the incidence ranging from 14.8% to 53%.[7] In general, it has been observed that hepatic dysfunction is more common in patients with severe COVID-19 compared with patients with mild illness. Presence of hepatic dysfunction in patients with COVID-19 has been associated with poor outcomes. Note that, although ACE-2 receptors in the liver are predominantly in cholangiocytes, a cholestatic pattern of injury with increase in alkaline phosphatase level is infrequent. Instead, a hepatocellular pattern of injury with increase in aminotransferase levels is commonly seen. Aspartate aminotransferase (AST) levels are usually higher than alanine aminotransferase (ALT) levels. Severe acute liver injury with significant increase in aminotransferase levels to more than 1000 U/L has been reported but is less common. Bilirubin level increases are uncommon and, if present, are usually mild, although higher levels of bilirubin may be seen in patients with severe COVID-19. Serum albumin level may be lower, especially in severe COVID-19 illness. Severe liver injury is uncommon in children and, even in severe illness, AST and ALT levels are only mildly increased (less than 2–3 times the upper limit of normal) in children. No cases of acute liver failure from COVID-19 have been reported to date. Patients with cirrhosis and COVID-19 infection may also present with new-onset hepatic decompensation. A substantial number of these patients have no respiratory symptoms at the time of diagnosis.

Mechanisms of Liver Injury

There seem to be several mechanisms for liver injury in patients with COVID-19 (**Fig. 1**).[8] Direct viral cytopathic effect on hepatocytes has been proposed.[8] However,

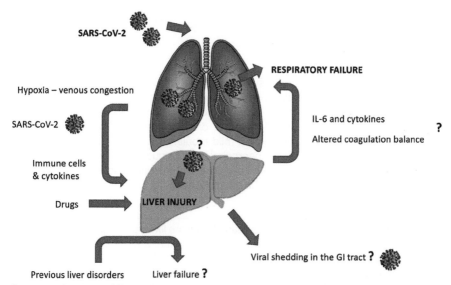

Fig. 1. Mechanisms of liver injury in patients with COVID-19 infection. GI, gastrointestinal; IL, interleukin. (*From* Sun J, et al. COVID-19 and liver diease. Liver Int 2020;40(6):1278-81; with permission.)

immune-mediated damage to hepatocytes during an inflammatory cytokine storm is an important mechanism of hepatic dysfunction in patients with severe COVID-19 illness. Several drugs, including antibiotics and antiviral agents that have been used empirically in the management of patients with COVID-19, are potentially hepatotoxic. Thus, drug-induced liver injury is an important contributor to increased liver enzyme levels in this setting. Often, it is not possible to determine whether increased liver enzyme levels are caused by the viral illness or medications. In addition, patients with severe COVID-19 infection may develop sepsis and septic shock, which can also contribute to increased aminotransferase levels.

Diagnosis

Diagnosis of COVID-19 involves a combination of clinical diagnosis through history/ physical examination, and real-time reverse transcription polymerase chain reaction (PCR) with nasal or oral swabs. Interestingly, the virus can also be isolated from stool.[9] The COVID-19 virus has been shown to remain in stool long after a negative respiratory sample.[9]

To date, it has been uncommon for patients with COVID-19 virus infection to have abnormal liver enzyme levels as the sole clinical manifestation. However, this is possibly because asymptomatic patients with incidentally diagnosed abnormal liver enzyme levels are not routinely tested for COVID-19. It may be reasonable to check for COVID-19 in patients with unexplained abnormal liver enzyme levels in the absence of other symptoms, although data are lacking in this regard. Patients with cirrhosis and new-onset hepatic decompensation should be considered for COVID-19 testing.

In patients with SARS-CoV-2 infection and abnormal liver enzyme levels, it is important to rule out other causes of abnormal liver enzyme levels such as viral hepatitis, autoimmune liver disease, and vascular disorders of the liver. Cholestatic increases in liver enzyme levels are uncommon; thus, an increase in alkaline phosphatase or gamma-glutamyl transferase levels would require thorough work-up for intrinsic liver diseases. In patients with chronic liver disease and COVID-19 virus infection, increase in liver enzyme levels must not be diagnosed and treated as flares of viral hepatitis or autoimmune hepatitis. Appropriate tests, including serology and liver biopsy, may be required for an accurate diagnosis.

Liver Histology

The first reported postmortem biopsy in a patient with COVID-19 showed moderate microvascular steatosis as well as mild lobular and portal inflammation (**Fig. 2**).[10] This pattern of liver injury seems to be nonspecific and may be seen with direct viral cytotoxic effect, immune-mediated injury, or drug-induced liver injury. Subsequent studies have reported similar findings of mild lobular infiltration but have also noted macrovesicular steatosis and focal necrosis.[11] Mild sinusoidal dilatation suggestive of hepatic vascular injury has also been observed. Interestingly, no evidence of significant biliary injury has been noted in histology specimens.

COVID-19 and Chronic Liver Disease

Patients with underlying chronic liver disease (CLD) are likely to be at increased risk for severe COVID-19. Up to 11% of patients with COVID-19 have preexisting CLD. A meta-analysis of observational studies has revealed that the prevalence of CLD in patients infected with SAR-CoV-2 is around 3%, although some studies have shown prevalence as high as 11%.[7,12] In patients with preexisting CLD, severe COVID-19 may cause worsening of liver disease, resulting in hepatic decompensation, acute-on-chronic liver disease, and death. In patients with preexisting untreated chronic

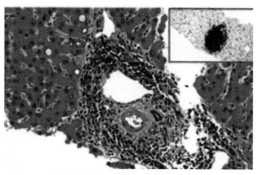

Fig. 2. Liver histology in a patient infected with COVID-19 showing atypical small lymphocytes infiltrating portal triads (CD20 immunostain). (*From* Tian S, et al. Pathological study of the 2019 novel coronavirus disease (COVID-19) through postmortem core biopsies. Mod Pathol 2020;33:1007-14; with permission.)

hepatitis B, immunosuppressive drugs that may be used for COVID-19 treatment may cause reactivation of hepatitis B infection, which can lead to acute liver injury or failure. In a meta-analysis by Kovalic and colleagues,[12] underlying CLD was significantly associated with a higher mortality and more severe COVID-19 than in patients without CLD. It seems that the more advanced the CLD, the higher the mortality with COVID-19. However, further studies are needed to determine the prognosis of patients with CLD who develop COVID-19.

Although liver-related mortality seems uncommon in patients with SARS-CoV-2 infection, even in severe cases, the COVID-19 pandemic may indirectly increase the risk of liver-related morbidity and mortality. The pandemic could lead to deferral of care for liver-related illness and may delay referral to advanced care centers for management of CLD.

COVID-19 and Hepatocellular Carcinoma

Patients with hepatocellular carcinoma (HCC) are at increased risk for COVID-19–related complications because of the presence of underlying CLD or cirrhosis and an associated immunosuppressed state. In addition, patients with HCC may be on immunotherapeutic treatments, which may worsen their immune response to COVID-19.

COVID-19 and Liver Transplant Recipients

The effect of SARS-CoV-2 infection on posttransplant immunosuppression in liver transplant recipients is not well known. High doses of immunosuppression used in the first few days after liver transplant may increase the risk of developing severe COVID-19. In addition, immunosuppression may also prolong viral shedding. A retrospective study on the outcomes of solid organ transplant recipients with COVID-19 revealed a 24% mortality.[11] Data from the European registry of liver transplant recipients on 103 patients with COVID-19 showed a 16% mortality with no deaths in patients less than 60 years old.[12] Despite the increased mortalities noted in liver transplant recipients with COVID-19, further data are required to conclusively determine whether posttransplant immunosuppression increases the risk of severe COVID-19 illness. Preemptive decrease in immunosuppression is thus not recommended at this time and may cause more harm (acute cellular rejection) than benefit in liver transplant recipients.

Treatment of COVID-19 in Patients with Liver Disease

Randomized clinical trials have not yet identified an effective treatment of patients with COVID-19 and liver disease. No specific treatment is currently recommended for patients with increased liver enzyme levels. Patients may receive experimental drug therapies in the setting of mildly increased liver enzyme levels; however, liver enzymes must be checked and closely monitored for all patients admitted with COVID-19. Checking hepatitis B surface antigen and core antibody status and initiation of appropriate antiviral therapy, especially in patients with hepatitis B surface antigen positivity, is crucial for patients who may receive corticosteroids or other immunosuppressive therapies.

Prognosis

Individuals at higher risk of COVID-19 complications include elderly patients and those with underlying chronic comorbidities, such as diabetes, cardiovascular disease, and cirrhosis. More intensive monitoring and individualized treatment is suggested for this group of patients with COVID-19.[11]

Prevention

Because patients with underlying liver disease may be susceptible to more serious complications, they are generally advised to follow general COVID-19 prevention guidelines, including social distancing, wearing face masks, and frequent hand washing or sanitizing.

ADENOVIRUS HEPATITIS

Human adenovirus infection is common but liver dysfunction from adenovirus infection is rare. It is most often a self-limiting disease in immunocompetent patients and typically causes mild upper respiratory, gastrointestinal, or ocular infections.[13] In immunosuppressed individuals, especially in children, it can lead to significant morbidity and mortality. Acute fulminant hepatitis from adenovirus infection has been described.[14]

Virology and Transmission

Human adenovirus is a double-stranded, nonenveloped DNA virus. Infection can be acquired via exposure to infected individuals or by reactivation of latent virus.[13] Transmission occurs via the respiratory route, exposure to infected tissue or blood, conjunctival inoculation, fomites, or a fecal-oral route.[15] In immunocompromised individuals such as recipients of solid organ transplants or stem cell transplants, patients on chemotherapy, or those with congenital immunodeficiency syndromes, adenovirus can cause severe infections, which can be localized or disseminated, involving the respiratory or gastrointestinal tracts, heart, pancreas, liver, conjunctiva, meninges, and brain.[13,14] Severe infections have also been reported in neonates who are not immunocompromised.[16]

Epidemiology

Adenoviruses are classified into subgroups (A–G) based on hemagglutination properties, DNA homology, and oncogenic potential in rodents. These subgroups are further divided into 67 serotypes.[17] There are 51 known serotypes, of which serotypes 1, 2, 3, 5, and 7 are most commonly associated with human disease.[18]

There is no seasonal variation in incidence of adenovirus infections.[15] They are endemic in children and in individuals living in close places.[15] Outbreaks of adenoviruses tend to occur in hospital or institutional settings.[19] Prevalence is higher in children compared with adults,[20] allogenic stem cell transplant recipients versus autologous grafts,[21] patients with T cell–depleted grafts,[22] and patients with acute graft-versus-host disease.[23] The incidence in solid organ transplant recipients is unclear; however, adenovirus has been isolated from 3.8% to 18% of bone marrow transplant recipients,[24] 8% to 18% of liver transplant patients,[25] and 12% of kidney transplant recipients.[26] The incidence in pediatric liver transplant recipients seems to be 2% to 4%.[27] Pediatric liver transplant patients are at increased risk for infection, which is partly related to the higher likelihood of primary infection in younger patients. Disseminated adenovirus infection can occur in immunocompromised patients with a case fatality rate as high as 60%.[28]

In immunocompromised hosts, the source of adenovirus infection is uncertain but there are 3 possibilities.[28] It is most likely caused by reactivation of latent adenovirus infection.[18] The second possibility is exogenous infection, which occurs via nosocomial transmission or community outbreak.[29] The third possibility is transmission via transplanted organ. A study showed that 67% of liver transplant recipients who were seronegative before transplant and received organs from seropositive donors developed adenovirus hepatitis.[30]

The proportion of infection caused by primary versus reactivation in immunosuppressed individuals is not known.[31] The overall survival rate of adenovirus hepatitis is approximately 15%[32,33] but mainly depends on severity of illness and degree of immunosuppression. Recipients of liver transplants have a higher likelihood of survival than recipients of bone marrow transplant (49% vs 10% survival).[14]

Clinical Features

The spectrum of illness ranges from asymptomatic viremia to pneumonia, enterocolitis, hepatitis, hemorrhagic cystitis, meningoencephalitis, and disseminated disease.[34,35] Adenovirus hepatitis is an uncommon manifestation of adenovirus infection. Common presenting symptoms include fever, malaise, and diarrhea. Jaundice and hepatomegaly are less common presenting symptoms.[14]

Adenovirus infection is defined as the presence of adenovirus as detected by diagnostic tests in the absence of clinical symptoms or signs.[36] Adenovirus disease is defined as the presence of organ-specific clinical signs and symptoms and the detection of the virus in the biopsy specimen or bronchoalveolar specimen or cerebrospinal fluid.[37] Disseminated disease is defined by the involvement of 2 or more organs other than viremia.[38]

In liver transplant recipients, hepatitis is the most common presentation. However, it can affect respiratory, gastrointestinal, and urinary tracts.[39] Risk factors in solid organ transplant recipients include age, allograft type, and degree of immunosuppression. Children less than 5 years of age who have received an organ transplant are at increased risk, likely because of higher exposure and being immunologically naive.[40] Similarly, intestinal transplant seems to have the highest risk compared with other allografts, which is likely related to the intense immunosuppression needed because of a large amount of lymphoid tissue.[36,40] High rates of infection during the first month or after rejection, and resolution of infection with reduced immunosuppression, suggest the degree of immunosuppression as an independent risk factor.[40,41] Risk factors for a progressive disease include early posttransplant infection, intense immunosuppression, and persistent infection of 1 site.[36,39] Asymptomatic viremia is common in adult solid organ transplant recipients (6.5%–22.5%). Risk of progression to adenoviral disease is low but not exactly known,[38] and routine screening is not recommended.[35]

Diagnosis of Adenovirus Hepatitis

Diagnosis is based on history, physical examination, laboratory testing, serology, PCR, histology, and imaging studies. In cases of adenovirus hepatitis, serum AST levels are typically higher than ALT levels.[14,42] Schaberg and colleagues[16] reported the consistent increase of serum AST levels more than serum ALT levels can be a clue to the diagnosis of adenovirus infection, although this may not always be the case.[42]

Serology has a limited role in immunosuppressed individuals because of a lack of sensitivity and the presence of serum antibodies from previous exposure.[34] Presence of adenovirus on PCR in the right clinical setting along with clinical and laboratory features of hepatitis favors a high likelihood of adenovirus hepatitis. The definitive diagnosis of adenovirus hepatitis may require a liver biopsy.[34] Histopathology is characterized by focal coagulative necrosis, which can be seen in up to 98% of cases; inflammatory changes; and glassy intranuclear inclusions within hepatocytes, with a smudged appearance (**Fig. 3**).[16] Intranuclear inclusions stain strongly with immunohistochemical stain for adenovirus.[16] Other histologic findings include focal portal lymphohistiocytic infiltrates and rarely granulomas.[16,43] Most cases do not have associated inflammation.[16] When present, it may be difficult to determine whether an inflammatory reaction is against the viral infection or whether it represents acute cellular rejection because most patients are liver transplant recipients and immunosuppression is withdrawn to treat the viral infection.

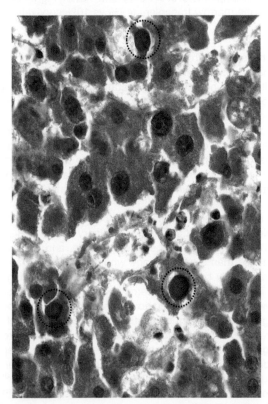

Fig. 3. Liver histology in a patient with adenovirus hepatitis. Dotted circle showing adenovirus intranuclear inclusions (hematoxylin-eosin, original magnification ×600).

Imaging findings on computed tomography (CT) scan or ultrasonography (US) include heterogeneous involvement of the liver parenchyma, and well-defined areas of low attenuation that could be mistaken for metastasis. CT scan sometimes shows an intrahepatic rim-enhancing lesion resembling an abscess.[14,44,45] US can be normal in affected patients and hence a CT scan may be necessary for identifying areas of attenuation[14] from which targeted liver biopsy can be performed to confirm diagnosis.

Treatment

There are currently no proven effective treatments available for adenovirus hepatitis.[34] Ribavirin, cidofovir, and intravenous immunoglobulin (IVIG) have been tried,[14,34] but their efficacy is unclear and requires further study. Reduction in immunosuppression is associated with better outcomes. In 1 study, patients receiving only antivirals without IVIG or without reducing immunosuppression did not survive.[14]

Prevention

The Centers for Disease Control and Prevention recommend contact and droplet precautions to prevent nosocomial spread.[19] A live oral vaccine (containing types 4 and 7) has been approved for those in the United States military[46] but is contraindicated in transplant recipients. It is also not recommended before transplant because it offers immunity against only 2 serotypes.

Adenovirus and Hepatocellular Carcinoma

Adenovirus has been studied extensively for its potential role in the treatment of HCC. Oncolytic virotherapy is a novel tumor gene therapy treatment strategy using viruses to induce tumor lysis. Adenovirus has been extensively studied to target tumor cells, including HCC, because of its high transduction efficiency and ability to insert large therapeutic genes in cancer cells.[47] Oncolytic adenovirus therapy is also being studied in combination with immunotherapy in the treatment of HCC and has been shown to be effective in in vitro studies.

In summary, early diagnosis, prompt testing including testing via serum PCR, reducing immunosuppression, and starting empiric antiviral therapy pending diagnostic confirmation can be lifesaving. Patients refractory to medical treatment require liver transplant.[14]

Herpes Simplex Virus and Hepatitis

HSV infection is a common infection in adults. HSV-1 is associated with herpes labialis, whereas HSV-2 infection is associated with genital lesions. HSV hepatitis occurs as a part of disseminated HSV infection. HSV hepatitis is a rare condition that is usually seen in immunocompromised patients and pregnant women. It is associated with high mortality if not identified and treated early.

Virology and Transmission

HSV is a linear double-stranded enveloped DNA virus surrounded by an icosahedral capsid.[48] Transmission occurs via direct contact with mucosal surfaces or skin during intimate or close contact with the infected individual.[49] HSV-1 infections are transmitted by respiratory droplets or saliva and are generally limited to the oropharynx. HSV-2 infections are transmitted via sexual contact.[50]

Epidemiology

HSV infection is widely prevalent in adults. In the Western world, most adults are infected with HSV-1 compared with HSV-2. HSV predominantly causes cutaneous lesions. HSV can persist in neurons and may cause recurrent infections. Reinfection by a different strain of the virus can also occur. Some strains are more virulent than others and have a greater tendency to cause hepatitis.[51]

Disseminated or isolated HSV-1 or HSV-2 hepatitis is sometimes seen in immunocompromised patients, typically recipients of organ transplants (especially liver transplants), those on immunosuppressive therapy, or those with immunodeficiency diseases such as human immunodeficiency virus (HIV). Pregnant women in the second and third trimesters are also at risk of a disseminated disease mainly because of low T-cell counts and low immunoglobulin (Ig) G levels at 27 to 33 weeks caused by hemodilution.[52–54]

Clinical Features

Both HSV-1 and HSV-2 serotypes can cause hepatitis.[55] HSV hepatitis has been documented in liver, kidney, pancreas, lung, and heart transplant recipients.[56,57] The source of infection in most cases is the reactivation of latent HSV in the recipient or new primary infection. Transmission from donor graft has also been identified.[58]

HSV hepatitis presents with nonspecific symptoms, often causing a delay in timely diagnosis and treatment. In addition, the typical mucocutaneous vesicular rash seen in HSV infection is only present in 18% to 50% of individuals with HSV hepatitis. Thus, its absence should not exclude HSV from the differential diagnosis. Typical presenting symptoms include fever, right upper quadrant pain, nausea, and/or vomiting. Hepatomegaly may be noted on examination. Laboratory tests usually reveal increased aminotransferase levels without significant increase in bilirubin level in patients with disseminated HSV. In patients with fulminant hepatitis, AST/ALT level can be more than 50 to 100 times the upper limit of normal. Leukopenia, thrombocytopenia, and coagulopathy with or without disseminated intravascular coagulation may be present. Acute kidney injury may develop quickly, and patients may progress rapidly into multiorgan failure resulting in death. Factors associated with higher mortality include male gender, age greater than 40 years, immunocompromised status, degree of AST level increase, coagulopathy, and encephalopathy.[54,55]

Although uncommon, HSV hepatitis may lead to acute liver failure. Less than 1% of all acute liver failures and less than 2% of all viral-related acute liver failures are caused by HSV hepatitis.[55] Patients developing HSV hepatitis and acute liver failure have a very high mortality, as high as 70%, especially in the absence of liver transplant.[55]

Diagnosis

Diagnosis is based on physical examination findings, serology, PCR, and liver biopsy if needed. Physical examination should include skin and pelvic examinations for herpetic lesions. Serology involves detecting IgG and IgM antibodies; however, its use is limited by poor sensitivity and specificity. PCR from blood samples to identify HSV DNA has high sensitivity and specificity. However, test results are often not available for 48 to 72 hours. Liver biopsy is a confirmatory test but has a higher risk of bleeding, especially in acute liver failure. If liver biopsy is deemed necessary, a transjugular approach is preferred to percutaneous because of its lower risk of bleeding.[59,60]

Histopathology is characterized by irregular zones of hemorrhagic or coagulative necrosis, scattered acidophilic bodies, and destruction of the reticulin network. There is a lack of inflammatory cells in the parenchyma or in the region of the portal vein. Hepatocytes infected with the virus typically have Cowdry type A bodies with ground-glass appearance, with chromatin squeezed to the margins (**Fig. 4**). Multinucleated giant cells are not common.[54]

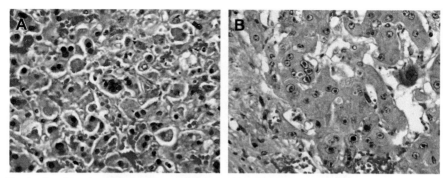

Fig. 4. Liver histology in a patient with HSV hepatitis (*A*) showing Cowdry type A inclusions (*B*) (hematoxylin-eosin, original magnification ×400).

CT imaging may reveal small, diffuse, hypodense liver lesions (**Fig. 5**). These lesions reflect the focal areas of necrosis. These lesions are not specific for HSV hepatitis and can be found in candida or histoplasma hepatitis, infection, sarcoidosis, and lymphoma.

Herpes Simplex Virus in Chronic Liver Disease and Hepatocellular Carcinoma

HSV infection has not been shown to result in CLD or liver cirrhosis, or to predispose to HCC. Similar to adenovirus, oncolytic HSVs have been studied against HCC and been found to be effective in vitro.[61] Further studies are needed to evaluate the role of HSV in the treatment of HCC.

Herpes Simplex Virus Hepatitis in Liver Transplant Recipients

HSV hepatitis in liver transplant recipients tends to occur in the very early postoperative period. Onset is usually 20 ± 12 days.[62] This short interval might suggest reactivation of the virus in the recipient caused by immunosuppression or possibly acquired from the donor. HSV hepatitis in recent liver transplant patients is associated with significantly increased mortality. Early detection and timely diagnosis improve survival.[63] HSV hepatitis may not be recognized promptly because evaluation for more common causes, such as acute cellular rejection or biliary complications, is prioritized. Empiric treatment with acyclovir should be initiated as soon as the diagnosis is suspected.[64] Prophylaxis against HSV is associated with a low incidence of clinical disease and has been recommended for HSV-1 and HSV-2 seropositive solid organ transplant recipients not receiving cytomegalovirus (CMV) prophylaxis that has activity against HSV.[65]

Treatment

There are no established guidelines for treatment of HSV hepatitis. Because of its high mortality and rapid deterioration to acute liver failure, it is advised to start treatment as soon as possible because the disease is curable. It has been reported that early treatment with acyclovir reduces mortality and the need for liver transplant. Keeping a high level of suspicion in populations at risk and starting early acyclovir until HSV is excluded as the cause of liver failure is critical. Experts recommend treating for 2 to 3 weeks, and up to 4 weeks in some cases.[55]

Resistance to acyclovir has been reported in 0.27% of immunocompetent and 7% of immunocompromised individuals.[66] Cidofovir and foscarnet have successfully been used for treatment in these cases.[67] In patients refractory to antiviral therapy, urgent liver transplant is indicated. Liver transplant recipients are at risk of recurrent HSV

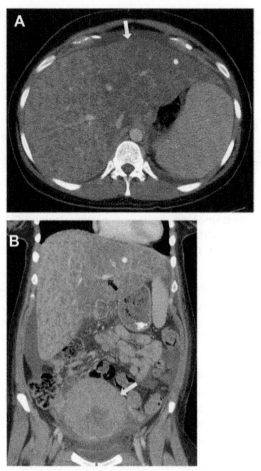

Fig. 5. CT findings of multiple hypodense lesions in the liver in patients with HSV hepatitis (*A*) Axial view; (*B*) Coronal view. (*From* Tripuraneni V, et al. Fulminant herpes simplex viral hepatitis: ultrasound and CT imaging appearance and a review of the imaging literature. Clin Imaging 2014;38:191-4; with permission.)

infection, which necessitates long-term acyclovir therapy; however, this can result in increased acyclovir resistance.[66,68,69]

Plasma exchange has been attempted for treatment of acute liver failure from HSV hepatitis.[70] The rationale is that it helps to remove HSV virions and infectious particles, decreasing viral burden and allowing time for the immune system to develop a stronger response. More studies are needed to further elaborate the role of plasma exchange in severe HSV hepatitis.

HEPATITIS CAUSED BY *COXIELLA BURNETII*

C burnetii is an intracellular gram-negative bacterium that causes a zoonotic disease known as Q fever.[71] Farm animals, such as cattle, sheep, and goats, and pets are the main reservoirs.[72] Transmission occurs through contact with livestock via inhalation of contaminated aerosols and dusts, or through ingestion of raw milk or unpasteurized goat cheese.[72,73] The disease has an incubation period of 2 to 3 weeks.[74]

Q fever has a variable clinical presentation. Many infections are subclinical and the infected are usually asymptomatic. About 50% of patients infected with Q fever become symptomatic. Acute Q fever usually manifests as flulike illness with symptoms of fever, chills, headache, fatigue, and muscle pain. Hepatitis and pneumonia may be seen in patients infected with Q fever.[75] Q fever can also cause acute acalculous cholecystitis. In less than 5% of patients, Q fever can present as chronic illness, which is usually manifested as endocarditis.[74]

Patients with acute Q fever may develop acute hepatitis, which may range in severity from mild to severe. About 85% of patients with acute Q fever have increased aminotransferase levels.[76] Most patients only have mild to moderate increases in aminotransferase and alkaline phosphatase levels. Significant hyperbilirubinemia is uncommon but, if present, may indicate severe illness.[73] Chronic Q fever can result in chronic granulomatous hepatitis.[77] These patients usually have hepatosplenomegaly.

Diagnosis of *C burnetii* hepatitis requires a high index of suspicion because the symptoms of Q fever are nonspecific. A triad of fever, hepatitis, and atypical pneumonia should raise a high suspicion of Q fever.[78] Serologic testing to detect antibodies to *C burnetii* using immunofluorescence assay is commonly performed to confirm the diagnosis of Q fever. The test may be negative in the first 2 weeks of acute illness because antibodies usually develop 2 to 3 weeks after infection. Quantitative PCR estimation of *C burnetii* is rapid and sensitive and may identify Q fever within 2 weeks of infection. However, PCR testing may not be easily accessible, and the specificity of the test may vary based on the gene target used for testing. Liver biopsy can assist in diagnosis in patients with acute hepatitis. Liver biopsy reveals inflammation predominantly with lymphocytes and neutrophils. Fibrin ring granulomas are classically associated with Q fever (**Fig. 6**).[76] Though not specific to Q fever, presence of fibrin ring granulomas should induce the physician to pursue the diagnosis of Q fever vigorously. Epithelioid granulomas with multinucleated giant cells may also be seen in liver biopsy specimens.

Acute infections are mostly subclinical and hence do not require treatment. In patients with acute illness, treatment with oral doxycycline 100 mg every 12 hours for 14 days should be initiated immediately following definite diagnosis.[77]

VIRAL HEPATITIS CAUSED BY FLAVIVIRUSES

Flaviviruses are positive, enveloped, single-stranded RNA viruses. They are primarily found in ticks and mosquitoes and occasionally infect humans. Although infections

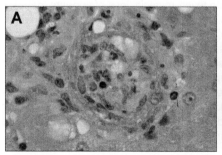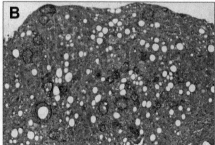

Fig. 6. Liver histology in a patient with *C burnetii* hepatitis showing fibrin ring granuloma.(*A*) Fibrin ring granuloma (hematoxylin-eosin, original magnification ×250). (*B*) Accentuated fibrin ring granulomas (PTAH, phosphotungstic acid hematoxylin, original magnification ×40).

from flaviviruses are not endemic in North America, North American travelers to areas endemic to flaviviruses may acquire the infection and should be advised of measures to minimize the risk of acquiring these infections.

Dengue

Dengue viruses belong to the genus Flavivirus and have 4 known serotypes. It is transmitted by a mosquito, either *Aedes aegypti* or *Aedes albopictus*.[79] Dengue can cause 4 spectra of disease ranging from asymptomatic infection, classic dengue fever, dengue hemorrhagic fever (DHF), and atypical infection. Only 1 of 4 patients infected with dengue virus becomes symptomatic. Severe dengue illness is uncommon but, when present, can be life threatening. Children (especially infants), pregnant women, and those with prior history of dengue infection are at increased risk for severe illness. Similar to other viral illness, fever, myalgia, and arthralgia are the most common symptoms. Severe illness can cause vomiting, hematemesis, hematochezia, bleeding from the gums and nasal cavity, and altered mental status.

Dengue can infect various cell types, including liver cells.[80] It can also present as acute hepatitis with right upper quadrant pain, hepatomegaly, jaundice, and increased liver enzyme levels.[81] Hepatic involvement is usually mild. Other laboratory findings usually include leukopenia with atypical lymphocytes, thrombocytopenia less than $100,000/mm^3$, and evidence of hemoconcentration.[79] Although rare, it can cause fulminant hepatitis,[82] and, in patients with DHF, it can cause severe hepatic dysfunction.[83] Treatment is mainly supportive because no specific treatment is available.

Zika Virus

Zika virus, belonging to the genus Flavivirus, is also transmitted by the *Aedes* mosquito.[84] Most infections are asymptomatic. In 20% of cases, it causes a mild, self-limited infection characterized by fever, sore throat, conjunctivitis, and skin rash that resolves in 1 to 2 weeks.[85] Occasionally, Zika virus infection has been associated with Guillain-Barré syndrome, transient hearing loss, retinal lesions, severe abdominal pain, and cardiovascular complications.[86] Very rarely, it can cause severe liver injury and coagulopathy.[87] Treatment is usually supportive.

YELLOW FEVER

Yellow fever virus is endemic to the tropical and subtropical areas of Africa and South America. Infection is transmitted through the bite of mosquitoes of the *Haemagogus*, *Sabethes*, and *Aedes* genera.[88] Incubation period is 3 to 6 days. Yellow fever infection is most often a mild, self-limited disease with fever, myalgia, loss of appetite, nausea, or vomiting. However, a small percentage of patients develop a severe form within 24 hours of recovery from initial symptoms, and this is associated with jaundice; coagulopathy; uncontrolled bleeding from eyes, nasal/oral cavity, or gastrointestinal tract; acute kidney injury; and shock. Yellow fever virus can also, rarely, result in acute liver failure.[89] It can also cause late-relapsing hepatitis after the resolution of the acute syndrome.[90] About 50% of patients with severe yellow fever infection succumb to the disease. Travelers to areas endemic to yellow fever should be offered yellow fever vaccine at least 10 days but preferably 30 days before travel. The vaccine is effective, and a single dose is enough to develop immunity.

VIRAL HEPATITIS CAUSED BY FILOVIRUSES

Marburg virus and Ebola virus belong to the Filovirus family and can cause an increase in liver enzyme levels during acute syndromes. Treatment is supportive.[91]

OTHER RARE INFECTIONS OF THE LIVER

Human herpesvirus 6 (HHV-6) and varicella-zoster viruses (VZV) typically produce a milder form of self-limited hepatitis in immunocompetent patients and possible fulminant hepatitis in immunocompromised patients.[92] Early clinical suspicion and testing are necessary to decrease mortality. Diagnosis of HHV-6 is seldom made in a timely fashion because it cannot be detected on blood samples and needs tissue biopsy. VZV hepatitis is usually associated with maculopapular eruptions and vesicles that provide a clue to the diagnosis of VZV infection. Serum PCR is also usually positive for VZV hepatitis, unlike HHV-6. Two forms of zoonotic viral hepatitis causing viral hemorrhagic fever are naviruses and bunyaviruses. Hepatitis ranges from uncommon and mild in the Argentine, Bolivian, and Venezuelan subtypes to moderately severe in Lassa fever.[93,94] When severe, bunyavirus hepatitis is associated with rapid hepatocellular destruction leading to extensive necrosis.[95] Brucellosis is an uncommon nonbacterial hepatitis that most commonly presents as granulomatous disease on biopsy.[96]

CLINICS CARE POINTS

- In patients with SARS-CoV-2 infection, the elevation in liver enzymes is most commonly from the infection itself or from the medications used to help manage the infection. However, alternative etiologies such as viral or autoimmune hepatitis and vascular disorders of the liver must be considered especially in patients with chronic liver disease.

- Pre-emptive decrease in immunosuppression in post-liver transplant patients with SARS-CoV-2 infection may not be necessary and may increase the risk of acute rejection.

- In patients suspected to have herpes simplex virus hepatitis, empiric treatment must be started at the earliest due to the high risk for mortality from progression to acute liver failure especially in pregnant women.

- Symptoms of Q fever are often non-specific and the triad of fever, pneumonia, and hepatitis may not always be seen. Fibrin ring granulomas on liver histology should strongly raise the suspicion for Q fever. Serologic testing may be negative in the first 2 weeks of infection and quantitative PCR estimation may be needed.

ACKNOWLEDGMENTS

The authors thank Kristina Greiner for her editing assistance in preparing this article and for obtaining permissions for reproducing images. The authors also thank Andrew Bellizzi, MD, and Frank Mitros, MD, for providing histology images.

DISCLOSURE

A.R. Murali receives research grants from Arrowhead and Eiger. None of the other authors have disclosures.

REFERENCES

1. Ahn DG, Shin HJ, Kim MH, et al. Current status of epidemiology, diagnosis, therapeutics, and vaccines for Novel Coronavirus Disease 2019 (COVID-19). J Microbiol Biotechnol 2020;30(3):313–24.
2. Park M, Cook AR, Lim JT, et al. A systematic review of COVID-19 epidemiology based on current evidence. J Clin Med 2020;9(4):967.

3. Jin Y, Yang H, Ji W, et al. Virology, epidemiology, pathogenesis, and control of COVID-19. Viruses 2020;12(4):372.

4. Jeong HW, Kim SM, Kim HS, et al. Viable SARS-CoV-2 in various specimens from COVID-19 patients. Clin Microbiol Infect 2020;26(11):1520-4.

5. Organization WH. WHO coronavirus disease (COVID-19) dashboard;2020. Geneva (Switzerland): World Health Organization. Available at: https://covid19whoint/. Accessed September 17, 2020.

6. Han C, Duan C, Zhang S, et al. Digestive symptoms in COVID-19 patients with mild disease severity: clinical presentation, stool viral RNA testing, and outcomes. Am J Gastroenterol 2020;115(6):916-23.

7. Mantovani A, Beatrice G, Dalbeni A. Coronavirus disease 2019 and prevalence of chronic liver disease: a meta-analysis. Liver Int 2020;40(6):1316-20.

8. Sun J, Aghemo A, Forner A, et al. COVID-19 and liver disease. Liver Int 2020; 40(6):1278-81.

9. Cheung KS, Hung IFN, Chan PPY, et al. Gastrointestinal manifestations of SARS-CoV-2 infection and virus load in fecal samples from a Hong Kong Cohort: systematic review and meta-analysis. Gastroenterology 2020;159(1):81-95.

10. Xu Z, Shi L, Wang Y, et al. Pathological findings of COVID-19 associated with acute respiratory distress syndrome. Lancet Respir Med 2020;8(4):420-2.

11. Tian S, Xiong Y, Liu H, et al. Pathological study of the 2019 novel coronavirus disease (COVID-19) through postmortem core biopsies. Mod Pathol 2020;33(6): 1007-14.

12. Kovalic AJ, Satapathy SK, Thuluvath PJ. Prevalence of chronic liver disease in patients with COVID-19 and their clinical outcomes: a systematic review and meta-analysis. Hepatol Int 2020;14(5):612-20.

13. Lynch J, Fishbein M, Echavarria M. Adenovirus. Seminars in respiratory and critical care medicine. Germany: Thieme Medical Publishers; 2011. p. 494-511.

14. Ronan B, Agrwal N, Carey E, et al. Fulminant hepatitis due to human adenovirus. Infection 2014;42(1):105-11.

15. Ruuskanen O, Meurman O, Akusjärvi G, et al. Clinical virology. New York: Churchill Livingstone Inc; 1997. p. 525-48.

16. Schaberg KB, Kambham N, Sibley RK, et al. Adenovirus hepatitis. Am J Surg Pathol 2017;41(6):810-9.

17. Lion T. Adenovirus infections in immunocompetent and immunocompromised patients. Clin Microbiol Rev 2014;27(3):441-62.

18. Anderson LJ, Patriarca PA, Hierholzer JC, et al. Viral respiratory illnesses. Med Clin North Am 1983;67(5):1009-30.

19. Siegel JD, Rhinehart E, Jackson M, et al, Committee HCICPA. 2007 guideline for isolation precautions: preventing transmission of infectious agents in health care settings. Am J Infect Control 2007;35(10):S65.

20. Ison MG, Hayden FG. Viral infections in immunocompromised patients: what's new with respiratory viruses? Curr Opin Infect Dis 2002;15(4):355-67.

21. Baldwin A, Kingman H, Darville M, et al. Outcome and clinical course of 100 patients with adenovirus infection following bone marrow transplantation. Bone Marrow Transplant 2000;26(12):1333-8.

22. Chakrabarti S, Mautner V, Osman H, et al. Adenovirus infections following allogeneic stem cell transplantation: incidence and outcome in relation to graft manipulation, immunosuppression, and immune recovery. Blood 2002;100(5):1619-27.

23. Runde V, Ross S, Trenschel R, et al. Adenoviral infection after allogeneic stem cell transplantation (SCT): report on 130 patients from a single SCT unit involved in a

prospective multi center surveillance study. Bone Marrow Transplant 2001; 28(1):51–7.

24. Shields AF, Hackman RC, Fife KH, et al. Adenovirus infections in patients undergoing bone-marrow transplantation. N Engl J Med 1985;312(9):529–33.

25. McGrath D, Falagas ME, Freeman R, et al. Adenovirus infection in adult orthotopic liver transplant recipients: incidence and clinical significance. J Infect Dis 1998;177(2):459–62.

26. Lecatsas G, Van Wyk J. DNA viruses in urine after renal transplantation. S Afr Med J 1978;53(20):787–8.

27. Kojaoghlanian T, Flomenberg P, Horwitz MS. The impact of adenovirus infection on the immunocompromised host. Rev Med Virol 2003;13(3):155–71.

28. Hierholzer JC. Adenoviruses in the immunocompromised host. Clin Microbiol Rev 1992;5(3):262–74.

29. Flomenberg PR, Chen M, Munk G, et al. Molecular epidemiology of adenovirus type 35 infections in immunocompromised hosts. J Infect Dis 1987;155(6): 1127–34.

30. Koneru B, Atchison R, Jaffe R, et al. Serological studies of adenoviral hepatitis following pediatric liver transplantation. Paper presented at: Transplantation proceedings. August 1990; USA.

31. Carrigan DR. Adenovirus infections in immunocompromised patients. Am J Med 1997;102(3):71–4.

32. Perez D, McCormack L, Petrowsky H, et al. Successful outcome of severe adenovirus hepatitis of the allograft following liver transplantation. Transpl Infect Dis 2007;9(4):318–22.

33. Kerensky T, Hasan A, Schain D, et al. Histopathologic resolution of adult liver transplantation adenovirus hepatitis with cidofovir and intravenous immunoglobulin: a case report. Paper presented at: Transplantation proceedings. January 2013; USA.

34. Echavarría M. Adenoviruses in immunocompromised hosts. Clin Microbiol Rev 2008;21(4):704–15.

35. Ison MG. Adenovirus infections in transplant recipients. Clin Infect Dis 2006; 43(3):331–9.

36. Pinchoff RJ, Kaufman SS, Magid MS, et al. Adenovirus infection in pediatric small bowel transplantation recipients. Transplantation 2003;76(1):183–9.

37. Ljungman P, Infectious Diseases Working Party of the European Group for Blood and Marrow Transplantation. Cidofovir for adenovirus infections after allogeneic hematopoietic stem cell transplantation: a survey by the Infectious Diseases Working Party of the European Group for Blood and Marrow Transplantation. Bone Marrow Transplant 2003;31:481–6.

38. Humar A, Kumar D, Mazzulli T, et al. A surveillance study of adenovirus infection in adult solid organ transplant recipients. Am J Transplant 2005;5(10):2555–9.

39. McLaughlin GE, Delis S, Kashimawo L, et al. Adenovirus infection in pediatric liver and intestinal transplant recipients: utility of DNA detection by PCR. Am J Transplant 2003;3(2):224–8.

40. Hoffman JA. Adenovirus infections in solid organ transplant recipients. Curr Opin Organ Transplant 2009;14(6):625–33.

41. Michaels MG, Green M, Wald ER, et al. Adenovirus infection in pediatric liver transplant recipients. J Infect Dis 1992;165(1):170–4.

42. Terasako K, Oshima K, Wada H, et al. Fulminant hepatic failure caused by adenovirus infection mimicking peliosis hepatitis on abdominal computed tomography

images after allogeneic hematopoietic stem cell transplantation. Intern Med 2012;51(4):405–11.

43. Koneru B, Jaffe R, Esquivel CO, et al. Adenoviral infections in pediatric liver transplant recipients. JAMA 1987;258(4):489–92.

44. Lo AA, Lo EC, Rao MS, et al. Concurrent acute necrotizing adenovirus hepatitis and enterocolitis in an adult patient after double cord blood stem cell transplant for refractory Crohn's disease. Int J Surg Pathol 2015;23(5):404–8.

45. Putra J, Suriawinata AA. Adenovirus hepatitis presenting as tumoral lesions in an immunocompromised patient. Ann Hepatol 2014;13(6):827–9.

46. US Food and Drug Administration. Adenovirus type 4 and type 7 vaccine, live, oral-package insert.(2019).

47. Wang Y-G, Huang P-P, Zhang R, et al. Targeting adeno-associated virus and adenoviral gene therapy for hepatocellular carcinoma. World J Gastroenterol 2016;22(1):326.

48. Arduino PG, Porter SR. Herpes simplex virus type 1 infection: overview on relevant clinico-pathological features. J Oral Pathol Med 2008;37(2):107–21.

49. Butel JS, Melnick JL, Brooks G, et al. Microbiología médica de Jawets, Melnick y Adelberg. 2005.

50. Rechenchoski DZ, Faccin-Galhardi LC, Linhares REC, et al. Herpesvirus: an underestimated virus. Folia Microbiol (Praha) 2017;62(2):151–6.

51. Miyazaki Y, Akizuki SI, Sakaoka H, et al. Disseminated infection of herpes simplex virus with fulminant hepatitis in a healthy adult: a case report. APMIS 1991; 99(7-12):1001–7.

52. Wertheim R, Brooks JB, Rodriguez JF, et al. Fatal herpetic hepatitis in pregnancy. Obstet Gynecol 1983;62(3 Suppl):38s–42s.

53. Bernstein CN, Minuk GY. Infectious mononucleosis presenting with cholestatic liver disease. Ann Intern Med 1998;128(6):509.

54. Kaufman B, Gandhi SA, Louie E, et al. Herpes simplex virus hepatitis: case report and review. Clin Infect Dis 1997;24(3):334–8.

55. Norvell JP, Blei AT, Jovanovic BD, et al. Herpes simplex virus hepatitis: an analysis of the published literature and institutional cases. Liver Transplant 2007; 13(10):1428–34.

56. Al Midani A, Pinney J, Field N, et al. Fulminant hepatitis following primary herpes simplex virus infection in renal transplant recipients. Saudi J Kidney Dis Transpl 2011;22(1):107.

57. Feugeas J, Mory S, Jeulin H, et al. Herpes simplex virus type 1 hepatitis due to primary infection in a pancreas-kidney transplant recipient. J Clin Virol 2016; 80:57–9.

58. Shaw BI, Nanavati AJ, Taylor V, et al. Donor derived HSV hepatitis in a kidney transplant recipient leading to liver fibrosis and portal hypertension. Transpl Infect Dis 2019;21(1):e13029.

59. Smith I, Peutherer J, Hunter J. Cervical infection with herpes simplex virus. Lancet 1981;317(8228):1051.

60. Down C, Mehta A, Salama G, et al. Herpes simplex virus hepatitis in an immunocompetent host resembling hepatic pyogenic abscesses. Case Rep Hepatol 2016;2016:8348172.

61. Song T-J, Eisenberg DP, Adusumilli PS, et al. Oncolytic herpes viral therapy is effective in the treatment of hepatocellular carcinoma cell lines. J Gastrointest Surg 2006;10(4):532–42.

62. Côté-Daigneault J, Carrier F, Toledano K, et al. Herpes simplex hepatitis after liver transplantation: case report and literature review. Transpl Infect Dis 2014;16(1): 130–4.

63. Navaneethan U, Lancaster E, Venkatesh P, et al. Herpes simplex virus hepatitis—it's high time we consider empiric treatment. J Gastrointestin Liver Dis 2011; 20(1):93–6.

64. Basse G, Mengelle C, Kamar N, et al. Disseminated herpes simplex type-2 (HSV-2) infection after solid-organ transplantation. Infection 2008;36(1):62.

65. Lee DH, Zuckerman RA, Practice AIDCo. Herpes simplex virus infections in solid organ transplantation: guidelines from the American Society of Transplantation Infectious Diseases Community of Practice. Clin Transplant 2019;33(9):e13526.

66. Stránská R, Schuurman R, Nienhuis E, et al. Survey of acyclovir-resistant herpes simplex virus in the Netherlands: prevalence and characterization. J Clin Virol 2005;32(1):7–18.

67. Chaudhary D, Ahmed S, Liu N, et al. Acute liver failure from herpes simplex virus in an immunocompetent patient due to direct inoculation of the peritoneum. ACG Case Rep J 2017;4:e23.

68. Shanley CJ, Braun DK, Brown K, et al. Fulminant hepatic failure secondary to herpes simplex virus hepatitis: successful outcome after orthotopic liver transplantation. Transplantation 1995;59(1):145–9.

69. Devictor D, Desplanques L, Debray D, et al. Emergency liver transplantation for fulminant liver failure in infants and children. Hepatology 1992;16(5):1156–62.

70. Holt EW, Guy J, Gordon SM, et al. Acute liver failure caused by herpes simplex virus in a pregnant patient: is there a potential role for therapeutic plasma exchange? J Clin Apher 2013;28(6):426–9.

71. Angelakis E, Raoult D. Q fever. Vet Microbiol 2010;140(3–4):297–309.

72. Fishbein DB, Raoult D. A cluster of Coxiella burnetii infections associated with exposure to vaccinated goats and their unpasteurized dairy products. Am J Trop Med Hyg 1992;47(1):35–40.

73. Maurin M, Raoult Df. Q fever. Clin Microbiol Rev 1999;12(4):518–53.

74. Bolaños M, Santana OE, Pérez-Arellano JL, et al. Q fever in Gran Canaria: 40 new cases. Enferm Infecc Microbiol Clin 2003;21(1):20–3.

75. Raoult D, Marrie T. Q fever. Clin Infect Dis 1995;20(3):489–95. Available at: http://www.jstor.org/stable/4458369. Accessed March 27, 2021.

76. Fournier P-E, Marrie TJ, Raoult D. Diagnosis of Q fever. J Clin Microbiol 1998; 36(7):1823–34.

77. Parker NR, Barralet JH, Bell AM. Q fever. Lancet 2006;367(9511):679–88.

78. Hartzell JD, Peng SW, Wood-Morris RN, et al. Atypical Q fever in US soldiers. Emerg Infect Dis 2007;13(8):1247.

79. Souza L, e Prevenção DDT. Rio de Janeiro (Brazil): Ed Rúbio. Dengue – Diagnóstico, Tratamento e Prevenção; 2007.

80. Havens W Jr. Hepatitis, yellow fever, and dengue. Annu Rev Microbiol 1954;8(1): 289–310.

81. Souza LJd, Alves JG, Nogueira RMR, et al. Aminotransferase changes and acute hepatitis in patients with dengue fever: analysis of 1,585 cases. Braz J Infect Dis 2004;8(2):156–63.

82. Ling L, Wilder-Smith A, Leo Y. Fulminant hepatitis in dengue haemorrhagic fever. J Clin Virol 2007;38(3):265–8.

83. Nguyen T, Nguyen T, Tieu N. The impact of dengue haemorrhagic fever on liver function. Res Virol 1997;148(4):273–7.

84. Dick G, Kitchen S, Haddow A. Zika virus (I). Isolations and serological specificity. Trans R Soc Trop Med Hyg 1952;46(5):509–20.

85. Triunfol M. Microcephaly in Brazil: confidence builds in Zika connection. Lancet Infect Dis 2016;16(5):527–8.

86. Calvet GA, dos Santos FB, Sequeira PC. Zika virus infection: epidemiology, clinical manifestations and diagnosis. Curr Opin Infect Dis 2016;29(5):459–66.

87. Wu Y, Cui X, Wu N, et al. A unique case of human Zika virus infection in association with severe liver injury and coagulation disorders. Sci Rep 2017;7(1):1–8.

88. Monath TP, Vasconcelos PF. Yellow fever. J Clin Virol 2015;64:160–73.

89. Johansson MA, Vasconcelos PF, Staples JE. The whole iceberg: estimating the incidence of yellow fever virus infection from the number of severe cases. Trans R Soc Trop Med Hyg 2014;108(8):482–7.

90. Rezende IM, Pereira LS, Fradico JRB, et al. Late-relapsing hepatitis after yellow fever. Viruses 2020;12(2):222.

91. Zuckerman AJ, Dih S. Exotic virus infections of the liver. 1979.

92. Cisneros-Herreros JM, Herrero-Romero M. Hepatitis due to herpes group viruses. Enferm Infecc Microbiol Clin 2006;24(6):392–7 [quiz: 398].

93. Pfau CJ. Chapter 57: Arenaviruses. In: Baron S, ed. Medical Microbiology. 3rd ed. Churchill Livingstone; 1991: 751-757.

94. Beier JI, Jokinen JD, Holz GE, et al. Novel mechanism of arenavirus-induced liver pathology. PLoS One 2015;10(3):e0122839.

95. Zeller H, Bouloy M. Bunyaviridae and Filoviridae. Rev Sci Tech 2000;19(1):79–91.

96. Akritidis N, Tzivras M, Delladetsima I, et al. The liver in brucellosis. Clin Gastroenterol Hepatol 2007;5(9):1109–12.

Acute Cholangitis
Causes, Diagnosis, and Management

Zhibo An, MD, PhD, Annie L. Braseth, MD, Nadav Sahar, MD*

KEYWORDS

- Acute cholangitis ● Ascending cholangitis ● Biliary obstruction ● Biliary infection
- ERCP

KEY POINTS

- Acute cholangitis classically presents with Charcot's triad (fever, jaundice, and abdominal pain) and can be a life-threatening condition if it is not recognized early.
- The mainstay of treatment consists of fluid resuscitation, antibiotics, and biliary drainage. Endoscopic retrograde cholangiopancreatography (ERCP) remains the preferred modality for biliary drainage.
- The most common pathogens isolated are gram negative bacteria (Escherichia coli in 25%–50% of cases, followed by Klebsiella species and Enterobacter species). Enterococcus species are the most common gram-positive bacteria (10%– 20% of cases) and the most commonly detected bacteria in patients with biliary stents.

INTRODUCTION

Acute cholangitis, also referred to as ascending cholangitis, is a clinical syndrome characterized by fever, jaundice, and abdominal pain (Charcot triad), which can be life-threatening, with mortality historically reported to be more than 50%.[1] Fortunately, recent advancements in diagnosis and management of patients with acute cholangitis have contributed to a significant reduction in mortality. Acute cholangitis occurs from infection in the biliary system usually from ductal obstruction.[2] The mainstay of treatment is fluid resuscitation, antibiotic therapy, and biliary drainage. Endoscopic retrograde cholangiopancreatography (ERCP) is the gold standard for biliary drainage, whereas percutaneous and surgical options are alternative modalities in select cases.[3] Ascending cholangitis is also the most frequent infectious complication of ERCP, thought to be secondary to incomplete drainage of an infected and obstructed biliary system.[4] This article provides an update on early diagnosis and management of acute cholangitis.

Division of Gastroenterology and Hepatology, Department of Internal Medicine, University of Iowa Hospitals and Clinics, 200 Hawkins Drive, 4608 JCP, Iowa City, IA 52242, USA
* Corresponding author.
E-mail address: nadav-sahar@uiowa.edu

Gastroenterol Clin N Am 50 (2021) 403–414
https://doi.org/10.1016/j.gtc.2021.02.005
0889-8553/21/© 2021 Elsevier Inc. All rights reserved.

CAUSES
Pathophysiology

Obstruction of bile is the most important factor for the development of acute cholangitis. Bile is normally sterile, but can become infected from ascending migration or portal bacteremia. Normally, there are several protective mechanisms in place to prevent infection in the bile duct. Typically, bile can flow freely in a nonobstructed duct flushing bacterium into the duodenum. Migration of bacteria from the small bowel into the bile ducts is prevented by the sphincter of Oddi. Bacterial reproductivity can be suppressed by bile salts. In addition, the epithelium in the biliary tree secretes IgA and mucous to act as antiadherent mechanisms, while tight junctions and Kupffer cells act to prevent translocation into the portal venous system.[2] When obstruction is present, these defensive mechanisms break down. The intraductal pressure increases secondary to bile stasis, which causes widening of tight junctions, malfunction of Kupffer cells, and decrease in local production of IgA. Increased pressure can also cause cholangiovenous reflux, which allows pathogens access to intrahepatic canicules in addition to hepatic veins and lymphatics. This leads to bacteremia, endotoxemia, and ultimately a systemic inflammatory response. Although there are many varieties of cholangitis, ascending cholangitis occurs most commonly from migration of bacteria into the common bile duct from the duodenum.[2,5]

Cause

There are multiple potential causes that lead to complete or partial biliary obstruction (**Box 1**). The most common risk factor for development of acute cholangitis is choledocholithiasis, representing about half of reported cases.[6] Risk factors for developing gallstones also increase the risk of development of acute cholangitis, and include a high-fat diet, obesity, sedentary lifestyle, and rapid weight loss.[2] The second most common cause of cholangitis is malignant obstruction, accounting for 10% to 30% of cases.[7]

Box 1
Causes for biliary duct obstruction

Choledocholithiasis

Pancreatic cancer

Porta hepatis tumor or metastasis

Primary sclerosing cholangitis

Mirizzi syndrome

Round worm (*Ascaris lumbricoides*) or tapeworm (*Taenia saginata*) infestation of the bile duct

Stricture of a bilioenteric anastomosis

Benign or malignant stricture of the bile/hepatic ducts

Ampullary cancer or adenoma

Biliary stent obstruction

Amyloid deposition in the biliary system

Lemmel syndrome

AIDS cholangiopathy

Post-ERCP-associated acute cholangitis

The reported incidence rate of acute cholangitis is 1% to 5% after ERCP.[8] In addition, the rate of developing cholangitis following biliary stent placement by ERCP is between 3.5% and 40%, with higher risks of developing acute cholangitis associated with hilar/multiple strictures (19.1%) and malignant biliary obstruction (15.6%).[9] A recent retrospective cohort study demonstrated that biliary stent placement by ERCP in patients with advanced malignant hilar biliary strictures may lead to acute cholangitis in up to 21.5% of patients, with Bismuth classification type IV and plastic stenting as independent risk factors for post-stenting cholangitis.[10]

DIAGNOSIS

The diagnosis of acute cholangitis is made by the presence of clinical features, laboratory results, and imaging studies.[2] Acute cholangitis should be suspected in patients with fever, abdominal pain, and jaundice (Charcot triad). In more severe cases patients may suffer from confusion and hypotension, known as Reynolds pentad. Although Charcot triad is not a sensitive tool, with studies reporting a sensitivity of 25%, it has a specificity greater than 90%.[11]

The Tokyo Guidelines, originally published in 2007 and most recently revised in 2018, are the most acceptable diagnostic criterion. These guidelines consist of a combination of clinical, laboratory, and imaging findings, and a grading system for disease severity (**Box 2**). The diagnosis is definite when there is systemic inflammation (fever and/or laboratory values), cholestasis, and imaging studies showing either biliary dilatation or evidence of a cause.[12] It has been shown that the Tokyo Guidelines provide accurate diagnosis in up to 90% of cases of acute cholangitis.[12]

Laboratory test findings in patients with acute cholangitis usually include an elevated white blood cell count and predominantly cholestatic liver test

---

Box 2
Tokyo guideline 2013/2018 diagnostic criteria

Criteria

A. Systemic inflammation
   A-1 Fever or chills
   • Greater than 38°C
   A-2 Biologic inflammatory syndrome
   • Leukocytes <4 or >10 G/L
   • CRP ≥10 mg/L

B. Cholestasis
   B-1 Icterus/jaundice
   B-2 Abnormal liver function test
   • Total bilirubin ≥34 μmol/L
   • AST, ALT, ALP, and γ-glutamyltransferase >1.5 × ULN

C. Imagery
   C-1 Bile duct dilatation
   C-2 Imagery providing proof of etiology

Suspected diagnosis
   • One item in A + one item in B or C

Certain diagnosis
   • One item in A, B, and C

Abbreviations: ALP, alkaline phosphatase; ALT, alanine aminotransferase; AST, aspartate aminotransferase; CRP, C-reactive protein; ULN, upper limit of normal.

abnormalities.[13] Procalcitonin is proposed as a marker to determine risk for clinical deterioration and need for more emergent biliary decompression. Lee and colleagues[14] showed that procalcitonin levels at presentation were strongly associated with severity of disease and a level greater than 3.77 ng/mL was indicative of clinical deterioration.

The 2018 Tokyo Guidelines also provide a grading system for severity (**Table 1**). Severe disease (grade III) is defined by the presence of any end-organ damage. Moderate disease (grade II) is determined when there is fever, white blood cell count greater than 12,000/mm^3 or less than 4000/mm^3, bilirubin greater than 5 mg/dL, low albumin, or advanced age. Mild disease (grade I) is defined by not meeting criteria for grade II or III. It is important to characterize the presentation based on severity, because moderate and severe disease require early biliary drainage.[15] For mild acute cholangitis antibiotic treatment is usually sufficient. However, biliary drainage should be considered if a patient with mild disease does not respond to antibiotics.

Disease Complications

The most common complications of acute cholangitis include acute pancreatitis (7.6% of cases), liver abscess (2.5%), and endocarditis (up to 0.26%).[16] Patients with acute cholangitis can also present with other complications including sepsis, multiple organ system dysfunction, portal vein thrombosis, gastrointestinal bleeding, and shock.[17,18]

Table 1
Tokyo guideline 2013/2018 severity criteria

Grade	Criteria
Grade 1: mild No criteria 2 or 3	

Grade 2: moderate
At least 2 criteria
	Leukocytes
	    <4 G/L or >12 G/L
	Fever
	    >39°C
	Age
	    >75 y
	Bilirubinemia
	    >85 μmol/L
	Hypoalbuminemia
	    <0.7 × ILN

Grade 3: severe
At least 1 criterium
	Cardiovascular dysfunction
	    Dopamine >5 μg/kg/min or
	        any dose of noradrenalin
	Neurologic dysfunction
	    Consciousness disorders
	Respiratory dysfunction
	    Pao_2/Fio_2 <300
	Renal dysfunction
	    Creatininuria >176 μmol/L or oliguria
	Liver dysfunction
	    INR >1.5
	Hematologic dysfunction
	    Platelets <100,000/mm^3

Abbreviations: Fio_2, fraction of inspired oxygen; ILN, inferior limit of the normal; INR, international normalized ratio.

Microbiology

Blood cultures in acute cholangitis may be positive in 21% to 71% of cases. Therefore, bile cultures should be obtained at the beginning of any procedure performed for acute cholangitis with grade II and III severity.[19] Culture of bile in patients with acute cholangitis but no biliary obstruction is rarely positive. In contrast, culture of bile taken from patients with acute cholangitis and ductal stones, or occluded biliary stents are positive in more than 90% of the cases,[20] yielding a mixed growth of gram-negative and gram-positive bacteria (**Table 2**).

Escherichia coli is the most common gram-negative bacterium isolated (25%–50% of cases), followed by *Klebsiella* species (15%–20%) and *Enterobacter* species (5%–10%). *Enterococcus* species are the most common gram-positive bacteria (10%–20%) and the most commonly detected bacteria in patients with biliary stents.[21] *Candida* is a rare cause of acute cholangitis, predominantly detected in patients with underlying malignancies.[20] A recent retrospective cohort study of 151 patients diagnosed with cholangitis or cholecystitis with bacterial septicemia demonstrated that history of a previous gastrectomy could be a helpful predictor for infection with gram-positive species.[22] An uncommon cause of cholangitis in developed countries, liver flukes may also lead to cholangitis; these flukes include *Clonorchis sinensis*, *Opisthorchis viverrini*, *Opisthorchis felineus*, *Fasciola hepatica*, and the North American liver fluke, *Metorchis conjunctus*.[23]

Imaging

Imaging studies may consist of ultrasound, computed tomography (CT), magnetic resonance cholangiopancreatography (MRCP), and/or endoscopic ultrasound (EUS). Abdominal ultrasound is the first-line diagnostic study because of its affordability, availability, and high specificity for detection of bile duct dilation and bile duct stones (94%–100%), but its sensitivity ranges widely from 38% to 91%. The accuracy of abdominal ultrasound is affected by technician experience and the patient's clinical conditions, such as obesity or interposed digestive gas.[24] Ultrasound findings suggestive of choledocholithiasis include direct visualization of a stone or filling defect, biliary tract dilation, or a dilated common bile duct greater than 8 mm.[25]

Abdominal CT scan is a highly sensitive test to identify bile duct dilation and biliary stenosis. The sensitivity for detecting choledocholithiasis depends on the amount of calcium phosphate or calcium carbonate in the stones. Some studies have reported that CT scans can detect stones in only 42% of patients.[12] CT scan findings of acute cholangitis include hyperdense areas on arterial phase imaging and peribiliary tract edema.[12]

Table 2	
Most common pathogens in ascending cholangitis	
More Common	**Less Common**
Escherichia coli (25%–50%)	*Bacteroides fragilis*[a]
Klebsiella species (15%–20%)	*Clostridium perfringens*[a]
Enterococcus species (10%–20%)	*Clonorchis sinensis*
Enterobacter species (5%–10%)	*Opisthorchis viverrini*
	Opisthorchis felineus
	Ascaris lumbricoides

[a] More common in patients in previous biliary surgery and elderly populations.

MRCP is used when a diagnosis is unclear despite the use of abdominal ultrasound or CT. MRCP is noninvasive and has the best diagnostic ability for determining the origin of biliary obstruction, either from malignant causes (sensitivity 96%, specificity 100%) including cholangiocarcinoma, periampullary carcinoma, pancreatic cancer, and cancer of gallbladder, or benign pathologies including choledocholithiasis, benign stricture, and cholangitis (sensitivity 100%, specificity 96%).[26] Some of the limitations of the procedure include inability to image patients that have MRI-incompatible metal implants, such as pacemakers or claustrophobia. In addition, the sensitivity of MRCP decreases when stones are 6 mm or smaller.[2] The most sensitive imaging modalities are MRCP and EUS. Although EUS is often considered a better test than MRCP for detection of stones, a comprehensive meta-analysis study showed that MRCP (sensitivity 93%, specificity 96%) and EUS (sensitivity 95%, specificity 97%) performed equally well for detection of common bile duct stones.[27] An advantage of EUS is that ERCP may be performed during the same anesthetic procedure as EUS, providing a needed therapeutic intervention coupled to a diagnostic test.

PROGNOSIS

Reported mortality rates for acute cholangitis are highly variable, ranging from 2% to 65%.[28] Studies of patients with severe cholangitis in the 1960s showed mortality rates in excess of 50%.[29] With advances in diagnosis and care, the mortality rate for acute cholangitis has dropped significantly to between 11% and 27% in the 1990s, and more recent studies showing mortality of 10% or less.[16]

Hypoalbuminemia is an independent predictor of mortality.[3] Serum procalcitonin level of greater than 0.5 and interleukin-7 level less than 6.0 is also associated with higher mortality.[30] In addition a high body mass index may be an independent mortality risk factor.[31]

Although mortality rates have improved, a recent retrospective cohort study showed a high (~21%) overall 30-day readmission rate. Causes for readmission included recurrent cholangitis, septicemia, and complications from prosthesis. Readmission was significantly lower in patients who underwent a cholecystectomy or ERCP (10%–17%) and higher in those who had undergone percutaneous biliary drainage.[32]

CLINICAL MANAGEMENT

Acute cholangitis must be recognized and treated early, because mortality rates rise with delays in treatment. The mainstay of treatment is aggressive fluid resuscitation, antibiotics, and biliary drainage.[2,3]

Antimicrobial Therapy

Current guidelines suggest initial antibiotic coverage for ascending cholangitis with a penicillin/β-lactamase inhibitor, third-generation cephalosporin, or carbapenem.[7] Further selection of antibiotics should take into consideration whether the infection is community-acquired versus health care–associated, and individual risk factors, local drug-resistance patterns, and risk for adverse outcomes. For patients with community-acquired cholangitis but no biliary prosthesis or intensive care admission, piperacillin/tazobactam normally provides excellent antibiotic coverage. In patients treated for acute cholangitis with risk factors, such as a high burden of comorbidity, the presence of biliary stenosis, or repeated biliary tract interventions for penicillin-resistant gram-negative bacteria (as determined by culture), use of carbapenems might be necessary.[33] In patients with biliary stents or with hospital-acquired infection, it is also best to start antifungal coverage.[19] Bile culture is important to enable early and targeted antibiotic treatment of acute cholangitis.[34] Stratification of antimicrobial therapy is emphasized in the 2018 Tokyo Guidelines, which recommends that patients with grade III community-acquired and health care–associated acute cholecystitis and cholangitis should be covered by broad-spectrum antibiotics, including agents with antipseudomonal activities and treatment of enterococci species with vancomycin.[19] The increasing prevalence of antimicrobial resistance, particularly because of extended-spectrum β-lactamase-producing Enterobacteriaceae, raises the importance of antimicrobial de-escalation when treating acute cholangitis with broad-spectrum regimens to limit further development of resistance.[35]

Consensus guidelines vary on length of antimicrobial therapy from 3 to up to 10 days. The 2018 Tokyo consensus guidelines recommend 4 to 7 days of antibiotics if adequate source control is achieved, although this is of low evidence. Antibiotics should be extended to 2 weeks for enterococci and streptococci because of the risk of endocarditis.[19,36] ERCP-obtained bile culture is a helpful guide antibiotic therapy in acute cholangitis and is able to shorten the course of antibiotics. A recent study from the Netherlands found that antibiotic duration of 3 days or less is sufficient in patients with acute cholangitis who underwent successful ERCP.[37] Similarly, a recent retrospective study in Japan found that in patients with mild to moderate acute cholangitis, clinical outcomes after successful ERCP did not differ following short-course (≤3 days) and long-course antibiotic treatment (≥4 days), suggesting that antibiotic treatment of less than or equal to 3 days may be adequate for these patients.[38] A multicenter, open-label, randomized trial is ongoing to compare the outcome between short-course antibiotic therapy (5 day) with conventional long-course therapy (>7 day) in patients with acute cholangitis.[39]

Endoscopic Procedures

The 2018 Tokyo Guidelines recommend urgent/emergent biliary drainage for moderate and severe cholangitis. Biliary drainage is only recommended in mild acute cholangitis if there is no response to antibiotics. Although the ideal timing is not specified, most experts would agree biliary decompression should be accomplished within 48 hours.[3] A retrospective study investigated the optimal timing of ERCP and found that early drainage (within 24–48 hours from onset of cholangitis) resulted in decreased incidence of organ failure, a shorter length of stay, and decreased mortality in comparison with delayed drainage, with most patients benefiting from prompt drainage within 24 hours.[3] Another recent meta-analysis found similar findings when ERCP was performed within 48 hours.[40] Khamaysi and Taha[41] recently showed that emergent ERCP performed with 12 hours further improves 30-day mortality rates. Current European guidelines also recommend ERCP within 12 hours in patients with septic shock.[42]

Prompt drainage of the biliary system provides source control for acute cholangitis thereby decreasing bile and serum endotoxin levels in addition to promoting the biliary excretion of IgA and antibiotics. When biliary drainage is performed promptly, clinical outcomes including 30-day mortality, length of hospital stay and intensive care unit stay, organ dysfunction, and duration of fever did not differ regardless of the sensitivity to empiric antibiotic coverage.[43] This suggests that source control with prompt biliary drainage rather than targeted antimicrobial coverage has the most impact on patient outcomes.

Endoscopic retrograde cholangiopancreatography

ERCP remains the gold standard for biliary decompression. Obstruction is managed with biliary sphincterotomy, biliary stenting, or nasobiliary tube placement. An added benefit to ERCP is that sphincterotomy and stone extraction are performed at the same time.[44] ERCP is successful at treating more than 90% of cases of cholangitis. The complication rate is about 5% with mortality only 1%. The only absolute contraindication to ERCP is known or suspected viscus perforation. Relative contraindications including cardiopulmonary instability, coagulopathy, pregnancy, and severe contrast allergy. If coagulopathy cannot be corrected before the procedure sphincterotomy is not recommended.[45]

Endoscopic nasobiliary drainage
In clinical practice this is performed less frequently compared with biliary stent placement because it is uncomfortable for patients and may dislodge if the patient is confused or delirious. Advantages include thick pus or purulent bile is drained more effectively, washing is performed if the tube becomes clogged, the bile is easily cultured, and a sphincterotomy is avoided.[2]

Percutaneous Transhepatic Cholangiography

Percutaneous drainage is typically considered a second-line treatment option either after a failed ERCP, in patients with multiple comorbidities, or in patients with surgically altered anatomy not amenable to endoscopic therapy. Because this procedure does not need intravenous sedation or anesthesia it may be safer in clinically unstable patients. This route also is best if the obstruction is above the common bile duct or when drainage of individual segments in the liver are needed.[44] Disadvantages include increased length of hospital stay; patient discomfort; and increased risk for complications that include intraperitoneal hemorrhage, biliary peritonitis, and sepsis. Contraindications included coagulopathies, ascites, and intrahepatic biliary obstructions.[2]

Surgery

Open surgical drainage is considered as a last resort when ERCP, percutaneous transhepatic cholangiography (PTC), and/or EUS are unsuccessful or contraindicated.

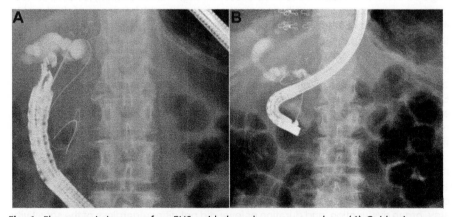

Fig. 1. Fluoroscopic images of an EUS-guided rendezvous procedure. (A) Guidewire access obtained into the extrahepatic bile duct under sonographic vision using a linear echoendoscope. A wire is advanced in retrograde fashion through the major papilla and allowed to coil in the duodenum. (B) After withdrawal of the echoendoscope while simultaneously leaving the wire in place, a therapeutic duodenoscope is advanced to the level of the major papilla. The wire is grasped with a forceps and advanced through the working channel of the duodenoscope. Wire access is then obtained into the bile duct with a standard traction sphincterotome.

It may be considered in patients undergoing a laparoscopic cholecystectomy with transcystic or transductal laparoscopic bile duct exploration.[44]

Newer Techniques

In the last 10 years EUS-guided drainage, transpapillary and transmural, has emerged as a new approach to allow access when ERCP has failed or the ampulla is inaccessible with conventional methods because of surgically altered anatomy. Therapeutic EUS can guide creation of a neofistula between the bile duct and stomach (hepaticogastrostomy) or duodenum (hepaticoduodenostomy) with a lumen-apposing metal stent. Creation of a gastrogastric fistula via an EGDE procedure (EUS-directed transgastric ERCP) can also assist in Billroth or Roux-en-Y anatomy. EUS can also guide placement of a stent in an antegrade manner across a stricture distal to the puncture site in cases when the papilla is inaccessible, and the intrahepatic duct is dilated. EUS-guided rendezvous (**Fig. 1**) gains access through intrahepatic or extrahepatic bile ducts to gain access by placing a guidewire through the papilla.[25] The high technical difficulty level of these procedures limits their use to high-volume centers with experienced endoscopists.

SUMMARY

Acute cholangitis should be suspected in patients with fever, abdominal pain, and jaundice. If acute changes of liver enzymes are also present, ERCP is warranted to confirm diagnosis and provide biliary drainage. Cultures and imaging studies contribute to the diagnosis. Management of acute cholangitis includes monitoring for and treating sepsis, providing antibiotic coverage, and establishing biliary drainage. A good understanding of the pathophysiology, diagnosis, and management of the disease permit making early and accurate diagnosis and selecting appropriate treatments in a timely fashion.

CLINICS CARE POINTS

- Acute cholangitis is very treatable when recognized and treated early. Failure to recognize and initiate early treatment leads to increased patient morbidity and mortality.

- Once a diagnosis is made prompt biliary drainage is the cornerstone of treatment. In the case of severe biliary sepsis drainage should be completed within 12 hours to reduce overall mortality.

- Penicillin/b-lactamase, third-generation cephalosporin, or carbapenem are all acceptable choices for first line treatment. Anti-fugal coverage should be added in patients with biliary stents or hospital-acquired infection.

DISCLOSURES

The authors have nothing to disclose.

REFERENCES

1. Sulzer JK, Ocuin LM. Cholangitis: causes, diagnosis, and management. Surg Clin North Am 2019;99(2):175–84.
2. Ahmed M. Acute cholangitis: an update. World J Gastrointest Pathophysiol 2018; 9(1):1–7.

3. Aboelsoud M, Siddique O, Morales A, et al. Early biliary drainage is associated with favourable outcomes in critically-ill patients with acute cholangitis. Prz Gastroenterol 2018;13(1):16–21.

4. Deviere J, Motte S, Dumonceau JM, et al. Septicemia after endoscopic retrograde cholangiopancreatography. Endoscopy 1990;22(2):72–5.

5. Lan Cheong Wah D, Christophi C, Muralidharan V. Acute cholangitis: current concepts. ANZ J Surg 2017;87(7–8):554–9.

6. Gigot JF, Leese T, Dereme T, et al. Acute cholangitis. Multivariate analysis of risk factors. Ann Surg 1989;209(4):435–8.

7. Yokoe M, Hata J, Takada T, et al. Tokyo Guidelines 2018: diagnostic criteria and severity grading of acute cholecystitis (with videos). J Hepatobiliary Pancreat Sci 2018;25(1):41–54.

8. Chen M, Wang L, Wang Y, et al. Risk factor analysis of post-ERCP cholangitis: a single-center experience. Hepatobiliary Pancreat Dis Int 2018; 17(1):55–8.

9. Everett BT, Naud S, Zubarik RS. Risk factors for the development of stent-associated cholangitis following endoscopic biliary stent placement. Dig Dis Sci 2019;64(8):2300–7.

10. Xia MX, Wang SP, Wu J, et al. The risk of acute cholangitis after endoscopic stenting for malignant hilar strictures: a large comprehensive study. J Gastroenterol Hepatol 2020;35(7):1150–7.

11. Rumsey S, Winders J, MacCormick AD. Diagnostic accuracy of Charcot's triad: a systematic review. ANZ J Surg 2017;87(4):232–8.

12. Kiriyama S, Kozaka K, Takada T, et al. Tokyo Guidelines 2018: diagnostic criteria and severity grading of acute cholangitis (with videos). J Hepatobiliary Pancreat Sci 2018;25(1):17–30.

13. Mosler P. Diagnosis and management of acute cholangitis. Curr Gastroenterol Rep 2011;13(2):166–72.

14. Lee YS, Cho KB, Park KS, et al. Procalcitonin as a decision-supporting marker of urgent biliary decompression in acute cholangitis. Dig Dis Sci 2018;63(9):2474–9.

15. Miura F, Okamoto K, Takada T, et al. Tokyo Guidelines 2018: initial management of acute biliary infection and flowchart for acute cholangitis. J Hepatobiliary Pancreat Sci 2018;25(1):31–40.

16. Gomi H, Takada T, Hwang TL, et al. Updated comprehensive epidemiology, microbiology, and outcomes among patients with acute cholangitis. J Hepatobiliary Pancreat Sci 2017;24(6):310–8.

17. Plessier A, Darwish-Murad S, Hernandez-Guerra M, et al. Acute portal vein thrombosis unrelated to cirrhosis: a prospective multicenter follow-up study. Hepatology 2010;51(1):210–8.

18. Sun G, Han L, Yang Y, et al. Comparison of two editions of Tokyo Guidelines for the management of acute cholangitis. J Hepatobiliary Pancreat Sci 2014;21(2):113–9.

19. Gomi H, Solomkin JS, Schlossberg D, et al. Tokyo Guidelines 2018: antimicrobial therapy for acute cholangitis and cholecystitis. J Hepatobiliary Pancreat Sci 2018;25(1):3–16.

20. Saradna A, Shankar S, Shamian B, et al. *Candida tropicalis* cholangitis in a patient without underlying malignancy. Cureus 2017;9(11):e1867.

21. Lubbert C, Wendt K, Feisthammel J, et al. Epidemiology and resistance patterns of bacterial and fungal colonization of biliary plastic stents: a prospective cohort study. PLoS One 2016;11(5):e0155479.

22. Jo IH, Kim YJ, Chung WC, et al. Microbiology and risk factors for gram-positive Cocci bacteremia in biliary infections. Hepatobiliary Pancreat Dis Int 2020; 19(5):461–6.
23. Xia J, Jiang SC, Peng HJ. Association between liver fluke infection and hepato-biliary pathological changes: a systematic review and meta-analysis. PLoS One 2015;10(7):e0132673.
24. Rickes S, Treiber G, Monkemuller K, et al. Impact of the operator's experience on value of high-resolution transabdominal ultrasound in the diagnosis of choledo-cholithiasis: a prospective comparison using endoscopic retrograde cholangiog-raphy as the gold standard. Scand J Gastroenterol 2006;41(7):838–43.
25. Nau P, Pauli EM, Sandler BJ, et al, SpringerLink (Online service). The SAGES manual of flexible endoscopy. 1st edition. Cham, Switzerland: Springer Nature Switzerland AG; 2020. https://doi.org/10.1007/978-3-030-23590-1.
26. Singh A, Mann HS, Thukral CL, et al. Diagnostic accuracy of MRCP as compared to ultrasound/CT in patients with obstructive jaundice. J Clin Diagn Res 2014; 8(3):103–7.
27. Giljaca V, Gurusamy KS, Takwoingi Y, et al. Endoscopic ultrasound versus mag-netic resonance cholangiopancreatography for common bile duct stones. Co-chrane Database Syst Rev 2015;(2):CD011549.
28. Kimura Y, Takada T, Kawarada Y, et al. Definitions, pathophysiology, and epidemi-ology of acute cholangitis and cholecystitis: Tokyo Guidelines. J Hepatobiliary Pan-creat Surg 2007;14(1):15–26.
29. Andrew DJ, Johnson SE. Acute suppurative cholangitis, a medical and surgical emergency. A review of ten years experience emphasizing early recognition. Am J Gastroenterol 1970;54(2):141–54.
30. Suwa Y, Matsuyama R, Goto K, et al. IL-7 and procalcitonin are useful biomarkers in the comprehensive evaluation of the severity of acute cholangitis. J Hepatobiliary Pancreat Sci 2017;24(2):81–8.
31. Akhtar F, Siddique MZ, Raza A, et al. Microbiology and clinical characteristics of acute cholangitis with their impact on mortality; a retrospective cross sectional study. J Pak Med Assoc 2020;70(4):607–12.
32. Parikh MP, Gupta NM, Thota PN, et al. Temporal trends in utilization and out-comes of endoscopic retrograde cholangiopancreatography in acute cholangitis due to choledocholithiasis from 1998 to 2012. Surg Endosc 2018;32(4):1740–8.
33. Kruis T, Guse-Jaschuck S, Siegmund B, et al. Use of microbiological and patient data for choice of empirical antibiotic therapy in acute cholangitis. BMC Gastro-enterol 2020;20(1):65.
34. Reiter FP, Obermeier W, Jung J, et al. Prevalence, resistance-rates and risk-factors of pathogens in routine bile cultures obtained during endoscopic retro-grade cholangiography. Dig Dis 2020;39(1):42–51.
35. Buckman SA, Mazuski JE. Review of the Tokyo Guidelines 2018: antimicrobial therapy for acute cholangitis and cholecystitis. JAMA Surg 2019;154(9):873–4.
36. Chandra S, Klair JS, Soota K, et al. Endoscopic retrograde cholangio-pancreatography-obtained bile culture can guide antibiotic therapy in acute chol-angitis. Dig Dis 2019;37(2):155–60.
37. Haal S, Ten Bohmer B, Balkema S, et al. Antimicrobial therapy of 3 days or less is sufficient after successful ERCP for acute cholangitis. United Eur Gastroenterol J 2020;8(4):481–8.
38. Satake M, Yamaguchi Y. Three-day antibiotic treatment for acute cholangitis due to choledocholithiasis with successful biliary duct drainage: a single-center retro-spective cohort study. Int J Infect Dis 2020;96:343–7.

39. Iwata K, Doi A, Oba Y, et al. Shortening antibiotic duration in the treatment of acute cholangitis: rationale and study protocol for an open-label randomized controlled trial. Trials 2020;21(1):97.
40. Iqbal U, Khara HS, Hu Y, et al. Emergent versus urgent ERCP in acute cholangitis: a systematic review and meta-analysis. Gastrointest Endosc 2020;91(4):753–60.e4.
41. Khamaysi I, Taha R. ERCP for severe acute cholangitis: the earlier, the better. Turk J Gastroenterol 2020;31(1):78–9.
42. Manes G, Paspatis G, Aabakken L, et al. Endoscopic management of common bile duct stones: European Society of Gastrointestinal Endoscopy (ESGE) guide-line. Endoscopy 2019;51(5):472–91.
43. Kawamura S, Karasawa Y, Toda N, et al. Impact of the sensitivity to empiric an-tibiotics on clinical outcomes after biliary drainage for acute cholangitis. Gut Liver 2020;14(6):842–9.
44. Navuluri R, Hoyer M, Osman M, et al. Emergent treatment of acute cholangitis and acute cholecystitis. Semin Intervent Radiol 2020;37(1):14–23.
45. Alexander CM. Management of pancreaticobiliary disease: endoscopic retro-grade cholangiopancreatography (ERCP). In: Narula VK, editor. The SAGES manual of flexible endoscopy. Cham, Switzerland: Springer Nature Switzerland AG; 2020.

Infectious Gastroenteritis in Transplant Patients

Lemuel R. Non, MD[a], Dilek Ince, MD[b],*

KEYWORDS

- Solid organ transplantation • Hematopoietic stem cell transplantation
- Gastrointestinal infection • Diagnostic workup

KEY POINTS

- Infectious diarrhea is common posttransplant with a prevalence of 20% to 50% in solid organ transplant and 20% to 44% in hematopoietic stem cell transplantation recipients.
- Infectious pathogens are similar to those in nontransplant populations, but their presentation can be more severe. Chronic infections or prolonged shedding are also more frequent in transplant recipients.
- *Clostridioides difficile* is the major bacterial pathogen in transplant recipients. In addition to risk factors applicable to general population, specific factors specific to transplant recipients exist and make prevention challenging.
- Cytomegalovirus and norovirus are the most common viral causes of diarrhea. Parasitic infections are common in developing countries and can be an important cause of morbidity and mortality among global transplant recipients.
- Newer, culture-independent tests have increased diagnostic yield in this patient population. A multistep diagnostic approach should be used in evaluation.

INTRODUCTION

Gastrointestinal (GI) infections occur commonly after both solid organ transplantation (SOT) and hematopoietic stem cell transplantation (HSCT). Prevalence of diarrhea is 20% to 50% in the SOT and 20% to 44% in the HSCT population.[1] Causes of diarrhea in transplant patients span infectious (**Table 1**) and noninfectious etiologies. Infectious causes are similar to those in nontransplant populations with some major differences, including more severe symptoms, higher incidence of opportunistic infections, higher likelihood of chronicity, and prolonged shedding.[2] Diarrhea in transplant recipients is associated with increased morbidity, including allograft loss and increased mortality.[3] This review emphasizes differences in epidemiology, risk factors, and management of gastrointestinal infections in transplant compared with nontransplant populations and provides a stepwise approach to diagnosis of diarrhea in transplant recipients.

[a] Department of Internal Medicine, University of Iowa, Carver College of Medicine, GH SW34, 200 Hawkins Drive, Iowa City, IA 52242, USA; [b] Department of Internal Medicine, University of Iowa, Carver College of Medicine, GH SE418, 200 Hawkins Drive, Iowa City, IA 52242, USA
* Corresponding author.
E-mail address: dilek-ince@uiowa.edu

Gastroenterol Clin N Am 50 (2021) 415–430
https://doi.org/10.1016/j.gtc.2021.02.013
0889-8553/21/© 2021 Elsevier Inc. All rights reserved.

Table 1 Common infectious causes of diarrhea in SOT and HSCT recipients[1,2,76,91]		
Bacteria	**Viruses**	**Parasites**
Clostridioides difficile	Cytomegalovirus	Cryptosporidium
Campylobacter spp	Norovirus	Cyclospora
Salmonella spp.	Rotavirus	Cystoisospora
Escherichia coli	Adenovirus	Microsporidium
Aeromonas spp	Sapovirus	Giardia
Yersinia enterocolitica	Enterovirus	Entamoeba
Shigella spp	SARS-CoV-2	
Bacterial overgrowth		

Abbreviations: HSCT, hematopoietic stem cell transplantation; SARS-CoV-2, severe acute respiratory syndrome coronavirus 2; SOT, solid organ transplantation.

BACTERIAL INFECTIONS

The Diarrhea Diagnosis Aid and Clinical Treatment study, a prospective study of 108 renal transplant patients, evaluated the etiology of posttransplant diarrhea. The most common cause of diarrhea was medications, with a bacterial infection identified in 20% of the patients, most frequently Campylobacter sp. In this study, bacterial overgrowth was suspected in 36% of the patients with improvement in symptoms with antibiotic treatment.[4]

Bacterial enterocolitis (excluding Clostridioides difficile) is a rare cause (0.9%) of both community-onset and hospital-onset diarrhea among SOT recipients.[3] Infections due to enteric pathogens were also rare (0.25%) in hospitalized patients with hematologic malignancies.[5] In a prospective study among autologous and allogeneic stem cell transplant recipients, an enteric pathogen was found in only 0.1% of patients, likely due to the inhibitory effects of routine use of antibiotic prophylaxis.[6]

A severe form of enterocolitis can occur in neutropenic patients, especially in the setting of chemotherapy and transplantation. Neutropenic enterocolitis is a life-threatening complication of HSCT and high-dose chemotherapy. It has been described in 5.3% of patients with hematologic malignancies hospitalized for chemotherapy and has been associated with mortality rates up to 38.8%.[7] Microbiologic cause is rarely determined but is presumed to be due to mostly gram-negative and anaerobic bacteria.[8] Sepsis due to translocation of intestinal bacteria, intra-abdominal abscesses, colon perforation, and pneumatosis intestinalis are among the complications of neutropenic enterocolitis.[9,10]

Clostridioides difficile Infection

C difficile is an urgent health care threat for both hospitalized and community patients and is the most frequently encountered bacteria leading to admissions for both community-onset and hospital-onset diarrhea in transplant patients.[3,11] Immunocompromised patients are disproportionately affected, with the incidence and prevalence of C difficile infection (CDI) depending on the immunocompromised population being evaluated.[12]

CDI in hematology and oncology populations ranges between 3% and 33%. It is most likely to occur in the first 100 days, with most cases in the first 30 days (preengraftment) after transplantation.[13,14] Risk factors for CDI in the general population, such as prior use of antibiotics, health care exposures, age older than 65, or use of proton pump inhibitor (PPI) also apply to immunocompromised patient population,[12,14,15] although one retrospective study in HSCT has shown PPI use to be protective.[16] Specific risk factors for CDI in HSCT recipients are shown in **Table 2**. Some studies have found an association between graft-versus-host disease (GVHD) leading to CDI or CDI leading to GVHD, whereas others have failed to show an association in either direction.[16–18]

Colonization with toxigenic *C difficile*, which increases the risk for development of CDI with an adjusted odds ratio of 11.6,[19] has been reported in 9% to 15% of HSCT patients on admission to transplant unit[19–22] and in 26% of patients within 72 hours of admission.[23] The use of antimicrobial prophylaxis in neutropenic patients in the setting of these high colonization rates makes prevention of CDI challenging in HSCT patients.

Prevalence of CDI in SOT recipients was estimated as 7.4% in a meta-analysis of studies from 1991 to 2014.[24] The incidence of CDI in SOT recipients varies based on type of transplanted organ, with the lowest incidence in kidney transplant recipients (2.6%–16%) and highest in lung transplant recipients (7%–31%).[11,25] Bimodal incidence of CDI is observed in SOT recipients: with highest incidence in the first 3 months posttransplantation due to more frequent antimicrobial exposures, health care exposure, and more intense chemotherapy.[25–27] Late-onset CDI occurring months to years later, is usually due to antimicrobial exposures or increased immunosuppression.[13]

Risk factors specific to SOT recipients are shown in **Table 2**. Many risk factors were identified in single retrospective studies using various *C difficile* testing methods. Consistently identified risk factors other than transplanted organ type include recent hospitalization and antibiotic use.[13]

As for immunocompetent patients, a multistep algorithm of diagnostic tests (enzyme immunoassays [EIAs] and nucleic acid amplification tests [NAATs]) is recommended for workup. EIAs have lower sensitivity in immunocompromised individuals[28] and NAAT may identify *C difficile* colonization in addition to infection,[12] indicating need for diagnostic stewardship.[25]

There are no specific treatment guidelines for immunocompromised patients, and treatment follows guidelines published in 2018.[12] Higher rates of colectomy have

Table 2
Risk factors for *Clostridioides difficile* infection[13,14,105]

HSCT	SOT
Antibiotic prophylaxis	Transplanted organ type
Acute allogeneic vs autologous	Immunosuppressive agents (steroids with highest risk)
Umbilical cord HSCT	Antithymocyte globulin
Total body irradiation	Gastrostomy/jejunostomy tube
Myeloablative conditioning	Surgical procedures
Chemotherapy	Retransplantation
Neutropenia	Antibiotic prophylaxis
Mucositis	Prolonged hospital stay
GVHD	Age >55
CMV reactivation	Prior episode of CDI
HSV or VZV reactivation	Deceased donor transplantation
Colonization with toxigenic strain	
VRE colonization	
Bacterial infection	
Mechanical ventilation	
Male gender	
Hypogammaglobulinemia	

Abbreviations: CDI, *Clostridioides difficile* infection; CMV, cytomegalovirus; GVHD, graft-versus-host disease; HSCT, hematopoietic stem cell transplantation; SOT, solid organ transplantation.

been reported in SOT recipients versus immunocompetent patients (13% vs <3%).[27] Recurrence is also a major problem, ranging from 8.0% to 41.0% in HSCT and 6.3% to 40.0% in SOT recipients.[13] There are limited data on use of fecal microbiota transfer (FMT) in immunocompromised hosts due to concerns for enteric bacteria translocation. In a retrospective multicenter study of 94 SOT recipients who underwent FMT, cure rate was 64% at 1 month with no episodes of FMT-related bacteremia and mild adverse events.[29] Bezlotoxumab is a humanized monoclonal antibody against C difficile toxin B approved for secondary prophylaxis of recurrent CDI in patients at high risk of recurrence. Although no trials have been performed in the HSCT population, based on clinical trials that included immunocompromised hosts, it can be considered for secondary prophylaxis in transplant recipients.[14,25]

Single-center retrospective studies in HSCT recipients or patients with hematologic malignancies have shown decreases in risk or recurrence of CDI rates with oral vancomycin[30,31] and, of confirmed CDI cases, with fidaxomicin prophylaxis.[32] Oral vancomycin prophylaxis was not found to be effective in primary or secondary prophylaxis of CDI in SOT recipients.[33,34] Due to lack of large prospective data, role of antimicrobials for prophylaxis of CDI in immunocompromised patients is unclear.

VIRAL INFECTIONS
Adenovirus

Adenovirus (AV) infections, usually mild and self-limiting in immunocompetent patients, can lead to severe and life-threatening diarrhea in immunocompromised hosts, especially in children and HSCT recipients.[35] Risk factors in the HSCT population include T-cell–depleting or myeloablative conditioning regimens, nonmatched related donor grafts, GVHD, lymphopenia, and cord blood as stem cell source.[36] Similar to HSCT, AV infection in SOT recipients is more common in children. Risk factors include allograft type, with intestinal transplantation having the highest risk, and degree of immunosuppression.[37]

AV can establish persistent infections in numerous cell types, particularly in T-lymphocytes in tonsils/adenoids and intestines, and in lung epithelial cells, leading to multiorgan manifestations due to reactivation from these sites. The intestine is possibly the main site of AV persistence and reactivation, and rising AV numbers in stool have been shown to precede invasive infection. In fact, monitoring of fecal viral load has been shown to predict the risk of viremia, especially in the pediatric HSCT recipients.[38] The European Conference on Infections in Leukemia recommends stool and blood screening for AV before conditioning and after HSCT in children, and blood monitoring in adults.[39]

Primary management of AV infection is reduction in immunosuppression. Cidofovir, associated in some series with improved survival in transplant recipients, has significant toxicity. In a survey among providers, reduction in immunosuppression and administration of cidofovir with probenecid were the most commonly cited strategies for AV infection after allogeneic HSCT.[40] Immunotherapy through adoptive transfer of specific anti-AV-cytotoxic-T-lymphocytes is a promising option, especially for patients unresponsive to antivirals.[41]

Cytomegalovirus

Gastrointestinal (GI) cytomegalovirus (CMV) disease presents with signs and symptoms attributed to CMV tissue invasion within the GI tract.[42] Upper GI CMV disease typically manifests as symptoms due to ulcerative lesions: oropharyngeal CMV with painful ulcers; esophagitis with dysphagia, odynophagia, epigastric pain, nausea, and vomiting; gastritis with epigastric pain, nausea, and vomiting; and enteritis with abdominal pain and diarrhea. Lower GI CMV manifestations include colitis, which presents with diarrhea, fever, abdominal pain, and hematochezia, and anorectal ulcerative lesions.[43,44]

Without preventive strategies, CMV infections typically occur during the first few months after SOT and HSCT, and incidence can be as high as 70% among at-risk groups. Risk factors in SOT include serologic mismatch between donor and recipient (positive donor/negative recipient portends highest risk), allograft rejection, and posttransplant immunosuppression.[42] Risk factors in HSCT include CMV-positive recipients, receipt of alemtuzumab, other T-cell–depleting agents, allogeneic and cord blood stem cell transplantation, use of mismatched or unrelated donors, high-dose steroids, and GVHD.[45] The main preventive strategies for CMV are universal antiviral chemoprophylaxis, the administration of prophylaxis during periods of highest risk posttransplantation (usually first 3–12 months after SOT, and first 100 days after HSCT), and preemptive therapy, administration of antiviral treatment based on weekly monitoring. Valganciclovir is generally used for prophylaxis in both SOT and HSCT, and letermovir in select HSCT populations.[46] Options for preemptive therapy are ganciclovir, valganciclovir, and foscarnet.[42,47] Although these preventive strategies have been effective, CMV disease following discontinuation of prophylaxis (delayed-onset or late-onset CMV disease) is common, with GI involvement being a frequent manifestation. Close clinical follow-up, viral surveillance for several months, extending duration of antiviral prophylaxis, and assessment of CMV-specific T-cell immunity before discontinuation of prophylaxis are options for prevention of late-onset CMV disease.[42]

GI CMV disease is diagnosed when upper and/or lower GI symptoms are accompanied by characteristic ulcerative lesions with CMV cytopathic effect in tissue as documented by histopathology, virus isolation, rapid culture, immunohistochemistry, or DNA hybridization techniques.[48] Negative CMV DNAemia or antigenemia does not rule out GI CMV disease. Management of CMV disease involves reduction in immunosuppression and administration of antivirals. First-line treatment is typically intravenous ganciclovir, although valganciclovir may be considered in mild-to-moderate disease. Other options include foscarnet, cidofovir, and use of CMV-specific T-cell therapy.[42,47]

Norovirus

Norovirus (NV) is one of the leading causes of gastroenteritis in the United States and worldwide.[49] Although NV usually causes a short-lived and self-limiting enteritis in immunocompetent patients, it can lead to severe chronic diarrheal disease in transplant recipients that can last for several weeks to months.[50] Nausea and vomiting are not always reported by patients and, if present, usually occur early on in the course. Diarrhea in chronic NV cases can be protracted, leading to significant debilitation, malnutrition, secondary lactose intolerance, kidney failure, weight loss, failure to thrive, and occasionally death.[2,51–53] NV diarrheal disease has also been associated with poor long-term graft survival in SOT.[54–56] Despite increasing recognition, NV remains underrecognized as a cause of chronic diarrhea in transplant recipients.

In a retrospective study among hospitalized SOT recipients, NV was identified in 3% of community-onset diarrhea and in 8.2% of hospital-onset diarrhea.[3] In other studies, NV has been identified in 18% of transplant patients presenting with severe diarrhea and in 40% with chronic diarrhea,[57,58] with an estimated cumulative incidence at 2 years of 13%.[59] Between 10% and 16% of transplant patients with NV infection develop chronic diarrhea.[54,60] In children with SOT and HSCT admitted for diarrhea, NV was found to cause diarrhea for ≥14 days in more than half of the cases.[61]

Risk factors for chronic NV infection include recipients of high-risk HLA-incompatible and/or ABO-incompatible transplants, plasmapheresis, antithymocyte globulin induction, steroid use, and antirejection therapy.[50,54] Specifically, use of cyclosporine-mycophenolate mofetil combination has been identified as a risk factor.[57] In a retrospective chart review among SOT recipients, nausea at presentation and CMV infection within the past 3 months were found to be associated with persistent diarrhea.[55] Among HSCT recipients, risk factors included use of peripheral blood or cord blood as stem cell source, and receipt of fludarabine and alemtuzumab.[59]

NV is commonly detected in stool samples using NV-specific reverse transcriptase polymerase chain reaction or the newer multiplex assays. Coinfection with other pathogens has been reported at 2%.[3] Viral shedding can be prolonged in transplant recipients, which can sometimes last for months to years (median 289 days).[58]

Rehydration and supportive care remain the cornerstones of management. Reduction in immune suppression is a key strategy in many transplant-associated infections, but whether this has significant impact on chronic NV diarrhea is unknown. Limited studies have shown potential benefit from nitazoxanide in reducing symptom duration and clearance of shedding,[62–64] likely by activation of cellular antiviral response through increased expression of interferon-stimulated genes, particularly interferon regulatory factor-1, which inhibits viral replication.[65] Administration of intravenous or oral immunoglobulin has also been suggested, especially in patients with hypogammaglobulinemia.[66]

Rotavirus

Rotavirus (RV) usually causes a mild, self-limiting gastroenteritis in immunocompetent adults, but can lead to severe disease in transplant recipients. The estimated incidence is approximately 3% and can occur at any point after the transplantation, and usually peaks during winter and spring seasons. Small bowel, liver, and HSCT recipients demonstrate the highest incidence of RV infection.[67] The median duration of diarrhea is 15 days (range 4 days to 4 months).[68] Risk factors include lymphopenia and immunosuppressive medications for GVHD.[68] Complications such as toxic megacolon, prolonged hospitalization, and development of acute cellular rejection and graft loss, especially in intestinal allografts, have been reported.[69–71] RV infections have been associated with increases in tacrolimus trough concentrations, possibly due to suppressive effect of inflammation on intestinal cytochrome P450 and P-glycoprotein, increased intestinal permeability, decreased hepatic metabolism, or decreased transit time in the GI tract, suggesting the need for close monitoring of tacrolimus levels.[67,72]

Vaccination against RV is recommended in children before transplantation. Management is nonspecific and is composed of supportive and rehydration strategies and nutritional support. Enteral immunoglobulins have been found to improve symptoms of RV gastroenteritis in pediatric HSCT recipients, and may be considered in severe cases.[73]

Severe Acute Respiratory Syndrome Coronavirus 2

Severe acute respiratory syndrome coronavirus 2 (SARS-CoV-2), the agent of the pandemic coronavirus disease 2019 (COVID-19) is primarily a respiratory virus. GI symptoms have been described more frequently in cohorts of both inpatient and outpatient SOT populations versus non-SOT populations (35%–54% vs 17%–20%).[74–76] Transplant status was not associated with increased mortality in hospitalized patients.

Gastrointestinal symptoms such as diarrhea may precede or occur simultaneously with respiratory symptoms.[77] SARS-CoV-2 uses the angiotensin-converting enzyme 2

(ACE2) for cellular entry and the serine protease TMPRSS2 for S protein priming, which are also both found in intestinal epithelia.[78] In fact, ACE2 is expressed at higher amounts in the intestines than in the lung.[79] Viral RNA has been found in stool for up to a month in more than 80% of patients and up to 20% can have detectable virus in the stool even after documented clearance from the respiratory tract.[80]

PARASITIC INFECTIONS

Intestinal parasitic infections are common in developing countries, and with increasing travel to and from these endemic areas and with an expanding global food trade, can be an important cause of morbidity and mortality among global transplant recipients.[81] Transplant patients may acquire intestinal parasites from the donor allograft, reactivation of a prior infection, or exposure after transplant.

Cryptosporidium, Cystoisospora belli, Giardia, and Cyclospora are usually acquired from contaminated food and water but may also be donor-derived, especially in the setting of intestinal transplantation.[82,83] They can lead to protracted diarrhea associated with significant complications.[84] Supportive care and reduction in immunosuppression are mainstays of treatment. Nitazoxanide has been used in transplant recipients with Cryptosporidium infections, based on experience from patients with human immunodeficiency virus. A meta-analysis on nitazoxanide use in immunocompromised hosts did not find any benefit; however, newer small, randomized, controlled trials in the general population have shown benefit in reducing diarrhea and oocyst shedding.[85–87]

Strongyloides stercoralis is an intestinal nematode with the potential to auto-infect perpetuating strongyloidosis.[88] In addition to de novo acquisition or reinfection in endemic areas, strongyloidosis can result from reactivation of chronic intestinal infection or may be donor-derived.[89] The most dreaded complication from Strongyloides infection is the hyperinfection syndrome, which can present with fever, dyspnea, wheezing, hemoptysis, acute respiratory distress–like syndrome, anorexia, nausea, vomiting, abdominal pain, diarrhea, ileus, obstruction, and gastrointestinal bleeding. Hyperinfection syndrome results from acceleration of the parasite's life cycle as a result of immunosuppression that can lead to bacteremia in up to 50% and septic shock in up to 40%, with mortality of more than 50%.[82,90] This high morbidity and mortality has led some centers to implement a screening strategy in SOT donors and recipients.[90]

Microsporidia, historically considered parasites but more recently classified as fungi, are emerging causes of gastroenteritis as well as occasionally genitourinary tract infection or disseminated infections (lungs, cornea, central nervous system) in transplant recipients, and it should be considered in transplant recipients in whom etiologies of diarrhea are not identified.[91] Identification requires special stains and main treatment is reduction of immunosuppression.

FUNGAL INFECTIONS

Invasive fungal infections (IFIs) are major causes of morbidity and mortality in both SOT and HSCT but rarely cause gastrointestinal disease. A prospective study among US transplant centers included in the Transplant-Associated Infections Surveillance Network (TRANSNET) demonstrated that among SOT recipients, small bowel transplant recipients were found to have the highest incidence, likely due to intestinal colonization, followed by lung, liver, heart, pancreas, and kidney. Among HSCT recipients, mismatched-related allogeneic transplant recipients had the highest 12-month cumulative incidence, followed by matched-unrelated, and matched-related HSCT recipients.[92,93]

Invasive candidiasis is the most common IFI among SOT recipients and the second most common among HSCT recipients.[92,93] Although peritonitis was encountered in 9% of SOT recipients, the exact incidence of gastrointestinal disease due to IFI is uncertain. Based on single-center studies, esophageal candidiasis has been reported in 10% to 16% of kidney and kidney-pancreas transplant recipients.[94,95] It should be noted that *Candida* species other than *Candida albicans* were identified in approximately half of the IFI in SOT recipients and in more than two-thirds of HSCT recipients in the TRANSNET database.[92,93] Isolated intestinal infection due to *Candida* sp is rare but has been reported in an autologous HSCT recipient.[96] Neutropenic enterocolitis or typhlitis can be a complication of chemotherapy and stem cell transplantation, and has been associated with candidemia.[7] Invasive gastrointestinal aspergillosis is also rare, and has been reported only a few times in autologous HSCT recipients.[97,98] Although not as common as candidiasis or aspergillosis, mucormycosis can also involve the gastrointestinal tract. In a systematic review and meta-analysis of case reports, gastrointestinal mucormycosis was found in 8% of patients with mucormycosis.[99]

Endemic mycoses, in particular histoplasmosis, can present with isolated gastrointestinal involvement in SOT and HSCT recipients. Presentations have varied and included lower GI bleeding, diarrhea, mesenteric mass, intra-abdominal lymphadenopathy, and ulcerative lesions.[100–102]

DIAGNOSTIC APPROACH TO INFECTIOUS DIARRHEA

The workup of diarrhea in transplant patients is different from immune-competent individuals, as it requires knowledge of timeline following transplantation, the multitude of risk factors associated with transplant, and the different, sometimes severe, presentation of, otherwise, self-limiting etiologies of infectious diarrhea in this patient population.

A stepwise approach to diagnosis of diarrhea is recommended (**Table 3**). A careful review of medications should be performed, and unnecessary medications should be discontinued. Medications with high likelihood of causing diarrhea should be switched if possible. Recommendations for first tier testing should include stool *C difficile* and bacterial pathogen testing, and whole blood or serum CMV viral load. Especially fever and bloody diarrhea should suggest invasive enteropathogens and CMV.

Traditional stool cultures are of low yield. Newer, culture-independent diagnostic tests, such as NAAT including polymerase chain reaction (PCR) (as individual PCRs

Table 3 Workup of diarrhea (>3 stools per day) in transplant patients[2,91]	
Step 1	Evaluate and discontinue potential medications *Clostridioides difficile* testing Blood/serum CMV PCR Stool culture and PCR (single or multiplex) for enteric pathogens
Step 2	Stool viral testing (if not performed in Step 1 as part of multiplex PCR assay) Stool ova and parasite Breath test for bacterial overgrowth
Step 3	Adjust/switch immunosuppressive medications implicated in diarrhea Upper and lower endoscopy for infectious causes or noninfectious causes (CMV, Mycobacteria, PTLD, IBD) Empiric therapy with antimotility drugs Evaluation for malabsorption

Abbreviations: CMV, cytomegalovirus; IBD, inflammatory bowel disease; PCR, polymerase chain reaction; PTLD, posttransplant lymphoproliferative disorder.

for single agents or multiplex PCRs for a range of pathogens) are increasingly used for detection of enteric pathogens with increased diagnostic yield and quick turnaround. NAAT permit identification of multiple pathogens in up to 28% of patients.[1] One disadvantage of these sensitive tests is their inability to differentiate between active disease, carrier state, or subclinical infection. Most centers perform multiplex PCR for enteric pathogens in the first tier. If not available, second-tier testing includes stool Norovirus or other viral PCR in stool, ova, and parasite examination, *Giardia* and *Cryptosporidium* enzyme immunoassay, and breath test for bacterial overgrowth.[2]

In HSCT recipients, a similar stepwise approach is recommended. In addition, if there is concern for neutropenic enterocolitis, blood and stool cultures should be obtained. In the early postengraftment period, CMV should be checked in addition to *C difficile*.[103,104] Second-tier testing includes ova and parasite examination, assays for adenovirus, CMV, rotavirus, and norovirus, and *Giardia* and *Cryptosporidium* EIA. In addition to infection, GVHD should be ruled out in the early postengraftment period and late postengraftment period, respectively.[104]

Finally, for both SOT and HSCT recipients, if the preceding testing is unrevealing, colonoscopy with or without esophagogastroduodenoscopy should be considered to evaluate for other potential etiologies, such as posttransplant lymphoproliferative disorder and mycobacterial diseases[2]

SUMMARY

Diarrhea is a common complication in transplant recipients, leading to significant morbidity and mortality. *C difficile*, CMV, and norovirus are among the most common infectious etiologies. Differential diagnosis should take clinical presentation, risk factors, and degree of immunosuppression into consideration and a stepwise approach to diagnosis should be undertaken.

CLINICS CARE POINTS

- Obtaining detailed history including medications, hobbies, pets, exposures and travel is extremely important as they might give important clues to infectious and noninfectious causes of gastroenteritis.
- Treatment for rejection leading to increased immunosuppression increases the likelihood of opportunistic infections, which might present with gastrointestinal symptoms.
- CMV viremia is not always present in cases of CMV gastroenteritis. Endoscopy might be needed for diagnosis.
- Highly sensitive, often multiplex molecular tests can identify colonizing organisms that are not the causative agents of the diarrhea illness. If treatment is given, patient should be followed closely for resolution of symptoms.

DISCLOSURE

The authors have nothing to disclose.

REFERENCES

1. Santoiemma PP, Ison MG, Angarone MP. Newer approaches in diagnosis of diarrhea in immunocompromised patients. Curr Opin Infect Dis 2019;32(5): 461–7.

2. Angarone M, Snydman DR, Practice AICo. Diagnosis and management of diarrhea in solid-organ transplant recipients: guidelines from the American Society of Transplantation Infectious Diseases Community of Practice. Clin Transplant 2019;33(9):e13550.

3. Echenique IA, Penugonda S, Stosor V, et al. Diagnostic yields in solid organ transplant recipients admitted with diarrhea. Clin Infect Dis 2015;60(5):729–37.

4. Maes B, Hadaya K, de Moor B, et al. Severe diarrhea in renal transplant patients: results of the DIDACT study. Am J Transplant 2006;6(6):1466–72.

5. Gorschluter M, Hahn C, Ziske C, et al. Low frequency of enteric infections by *Salmonella, Shigella, Yersinia* and *Campylobacter* in patients with acute leukemia. Infection 2002;30(1):22–5.

6. van Kraaij MG, Dekker AW, Verdonck LF, et al. Infectious gastro-enteritis: an uncommon cause of diarrhoea in adult allogeneic and autologous stem cell transplant recipients. Bone Marrow Transplant 2000;26(3):299–303.

7. Duceau B, Picard M, Pirracchio R, et al. Neutropenic enterocolitis in critically ill patients: spectrum of the disease and risk of invasive fungal disease. Crit Care Med 2019;47(5):668–76.

8. Nathan S, Ustun C. Complications of stem cell transplantation that affect infections in stem cell transplant recipients, with analogies to patients with hematologic malignancies. Infect Dis Clin North Am 2019;33(2):331–59.

9. Abu-Sbeih H, Ali FS, Chen E, et al. Neutropenic enterocolitis: clinical features and outcomes. Dis Colon Rectum 2020;63(3):381–8.

10. Batlle M, Vall-Llovera F, Bechini J, et al. Neutropenic enterocolitis in adult patients with acute leukemia or stem cell transplant recipients: study of 7 cases. Med Clin (Barc) 2007;129(17):660–3 [in Spanish].

11. Wong D, Nanda N. *Clostridium difficile* disease in solid organ transplant recipients: a recommended treatment paradigm. Curr Opin Organ Transplant 2020; 25(4):357–63.

12. McDonald LC, Gerding DN, Johnson S, et al. Clinical practice guidelines for *Clostridium difficile* infection in adults and children: 2017 update by the Infectious Diseases Society of America (IDSA) and Society for Healthcare Epidemiology of America (SHEA). Clin Infect Dis 2018;66(7):e1–48.

13. Revolinski SL, Munoz-Price LS. *Clostridium difficile* in immunocompromised hosts: a review of epidemiology, risk factors, treatment, and prevention. Clin Infect Dis 2019;68(12):2144–53.

14. Misch EA, Safdar N. *Clostridioides difficile* infection in the stem cell transplant and hematologic malignancy population. Infect Dis Clin North Am 2019;33(2): 447–66.

15. D'Silva KM, Mehta R, Mitchell M, et al. Proton pump inhibitor use and risk for recurrent *Clostridioides difficile* infection: a systematic review & meta-analysis. Clin Microbiol Infect 2021. https://doi.org/10.1016/j.cmi.2021.01.008.

16. Alonso CD, Treadway SB, Hanna DB, et al. Epidemiology and outcomes of *Clostridium difficile* infections in hematopoietic stem cell transplant recipients. Clin Infect Dis 2012;54(8):1053–63.

17. Dubberke ER, Reske KA, Srivastava A, et al. *Clostridium difficile*-associated disease in allogeneic hematopoietic stem-cell transplant recipients: risk associations, protective associations, and outcomes. Clin Transplant 2010;24(2):192–8.

18. Chakrabarti S, Lees A, Jones SG, et al. *Clostridium difficile* infection in allogeneic stem cell transplant recipients is associated with severe graft-versus-host disease and non-relapse mortality. Bone Marrow Transplant 2000;26(8):871–6.

19. Cannon CM, Musuuza JS, Barker AK, et al. Risk of *Clostridium difficile* infection in hematology-oncology patients colonized with toxigenic *C. difficile*. Infect Control Hosp Epidemiol 2017;38(6):718–20.

20. Jain T, Croswell C, Urday-Cornejo V, et al. *Clostridium difficile* colonization in hematopoietic stem cell transplant recipients: a prospective study of the epidemiology and outcomes involving toxigenic and nontoxigenic strains. Biol Blood Marrow Transplant 2016;22(1):157–63.

21. Bruminhent J, Wang ZX, Hu C, et al. *Clostridium difficile* colonization and disease in patients undergoing hematopoietic stem cell transplantation. Biol Blood Marrow Transplant 2014;20(9):1329–34.

22. Cho J, Seville MT, Khanna S, et al. Screening for *Clostridium difficile* colonization on admission to a hematopoietic stem cell transplant unit may reduce hospital-acquired *C difficile* infection. Am J Infect Control 2018;46(4):459–61.

23. Kamboj M, Sheahan A, Sun J, et al. Transmission of *Clostridium difficile* during hospitalization for allogeneic stem cell transplant. Infect Control Hosp Epidemiol 2016;37(1):8–15.

24. Paudel S, Zacharioudakis IM, Zervou FN, et al. Prevalence of *Clostridium difficile* infection among solid organ transplant recipients: a meta-analysis of published studies. PLoS One 2015;10(4):e0124483.

25. Mullane KM, Dubberke ER, Practice AICo. Management of *Clostridioides* (formerly *Clostridium*) *difficile* infection (CDI) in solid organ transplant recipients: guidelines from the American Society of Transplantation Community of Practice. Clin Transplant 2019;33(9):e13564.

26. Boutros M, Al-Shaibi M, Chan G, et al. *Clostridium difficile* colitis: increasing incidence, risk factors, and outcomes in solid organ transplant recipients. Transplantation 2012;93(10):1051–7.

27. Dallal RM, Harbrecht BG, Boujoukas AJ, et al. Fulminant *Clostridium difficile*: an underappreciated and increasing cause of death and complications. Ann Surg 2002;235(3):363–72.

28. Erb S, Frei R, Stranden AM, et al. Low sensitivity of fecal toxin A/B enzyme immunoassay for diagnosis of *Clostridium difficile* infection in immunocompromised patients. Clin Microbiol Infect 2015;21(11):998.e9-e15.

29. Cheng YW, Phelps E, Ganapini V, et al. Fecal microbiota transplantation for the treatment of recurrent and severe *Clostridium difficile* infection in solid organ transplant recipients: a multicenter experience. Am J Transplant 2019;19(2):501–11.

30. Morrisette T, Van Matre AG, Miller MA, et al. Oral vancomycin prophylaxis as secondary prevention against *Clostridioides difficile* infection in the hematopoietic stem cell transplantation and hematologic malignancy population. Biol Blood Marrow Transplant 2019;25(10):2091–7.

31. Ganetsky A, Han JH, Hughes ME, et al. Oral vancomycin prophylaxis is highly effective in preventing *Clostridium difficile* infection in allogeneic hematopoietic cell transplant recipients. Clin Infect Dis 2019;68(12):2003–9.

32. Mullane KM, Winston DJ, Nooka A, et al. A randomized, placebo-controlled trial of fidaxomicin for prophylaxis of *Clostridium difficile*-associated diarrhea in adults undergoing hematopoietic stem cell transplantation. Clin Infect Dis 2019;68(2):196–203.

33. Splinter LE, Kerstenetzky L, Jorgenson MR, et al. Vancomycin prophylaxis for prevention of *Clostridium difficile* infection recurrence in renal transplant patients. Ann Pharmacother 2018;52(2):113–9.

34. Bajrovic V, Budev M, McCurry KR, et al. Vancomycin prophylaxis for *Clostridium difficile* infection among lung transplant recipients. J Heart Lung Transplant 2019;38(8):874–6.
35. Lee YJ, Huang YT, Kim SJ, et al. Adenovirus viremia in adult CD34(+) selected hematopoietic cell transplant recipients: low incidence and high clinical impact. Biol Blood Marrow Transplant 2016;22(1):174–8.
36. Fowler CJ, Dunlap J, Troyer D, et al. Life-threatening adenovirus infections in the setting of the immunocompromised allogeneic stem cell transplant patients. Adv Hematol 2010;2010:601548.
37. Florescu DF, Schaenman JM, Practice ASTIDCo. Adenovirus in solid organ transplant recipients: guidelines from the American Society of Transplantation Infectious Diseases Community of Practice. Clin Transplant 2019;33(9):e13527.
38. Hum RM, Deambrosis D, Lum SH, et al. Molecular monitoring of adenovirus reactivation in faeces after haematopoietic stem-cell transplantation to predict systemic infection: a retrospective cohort study. Lancet Haematol 2018;5(9):e422–9.
39. Hiwarkar P, Kosulin K, Cesaro S, et al. Management of adenovirus infection in patients after haematopoietic stem cell transplantation: state-of-the-art and real-life current approach: a position statement on behalf of the Infectious Diseases Working Party of the European Society of Blood and Marrow Transplantation. Rev Med Virol 2018;28(3):e1980.
40. Cesaro S, Berger M, Tridello G, et al. A survey on incidence and management of adenovirus infection after allogeneic HSCT. Bone Marrow Transplant 2019;54(8):1275–80.
41. Qian C, Campidelli A, Wang Y, et al. Curative or pre-emptive adenovirus-specific T cell transfer from matched unrelated or third party haploidentical donors after HSCT, including UCB transplantations: a successful phase I/II multicenter clinical trial. J Hematol Oncol 2017;10(1):1–14.
42. Razonable RR, Humar A. Cytomegalovirus in solid organ transplant recipients-Guidelines of the American Society of Transplantation Infectious Diseases Community of Practice. Clin Transplant 2019;33(9):e13512.
43. O'Hara KM, Pontrelli G, Kunstel KL. An introduction to gastrointestinal tract CMV disease. JAAPA 2017;30(10):48–52.
44. Marques S, Carmo J, Pinto D, et al. Cytomegalovirus disease of the upper gastrointestinal tract: a 10-year retrospective study. GE Port J Gastroenterol 2017;24(6):262–8.
45. Pande A, Dubberke ER. Cytomegalovirus infections of the stem cell transplant recipient and hematologic malignancy patient. Infect Dis Clin North Am 2019;33(2):485–500.
46. Marty FM, Ljungman P, Chemaly RF, et al. Letermovir prophylaxis for cytomegalovirus in hematopoietic-cell transplantation. N Engl J Med 2017;377(25):2433–44.
47. Ljungman P, de la Camara R, Robin C, et al. Guidelines for the management of cytomegalovirus infection in patients with haematological malignancies and after stem cell transplantation from the 2017 European Conference on Infections in Leukaemia (ECIL 7). Lancet Infect Dis 2019;19(8):e260–72.
48. Ljungman P, Boeckh M, Hirsch HH, et al. Definitions of cytomegalovirus infection and disease in transplant patients for use in clinical trials. Clin Infect Dis 2017;64(1):87–91.
49. Centers for Disease C, Prevention. Emergence of new norovirus strain GII.4 Sydney–United States, 2012. MMWR Morb Mortal Wkly Rep 2013;62(3):55.

50. Avery RK, Lonze BE, Kraus ES, et al. Severe chronic norovirus diarrheal disease in transplant recipients: clinical features of an under-recognized syndrome. Transpl Infect Dis 2017;19(2).
51. Bonani M, Pereira RM, Misselwitz B, et al. Chronic norovirus infection as a risk factor for secondary lactose maldigestion in renal transplant recipients: a prospective parallel cohort pilot study. Transplantation 2017;101(6):1455–60.
52. Petrignani M, Verhoef L, de Graaf M, et al. Chronic sequelae and severe complications of norovirus infection: a systematic review of literature, vol. 105. Elsevier B.V.; J Clin Virol 2018; 105: 1-10.
53. Roddie C, Paul JPV, Benjamin R, et al. Allogeneic hematopoietic stem cell transplantation and norovirus gastroenteritis: a previously unrecognized cause of morbidity. Clin Infect Dis 2009;49(7):1061–8.
54. Brakemeier S, Taxeidi SI, Dürr M, et al. Clinical outcome of norovirus infection in renal transplant patients. Clin Transplant 2016;30(10):1283–93.
55. Chong PP, van Duin D, Sonderup JL, et al. Predictors of persistent diarrhea in norovirus enteritis after solid organ transplantation. Clin Transplant 2016; 30(11):1488–93.
56. Rolak S, Di Bartolomeo S, Jorgenson MR, et al. Outcomes of Norovirus diarrheal infections and *Clostridioides difficile* infections in kidney transplant recipients: a single-center retrospective study. Transpl Infect Dis 2019;21(2):e13053.
57. Coste JF, Vuiblet V, Moustapha B, et al. Microbiological diagnosis of severe diarrhea in kidney transplant recipients by use of multiplex PCR assays. J Clin Microbiol 2013;51(6):1841–9.
58. Roos-Weil D, Ambert-Balay K, Lanternier F, et al. Impact of norovirus/sapovirus-related diarrhea in renal transplant recipients hospitalized for diarrhea. Transplantation 2011;92(1):61–9.
59. Robles JDF, Cheuk DKL, Ha SY, et al. Norovirus infection in pediatric hematopoietic stem cell transplantation recipients: incidence, risk factors, and outcome. Biol Blood Marrow Transplant 2012;18(12):1883–9.
60. Swartling L, Ljungman P, Remberger M, et al. Norovirus causing severe gastrointestinal disease following allogeneic hematopoietic stem cell transplantation: a retrospective analysis. Transpl Infect Dis 2018;20(2):e12847.
61. Ye X, Van JN, Munoz FM, et al. Noroviruses as a cause of diarrhea in immunocompromised pediatric hematopoietic stem cell and solid organ transplant recipients. Am J Transplant 2015;15(7):1874–81.
62. Haubrich K, Gantt S, Blydt-Hansen T. Successful treatment of chronic norovirus gastroenteritis with nitazoxanide in a pediatric kidney transplant recipient. Pediatr Transplant 2018;22(4):e13186.
63. Rossignol JF, El-Gohary YM. Nitazoxanide in the treatment of viral gastroenteritis: a randomized double-blind placebo-controlled clinical trial. Aliment Pharmacol Ther 2006;24(10):1423–30.
64. Siddiq DM, Koo HL, Adachi JA, et al. Norovirus gastroenteritis successfully treated with nitazoxanide. J Infect 2011;63(5):394–7.
65. Dang W, Xu L, Ma B, et al. Nitazoxanide inhibits human norovirus replication and synergizes with ribavirin by activation of cellular antiviral response. Antimicrob Agents Chemother 2018;62(11):e00707–18.
66. Jurgens PT, Allen LA, Ambardekar AV, et al. Chronic norovirus infections in cardiac transplant patients: considerations for evaluation and management. Prog Transplant 2017;27(1):69–72.
67. Yin Y, Metselaar HJ, Sprengers D, et al. Rotavirus in organ transplantation: drug-virus-host interactions. Am J Transplant 2015;15(3):585–93.

68. Liakopoulou E, Mutton K, Carrington D, et al. Rotavirus as a significant cause of prolonged diarrhoeal illness and morbidity following allogeneic bone marrow transplantation. Bone Marrow Transplant 2005;36(8):691–4.

69. Adeyi OA, Costa G, Abu-Elmagd KM, et al. Rotavirus infection in adult small intestine allografts: a clinicopathological study of a cohort of 23 patients. Am J Transplant 2010;10(12):2683–9.

70. Stelzmueller I, Dunst KM, Hengster P, et al. A cluster of rotavirus enteritis in adult transplant recipients. Transpl Int 2005;18(4):470–4.

71. Stelzmueller I, Wiesmayr S, Swenson BR, et al. Rotavirus enteritis in solid organ transplant recipients: an underestimated problem? Transpl Infect Dis 2007;9(4): 281–5.

72. Maezono S, Sugimoto KI, Sakamoto KI, et al. Elevated blood concentrations of calcineurin inhibitors during diarrheal episode in pediatric liver transplant recipients: involvement of the suppression of intestinal cytochrome P450 3A and P-glycoprotein. Pediatr Transplant 2005;9(3):315–23.

73. Williams D. Treatment of rotavirus-associated diarrhea using enteral immunoglobulins for pediatric stem cell transplant patients. J Oncol Pharm Pract 2014;21(3):238–40.

74. Molnar MZ, Bhalla A, Azhar A, et al. Outcomes of critically ill solid organ transplant patients with COVID-19 in the United States. Am J Transplant 2020;20(11): 3061–71.

75. Chaudhry ZS, Williams JD, Vahia A, et al. Clinical characteristics and outcomes of COVID-19 in solid organ transplant recipients: a cohort study. Am J Transplant 2020;20(11):3051–60.

76. Kates OS, Haydel BM, Florman SS, et al. COVID-19 in solid organ transplant: a multi-center cohort study. Clin Infect Dis 2020;ciaa1097.

77. Chan JF, Yuan S, Kok KH, et al. A familial cluster of pneumonia associated with the 2019 novel coronavirus indicating person-to-person transmission: a study of a family cluster. Lancet 2020;395(10223):514–23.

78. D'Amico F, Baumgart DC, Danese S, et al. Diarrhea during COVID-19 infection: pathogenesis, epidemiology, prevention, and management. Clin Gastroenterol Hepatol 2020;18(8):1663–72.

79. Li XY, Dai WJ, Wu SN, et al. The occurrence of diarrhea in COVID-19 patients. Clin Res Hepatol Gastroenterol 2020;44(3):284–5.

80. Jiehao C, Jin X, Daojiong L, et al. A case series of children with 2019 novel coronavirus infection: clinical and epidemiological features. Clin Infect Dis 2020; 71(6):1547–51.

81. Silvia F, Simona F, Fabrizio B. Solid organ transplant and parasitic diseases: a review of the clinical cases in the last two decades, vol. 7. MDPI AG; Pathogens 2018;7(3); 65.

82. La Hoz RM, Morris MI, AST Infectious Diseases Community of Practice. Intestinal parasites including *Cryptosporidium, Cyclospora, Giardia*, and *Microsporidia, Entamoeba histolytica, Strongyloides, Schistosomiasis*, and *Echinococcus*: guidelines from the American Society of Transplantation Infectious Diseases Community of Practice. Clin Transplant 2019;33(9):e13618.

83. Pozio E, Rivasi F, Cacciò SM. Infection with *Cryptosporidium hominis* and reinfection with *Cryptosporidium parvum* in a transplanted ileum. APMIS 2004; 112(4–5):309–13.

84. Chen XM, Keithly JS, Paya CV, et al. Cryptosporidiosis. N Engl J Med 2002; 346(22):1723–31.

85. Abubakar I, Aliyu SH, Arumugam C, et al. Treatment of cryptosporidiosis in immunocompromised individuals: systematic review and meta-analysis. Br J Clin Pharmacol 2007;63:387–93.
86. Rossignol JF, Kabil SM, El-gohary Y, et al. Effect of nitazoxanide in diarrhea and enteritis caused by *Cryptosporidium* species. Clin Gastroenterol Hepatol 2006; 4(3):320–4.
87. Rossignol JFA, Ayoub A, Ayers MS. Treatment of diarrhea caused by *Cryptosporidium parvum*: a prospective randomized, double-blind, placebo-controlled study of nitazoxanide. J Infect Dis 2001;184(1):103–6.
88. Nutman TB. Human infection with Strongyloides stercoralis and other related Strongyloides species, vol. 144. Cambridge University Press; Parasitology. 2017; 144 (3): 263-73.
89. Abanyie FA, Gray EB, Delli Carpini KW, et al. Donor-derived strongyloides stercoralis infection in solid organ transplant recipients in the United States, 2009-2013. Am J Transplant 2015;15(5):1369–75.
90. Camargo JF, Simkins J, Anjan S, et al. Implementation of a *Strongyloides* screening strategy in solid organ transplant donors and recipients. Clin Transplant 2019;33(4):e13497.
91. Florescu DF. The evaluation of critically ill transplant patients with infectious diarrhea. Curr Opin Crit Care 2017;23(5):364–71.
92. Kontoyiannis DP, Marr KA, Park BJ, et al. Prospective surveillance for invasive fungal infections in hematopoietic stem cell transplant recipients, 2001-2006: overview of the Transplant-Associated Infection Surveillance Network (TRANS-NET) Database. Clin Infect Dis 2010;50(8):1091–100.
93. Pappas PG, Alexander BD, Andes DR, et al. Invasive fungal infections among organ transplant recipients: results of the Transplant-Associated Infection Surveillance Network (TRANSNET). Clin Infect Dis 2010;50(8):1101–11.
94. Veroux M, Macarone M, Fiamingo P, et al. Caspofungin in the treatment of azole-refractory esophageal candidiasis in kidney transplant recipients. Transplant Proc 2006;38(4):1037–9.
95. Gupta KL, Ghosh AK, Kochhar R, et al. Esophageal candidiasis after renal transplantation: comparative study in patients on different immunosuppressive protocols. Am J Gastroenterol 1994;89(7):1062–5.
96. Direkze S, Mansour M, Rodriguez-Justo M, et al. *Candida kefyr* fungal enteritis following autologous BMT. Bone Marrow Transplant 2012;47(3):465–6.
97. Kennes S, Van de Putte D, Van Dorpe J, et al. Primary intestinal aspergillosis resulting in acute intestinal volvulus after autologous stem cell transplantation in a patient with relapsed non-Hodgkin lymphoma: report on a rare infectious complication and a review of the literature. Acta Clin Belg 2019;74(5):359–63.
98. Lehrnbecher T, Becker M, Schwabe D, et al. Primary intestinal aspergillosis after high-dose chemotherapy and autologous stem cell rescue. Pediatr Infect Dis J 2006;25(5):465–6.
99. Jeong W, Keighley C, Wolfe R, et al. The epidemiology and clinical manifestations of mucormycosis: a systematic review and meta-analysis of case reports. Clin Microbiol Infect 2019;25(1):26–34.
100. Agrawal N, Jones DE, Dyson JK, et al. Fatal gastrointestinal histoplasmosis 15 years after orthotopic liver transplantation. World J Gastroenterol 2017;23(43): 7807–12.
101. Mohan M, Fogel B, Eluvathingal T, et al. Gastrointestinal histoplasmosis in a patient after autologous stem cell transplant for multiple myeloma. Transpl Infect Dis 2016;18(6):939–41.

102. Syed TA, Salem G, Kastens DJ. Lower gastrointestinal bleeding secondary to intestinal histoplasmosis in a renal transplant patient. ACG Case Rep J 2017; 4:e93.

103. Shadi Hamdeh AAMA, Elsallabi O, Pathak R, et al. Clinical approach to diarrheal disorders in allogeneic hematopoietic stem cell transplant recipients. World J Hematol 2016;5:23–30.

104. Robak K, Zambonelli J, Bilinski J, et al. Diarrhea after allogeneic stem cell transplantation: beyond graft-versus-host disease. Eur J Gastroenterol Hepatol 2017; 29(5):495–502.

105. Majeed A, Larriva MM, Iftikhar A, et al. A single-center experience and literature review of management strategies for *Clostridium difficile* infection in hematopoietic stem cell transplant patients. Infect Dis Clin Pract (Baltim Md) 2020; 28(1):10–5.

Potential Prenatal Origins of Necrotizing Enterocolitis

Sarah N. Watson, MD[a], Steven J. McElroy, MD[b,c],*

KEYWORDS

- Necrotizing enterocolitis • Fetal exposure to maternal inflammation
- Fetal inflammatory response syndrome • Intrauterine infection and inflammation
- Maternal origins of neonatal disease • Preeclampsia • Growth restriction

KEY POINTS

- Although several postnatal risk factors for necrotizing enterocolitis have been identified clearly, prenatal exposures to maternal disease and medications have also been implicated in disease development.
- Intrauterine infection and inflammation, preeclampsia, and intrauterine growth restriction are common obstetric complications that have been associated with necrotizing enterocolitis.
- Several medications given routinely when preterm birth is anticipated may impact the risk of necrotizing enterocolitis.
- Prenatal therapies may play a role in risk of developing necrotizing enterocolitis, although the corner stone of prevention remains prevention of preterm birth.
- Although mechanistic links between chorioamnionitis and intestinal susceptibility to injury remain incomplete, it is clear that fetal exposure to maternal inflammation has significant impacts on several aspects of intestinal homeostasis.

INTRODUCTION

Necrotizing enterocolitis (NEC) is a life-threatening disorder impacting the intestinal tract of the neonate. Despite decades of research, NEC remains one of the most serious and lethal conditions encountered in the neonatal intensive care unit. Currently, NEC lacks diagnostic biomarkers or targeted therapies, making clinical determination and management challenging. Much of the focus on understanding

[a] Obstetrics and Gynecology, Department of Obstetrics and Gynecology, University of Iowa, 200 Hawkins Drive, Iowa City, IA 52242-1080, USA; [b] Stead Family Department of Pediatrics, University of Iowa, 200 Hawkins Drive, Iowa City, IA 52242-1080, USA; [c] Department of Microbiology and Immunology, University of Iowa, 200 Hawkins Drive, Iowa City, IA 52242-1080, USA
* Corresponding author. Department of Microbiology and Immunology, University of Iowa, 200 Hawkins Drive, Iowa City, IA 52242-1080.
E-mail address: steven-mcelroy@uiowa.edu

Gastroenterol Clin N Am 50 (2021) 431–444
https://doi.org/10.1016/j.gtc.2021.02.006
0889-8553/21/© 2021 Elsevier Inc. All rights reserved.

susceptibility to NEC comes from the evaluation of postnatal risk factors, such as gestational age, birth weight, the food the infant eats, and the volumes of their feedings. However, less is understood about potential prenatal risk factors. This review focuses on these prenatal risk factors and how they may contribute to the pathogenesis of NEC. We also discuss several potential prenatal targets and therapeutic strategies that may be used to decrease the risk of NEC.

OVERVIEW OF NECROTIZING ENTEROCOLITIS

NEC is a life-threatening condition, with a mortality rate that reaches 30% in very low birth weight infants.[1] The incidence of NEC is inversely correlated with the degree of prematurity, making the most premature infants the most susceptible.[2] Neonatal risk factors for development of NEC are well-established and include prematurity, decreasing birth weight, rapid advancement of enteral feeding, feeding with infant formula instead of human milk, and intestinal dysbiosis. In addition, African American infants have a 4.40 times higher risk of NEC compared with their White peers.[3] Although the vast majority of affected infants are preterm, children born at term can also be affected, and certain conditions including sepsis, neonatal abstinence syndrome, and especially cardiac disease, seem to increase the risk.[4–7]

NEC can manifest in several different clinical presentations: it can have an insidious onset with mild symptoms that may overlap with other diseases of prematurity (sepsis, apnea of prematurity, intestinal dysmotility) and can take days to fully present; or it can have a sudden severe onset with acute intestinal dysfunction and injury that rapidly progresses over hours. Despite vigilance, the early detection of NEC is difficult owing to the lack of defined early warning signs or effective biomarkers. Early detection also remains elusive and definitive diagnosis is not currently possible until the appearance of radiographic evidence of pneumatosis intestinalis (a sign that intestinal tissue death has occurred after bacterial translocation and subsequent fermentation of the intestinal substrate) in combination with signs of clinical deterioration.[8] Currently, the tissue destruction seen in NEC is believed to be a final end point after the initiation of inflammation.[9] Key differences in the intestinal integrity and in the immune response in the preterm infant as compared with the more mature adult physiology are suspected to lead to the induction of inflammatory dysregulation, which ultimately culminates in intestinal tissue destruction and subsequent fulminant bowel necrosis, multiorgan dysfunction, and death.[10]

The current treatment for NEC includes conservative management with bowel rest, decompression, broad spectrum antibiotics, and, when required, surgical management.[11] In addition to a high mortality rate, NEC survivors experience high rates of morbidity, including short gut syndrome and neurodevelopmental delays.[12,13] Despite the stakes, advances in the treatment of NEC remain limited.[14] Given the severity and sequalae of the disease as well as the current lack of targeted treatment options, many investigators have focused on targeting and capitalizing on preventive strategies.[2] Several reviews have already discussed postnatal risk factors and the mainstays for prevention in the neonatal period including the impact of breastmilk, probiotics, avoidance of antacids, gradual and early introduction of enteral nutrition, and other potential interventions.[15–19]

One of the most significant risk factors for development of NEC is prematurity. This increased risk is attributed to the degree of structural and immunologically immaturity found in the premature infant.[10] However, preterm birth often results as a complication of maternal disease. As such, it is reasonable that maternal risk factors may also play a role in development of NEC. We focus here on common pregnancy complications associated with preterm birth and the evidence for a potential association with NEC (**Fig. 1**).

Intrauterine Inflammation and Infection as a Risk Factor for Necrotizing Enterocolitis

A significant risk factor for preterm delivery is the development of infection and inflammation within the uterus, commonly known as chorioamnionitis.[20] Chorioamnionitis encompasses diagnoses based on clinical symptoms and inflammatory pathology of the placenta. Diagnosis can therefore range from clinical symptoms with no placental pathology to the most severe forms, which include inflammatory pathologic involvement extending from the maternal tissues into the fetus itself.[21] NEC is one of the many neonatal sequalae associated with maternal chorioamnionitis.[20,22–24] A metanalysis of 12 cohort and case control studies including 22,601 pregnancies found a clinical diagnosis of intrauterine infection was associated with an increased risk of NEC (odds ratio [OR], 1.24; confidence interval, 1.01–1.52),[25] and that as chorioamnionitis severity increased, so did the association with NEC. In the subanalysis, 3 studies including 1641 pregnancies found that evidence of umbilical cord infiltration (funisitis) was associated with more than 3 times the risk of NEC (OR, 3.29; 95% confidence interval, 1.87–5.78).[25] Since this metanalysis was published, multiple additional studies have confirmed that fetal exposure to chorioamnionitis is associated with an increased risk of NEC.[22,24,26–28] In addition, severe histologic chorioamnionitis may be prognostic of severity and the need for surgical treatment, including the placement of a peritoneal drain and/or an exploratory laparotomy with excision of necrotic bowel followed by primary anastomosis or enterostomy.[29] Duci and colleagues[28] performed a case control study of 136 patients with NEC and gestational age–matched controls and examined the association of maternal factors. Eighty percent of infants requiring surgical treatment had mothers diagnosed with histologic chorioamnionitis, compared with only 38% of those successfully treated medically.[28] This association has been

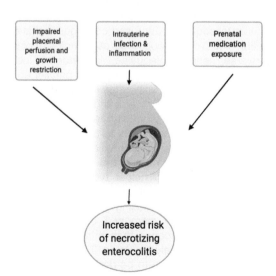

Fig. 1. The potential contribution of prenatal factors to the development of NEC. Contribution of obstetric complications (including intrauterine inflammation and infection, growth restriction, preeclampsia, and prenatal medications) to an increased risk of NEC.

seen in animal models of chorioamnionitis as well. Pregnant animals that developed intrauterine inflammation after exposure to bacterial lipopolysaccharide (LPS, endo-toxin) or polyI:C (a mimic of viral infection and an inflammatory mediator) have demon-strated an increased risk of neonatal intestinal injury, independent of microbial infection.[30–32] Our laboratory has shown in mice that fetal exposure to maternal inflam-mation induces intestinal injury, elevated baseline serum inflammatory cytokine levels, and a loss of Paneth cell and goblet cell density in the exposed offspring.[31] Whether the inflammation disrupted the development of these specialized intestinal cells or led to cellular death remains under investigation. These findings seem to be dose depen-dent, with increasing inflammation and injury seen with an increasing dose of LPS.[30,31] Wolfs and colleagues[32,33] found disrupted tight junction distribution in the intestines of preterm and near-term lamb fetuses exposed to intrauterine endotoxin for more than 6 days, but not in fetuses exposed for only 2 days. In addition to epithelial effects, in-testinal vascular development may also be altered by fetal exposure to maternal inflammation. Yan and colleagues[34] found a decreased density of the intestinal sub-mucosal vascular network, decreased intestinal villous endothelial cell proliferation, increased microvascular permeability, and decreased intestinal vascular endothelial growth factor and vascular endothelial growth factor receptor 2 protein expression in a mouse model. In addition, Wolfs and colleagues[33] found that acetylcholine-induced relaxation of the mesenteric arteries was inhibited and thromboxane receptor agonist-induced contraction of jejunal mesenteric arteries was augmented in preterm lambs after prenatal endotoxin exposure. Thus, although the mechanistic links be-tween chorioamnionitis and intestinal susceptibility to injury remain incomplete, it is clear that fetal exposure to maternal inflammation has significant impacts on several aspects of intestinal homeostasis.

Although chorioamnionitis is associated with bacterial infection, it is common for women who meet the clinical diagnostic criteria for chorioamnionitis to have symp-toms of infection without a positive bacterial culture of the amniotic fluid.[35] In fact, the term intrauterine infection and inflammation has been instituted to make clear the equally important and potentially independent role of intrauterine inflammation on neonatal outcomes.[36] Therefore, the inflammatory cascade itself may be critical in development of neonatal sequalae. Jung and colleagues[37] have published exten-sively on the association of IL-6 cord blood levels as an indicator of IL-6 content in fetal circulation, with adverse neonatal sequalae. Importantly, increasing levels of chorioamnionitis-induced IL-6 in umbilical cord blood parallel an increasing risk of composite neonatal morbidity and mortality rates independent of evidence of direct microbial invasion of the uterine cavity.[35,38] This finding supports a direct mechanistic role for IL-6 in development of neonatal morbidity. Multiple immunologic changes have also been described in the fetal immune system as a response of intrauterine infection and inflammation.[39,40] In addition to IL-6, maternal serum levels of IL-1β, IL-19, IL-10, and intra-amniotic neutrophils of maternal and fetal origin are all significantly increased after chorioamnionitis.[41,42] T-helper type 17 cell density (implicated in many chronic inflammatory conditions) is also increased in the setting of chorioamnio-nitis with increasing proportions at decreasing gestational ages.[43] Increased T-cell activation and increased numbers of memory T cells that, upon rechallenge, are capable of a stronger cytokine response than primary responder T lymphocytes have also been observed.[44] Conversely regulatory T cells (important in inflammatory response modulation) have been shown to be decreased in number or function in a majority of studies.[43,45]

Animal models examining the mechanisms behind intrauterine inflammation-related NEC-like injury suggest that fetal inflammatory exposure induces changes in both innate and adaptive immunity (**Table 1**). It has been well-established in multiple models that both the mother and her offspring mount a robust cytokine response, particularly IL-6, as well as IL-1β and tumor necrosis factor-α after exposure to maternal inflammation or intrauterine inflammation.[31,32,46] IL-6 in particular seems to play a critical role, because mice lacking IL-6 were spared from both intestinal and neurologic morbidity after fetal exposure to maternal inflammation.[31,47] Endotoxin exposure in preterm lambs also impacts inflammatory signaling pathways and has been shown to downregulate the expression of the pattern recognition receptor proteins Toll-like receptors (TLR) 1, 2, 4, and 6 after both acute and chronic exposure.[32] In addition, offspring exposed to intrauterine endotoxin have been shown to have increased polymorphonuclear cells, CD3[+] T cells, including gamma-delta T lymphocytes, whereas regulatory T cells have been shown to be downregulated in the ileum of lambs after 2 days of LPS or endotoxin exposure with normalization after 6 days.[32,33]

Genetic association studies provide additional evidence that variations in the immune system may be important in the pathogenesis of NEC. Franklin and colleagues[48] found that Caucasian infants with a single nucleotide polymorphism variant of IL-6 (rs1800795) had more than 6 times the odds of developing NEC and more than 7 times the odds of developing stage 3 NEC based on modified Bell's criteria compared with matched controls. In addition to IL-6, genetic variations of IL-17a and IL-23 have also been implicated in the development of NEC. In a Chinese cohort, NEC was significantly associated with variants in IL-17 (OR, 1.89) and IL-23 (OR, 1.82).[49] However, these associations have not been confirmed by other groups.[50] One additional area that has shown promise is genetic disturbances in regulation of expression of pattern recognition receptors including TLR4 and nucleotide binding oligomerization domains (NOD) receptor proteins. Upon recognition of the microbial cell wall component LPS, the TLR4 receptor complex signaling pathways upregulate proinflammatory cytokine gene expression with the potential for pathologic inflammatory responses.[51,52] NOD 1 and 2 proteins intracellularly recognize other components of bacterial cell wall and similarly activate key transcription factors for immune activation.[53,54] Zhou and colleagues[55] found an increased risk of severe NEC in neonates with a single nucleotide polymorphism in the MD2 co-receptor of TLR4 which is necessary for TLR4 function. In addition, TLR4 is downregulated by the single immunoglobulin and toll-interleukin 1 receptor gene. Sampath and colleagues[56,57] found that genetic variants in both the

Table 1
Fetal immune changes seen in association with neonatal intestinal injury after acute and chronic exposure to inflammation in animal models

	Immune Change	Acute Exposure Effect	Chronic Exposure Effect	Study Type
Innate immune system	Decrease in TLR expression	Yes	Yes	Lambs[32,33]
	Decrease in Paneth cells	Unknown	Yes	Mice[31]
	Decrease in goblet cells	Unknown	Yes	Mice[31]
	Increase in IL-6	Yes	Yes	Lambs, mice[30–32]
	Increase in IL-1β	Yes	Yes	Lambs, mice[30–32]
	Increase in TNFα	Yes	Yes	Lambs, mice[30–32,34]
	Increase in fetal neutrophils	No	Yes	Lambs[33]
Adaptive immune system	Increase in CD-3+ T cells	No	Yes	Lambs[33]
	Decrease in regulatory T cells	Yes	No	Lambs[32]

single immunoglobulin and toll-interleukin 1 receptor gene and in NOD1 were associated with an increase in NEC development. Hartel and colleagues[58] also found that infants carrying a loss-of-function variant of NOD2 had an increase in surgical NEC. These studies support the idea that maternal factors and exposures can impact the complex immunologic cascade that occurs during pathogenesis of NEC.

Other Prenatal Risk Factors for Necrotizing Enterocolitis

Although chorioamnionitis is clearly implicated in development of NEC, the impact of other causes of prematurity is not so well-defined (**Table 2**). Several well-defined demographic risk factors associated with preterm birth are clearly not associated with the development of NEC. These include maternal age, weight, smoking status, and socioeconomic status.[59] Ahle and colleagues[60] notably describe a Swedish case control study including maternal risk factors and NEC in 720 cases where no associations were found between NEC development and maternal age, smoking status, education, or income, and March and colleagues[26] found similar results in a smaller US case control study. Although these demographic risk factors do not seem to impact NEC risk, diagnosis of fetal growth restriction, another common cause of preterm birth, has been found to be an independent risk factor for NEC.[61] In a larger retrospective study of 29,916 neonates admitted to the neonatal intensive care unit between 23 and 34 weeks of gestation, the 2512 growth-restricted infants had a 3.9% risk of NEC compared with a 2.9% of infants without growth restriction (OR, 1.5).[62] This association is particularly compelling because increased severity of growth restriction is associated with more significant risk of NEC. Abnormal blood flow in the umbilical cord of growth restricted fetuses (measured by umbilical artery Doppler) is a mainstay of surveillance for fetal well-being.[63] Two smaller studies in 1987 and 1991 documented an increased risk of NEC in growth restricted infants with abnormal Doppler measurements compared with growth restricted controls with normal Doppler studies.[64,65] These findings were confirmed by a larger study of 206 infants that found infants born less then 32 weeks with abnormal umbilical artery Doppler measurements to have a fivefold increased risk of NEC, and an increase in NEC severity, when adjusted for gestational age, and birth weight compared to controls.[66] Last, 2 additional case control studies (which include 57 and 136 infants) examined infants with NEC

Table 2
Prenatal risk factors and medications for preterm birth and their association with NEC

Condition	Association with NEC	Type of Evidence
Intrauterine infection and inflammation	Increased	Retrospective[25]
Preeclampsia	Conflicting evidence for risk	Retrospective[67–70]
Preeclampsia with fetal growth restriction	Increased risk	Retrospective and prospective studies[69,70]
Fetal growth restriction with abnormal umbilical artery blood flow	Increased risk	Retrospective[64–66]
Amoxicillin–clavulanic acid	Concern for increased risk	Retrospective[78–80]
Indomethacin	Concern for increased risk	Retrospective[87–89]
Magnesium	Conflicting evidence for risk	Secondary analysis of a randomized controlled trial, retrospective[82–84]

compared with matched controls. In both studies, approximately 30% of infants with NEC had an associated prenatal diagnosis of fetal growth restriction.[26,28] This association is reasonable considering low birthweight is a well-established risk factor for NEC and a leading cause of low birthweight is fetal growth restriction.

Although fetal growth restriction is associated with NEC, the association between NEC and preeclampsia is less clear. Preeclampsia is a hypertensive disease specific to pregnancy that is estimated to be the primary cause of 11.8% of premature births.[61] Many but not all studies have found a modest increased risk of NEC in the infants of women with hypertensive disorders of pregnancy, particularly preeclampsia.[26,28,67,68] In addition, a large retrospective case control study performed by Yang and colleagues[69] of 29,013 Taiwanese women found that preeclamptic mothers had 1.86 times the odds of having an infant impacted by NEC as diagnosed by ICD-9 codes compared with matched controls. However, not all studies have found an association between NEC and preeclampsia.[26] A large multicenter prospective study of preterm infants in Germany by Bossung and colleagues[70] found a decreased risk of NEC requiring surgery in infants of preeclamptic mothers. This conflicting association between preeclampsia and NEC may be due to the significant overlap between pregnancies affected by preeclampsia and growth restriction.[63] Although the association between NEC and preeclampsia was modest in the large Taiwanese case control study, a prenatal diagnosis of growth restriction in preeclamptic mothers was associated with a more than 3-fold increased risk of NEC. A similar increased risk of NEC in growth-restricted infants of preeclamptic mothers was seen in the multicenter prospective study published by Bossung and colleagues,[70] even though they found no association between preeclampsia and NEC alone. The association between preeclampsia and NEC is more compelling when concurrent growth restriction is present based on current evidence, although whether the preeclamptic state compounds NEC risk beyond its contribution to growth restriction remains unclear.

Unfortunately, there are few additional mechanistic data from animal models to help understand the impact of hypertensive disorders and growth restriction on neonatal intestinal injury. Our laboratory has shown that mice exposed to thromboxane inhibitors to induce fetal growth restriction induced several structural changes in the offspring intestine, including a loss of Paneth and goblet cells, and a decrease in intestinal epithelial proliferation.[71] The decrease in Paneth cells was associated with increasing severity of growth restriction. These findings were consistent with the decreased number of Paneth cells per crypt seen in intestinal samples from growth restricted human infants compared with age matched controls with noninflammatory gastrointestinal diseases.[71] Given these findings, additional studies examining the role of growth restriction and NEC induction are warranted.

Prenatal Medications and Necrotizing Enterocolitis

Multiple medications are used routinely before an anticipated preterm delivery, many of which have anti-inflammatory or antimicrobial properties. An example of this is the use of antenatal steroids. Administration of a 48-hour course of either betamethasone or dexamethasone is currently the standard of care in the setting of preterm labor. Maternal steroid administration has been shown to decrease several postnatal complications, including developing NEC.[72] In the most recent Cochrane review, steroid use was found to have a risk ratio of 0.50 for NEC as a secondary outcome in a metanalysis of 4702 participants across 10 randomized controlled studies.[73] The mechanism behind this risk reduction, however, is not well-understood. One study using a rat model of NEC found that prenatal corticosteroid exposure decreased NEC-like injury and mortality and had an associated decrease in bacterial translocation.[74]

However, a detailed understanding of the mechanisms of action for the potential protective effect of maternal steroids requires further study.

Antibiotic exposure is common in pregnancy, whether for routine prophylaxis or for the treatment of maternal infections, and prophylactic antibiotic administration in pregnancy has been associated with a decreased risk of NEC in multiple studies. In a randomized controlled trial of 614 women who received a regimen involving ampicillin, erythromycin, and amoxicillin after rupture of the membranes, infants of mothers treated with antibiotics had less than one-half the risk of NEC as compared with controls.[75] In a second retrospective cohort of 580 infants born before 32 weeks of gestation, antibiotic use for prophylaxis or for treatment administered within 72 hours of delivery was associated with a decreased risk of Bell stage 2 or 3 NEC (OR, 0.28).[76] However, there has been concern that use of certain antibiotics may actually increase the risk of NEC. A randomized controlled trial of antibiotic administration for preterm labor that compared amoxicillin–clavulanic acid with erythromycin and placebo in 6295 women found 2% of infants exposed to amoxicillin–clavulanic acid developed NEC compared with 0.8% of infants whose mothers received placebo.[77] Although the relationship was not statistically significant, some but not all subsequent retrospective case control studies have found an increase in risk.[78–80] As a result, national obstetric guidelines do not recommend the use of amoxicillin–clavulanic acid[81] (see **Table 2**).

Magnesium sulfate is used routinely in the setting of anticipated preterm delivery less than 32 weeks of gestation to decrease the risk of cerebral palsy and to decrease the risk of maternal seizures owing to preeclampsia. However, a secondary analysis of a multicenter randomized trial raised concerns that magnesium may increase the risk of NEC in extremely low birth weight infants born at less than 26 weeks gestation.[82] Subsequent retrospective studies, however, have shown no increase in risk, and in fact have suggested a potential dose-dependent benefit.[83,84] Although magnesium sulfate has been protective for the brain and other organ systems in animals, particularly those exposed to prenatal inflammation,[85,86] its impact on the neonatal intestine has not been well-studied, leaving the impact of magnesium sulfate on development of NEC unclear. A similar concern has been raised about indomethacin, a nonsteroidal anti-inflammatory medication that impacts prostaglandin synthesis. Indomethacin is used in the setting of preterm labor for tocolysis to attempt to stall or arrest labor, but its use has been associated with an increased risk of NEC in some retrospective observational studies,[87,88] and in a meta-analysis of 21 observational studies.[89] However, as with magnesium, the causality and mechanisms behind these associations remain unclear and require further investigation.

SUMMARY

NEC remains one of the most significant causes of morbidity and mortality in preterm infants. Although much attention has been paid to neonatal risk factors, there is an increasing interest in understanding ways that the mother may impact an infant's risk of developing NEC. Maternal complications and medication exposures in pregnancy may predispose infants to future intestinal injury and NEC. Given the preliminary associations and findings in animal models, further study is warranted and may help to identify potential targets and therapeutics that can be used prenatally to prevent disease after birth. Although the potential for targeted therapeutics is of interest, the most pragmatic and evidence-based approach at this time to prevent NEC should include the optimization of maternal health to decrease the risks of obstetric complications and subsequent preterm birth. Counseling should begin before pregnancy to optimize maternal health, identify women with an increased risk of giving birth preterm, and encourage women to wait at least 6 months between pregnancies, because shorter interpregnancy intervals have been shown to increase the risk of preterm birth.[90] In addition, prenatal counseling should include the benefits of breastfeeding, because professional breastfeeding education has been shown to increase the rate of breast-feeding initiation and should be part of standard prenatal care.[91] Last, the effective use of antenatal corticosteroids and antibiotics when indicated in the setting of threatened preterm birth should be encouraged. Further study of intrauterine exposures, especially of intrauterine inflammation and infection, preeclampsia, and fetal growth restriction, hold significant promise in furthering our understanding of the etiology of NEC. Future preclinical and clinical studies are critically needed to identify additional prenatal targets that may be of benefit in preventing NEC.

CLINICS CARE POINTS

- NEC risk reduction begins with identifying and managing women at risk of preterm birth.
- Prenatal breastfeeding support and education is a crucial preventive strategy for NEC.
- Antenatal corticosteroids should be administered in the setting of increased risk of preterm birth within 7 days.
- The judicious use of antibiotics in pregnancy and in the neonatal period is warranted with regard to NEC prevention.
- Avoid the use of amoxicillin–clavulanic acid for prophylaxis in the setting of premature rupture of membranes.
- Limit the use of indomethacin for tocolysis when other agents are available, particularly when multiple risk factors for NEC are present.
- A multidisciplinary discussion to identify risk factors before preterm birth may risk stratify infants for NEC.

ACKNOWLEDGMENTS

Figure created using www.Biorender.com.

DISCLOSURE

The authors have nothing to disclose.

REFERENCES

1. Fitzgibbons SC, Ching Y, Yu D, et al. Mortality of necrotizing enterocolitis expressed by birth weight categories. J Pediatr Surg 2009;44(6):1072–6.
2. Neu J, Walker WA. Necrotizing Enterocolitis. N Engl J Med 2011;364(3):255–64.
3. Janevic T, Zeitlin J, Auger N, et al. Association of race/ethnicity with very preterm neonatal morbidities. JAMA Pediatr 2018;172(11):1061–9.
4. Andrews L, Davies TH, Haas J, et al. Necrotizing enterocolitis and its association with the neonatal abstinence syndrome. J Neonatal Perinatal Med 2020; 13(1):81–5.
5. Velazco CS, Fullerton BS, Hong CR, et al. Morbidity and mortality among "big" babies who develop necrotizing enterocolitis: a prospective multicenter cohort analysis. J Pediatr Surg 2017. https://doi.org/10.1016/j.jpedsurg.2017.10.028.

6. Lambert DK, Christensen RD, Henry E, et al. Necrotizing enterocolitis in term neonates: data from a multihospital health-care system. J Perinatol 2007;27(7): 437–43.

7. Christensen RD, Lambert DK, Baer VL, et al. Necrotizing enterocolitis in term infants. Clin Perinatol 2013;40(1):69–78.

8. Patel RM, Ferguson J, McElroy SJ, et al. Defining necrotizing enterocolitis: current difficulties and future opportunities. Pediatr Res 2020;88(Suppl 1):10–5.

9. Lueschow SR, McElroy SJ. The Paneth cell: the curator and defender of the immature small intestine. Front Immunol 2020;11:587.

10. McElroy SJ, Frey MR, Torres BA, Maheshwari A. 72 - Innate and Mucosal Immunity in the Developing Gastrointestinal Tract. In: Gleason CA, Juul SE, eds. Avery's Diseases of the Newborn (Tenth Edition). Philadelphia: Elsevier; 2018:1054-1067.e1055.

11. Frost BL, Modi BP, Jaksic T, et al. New Medical and Surgical Insights Into Neonatal Necrotizing Enterocolitis. JAMA Pediatr 2017;171(1):83.

12. Han SM, Knell J, Henry O, et al. Long-term outcomes of severe surgical necrotizing enterocolitis. J Pediatr Surg 2020;55(5):848–51.

13. Han SM, Hong CR, Knell J, et al. Trends in incidence and outcomes of necrotizing enterocolitis over the last 12years: a multicenter cohort analysis. J Pediatr Surg 2020;55(6):998–1001.

14. Caplan MS, Underwood MA, Modi N, et al. Necrotizing enterocolitis: using regulatory science and drug development to improve outcomes. J Pediatr 2019;212: 208–215 e1.

15. Hackam DJ, Sodhi CP, Good M. New insights into necrotizing enterocolitis: from laboratory observation to personalized prevention and treatment. J Pediatr Surg 2019;54(3):398–404.

16. Nolan LS, Rimer JM, Good M. The role of human milk oligosaccharides and probiotics on the neonatal microbiome and risk of necrotizing enterocolitis: a narrative review. Nutrients 2020;12(10):3052.

17. Elgin TG, Kern SL, McElroy SJ. Development of the neonatal intestinal microbiome and its association with necrotizing enterocolitis. Clin Ther 2016;38(4): 706–15.

18. Underwood MA. Probiotics and the prevention of necrotizing enterocolitis. J Pediatr Surg 2019;54(3):405–12.

19. Alsaied A, Islam N, Thalib L. Global incidence of necrotizing enterocolitis: a systematic review and meta-analysis. BMC Pediatr 2020;20(1):344.

20. Yoon BH, Romero R, Moon JB, et al. Clinical significance of intra-amniotic inflammation in patients with preterm labor and intact membranes. Am J Obstet Gynecol 2001;185(5):1130–6.

21. Kim CJ, Romero R, Chaemsaithong P, et al. Acute chorioamnionitis and funisitis: definition, pathologic features, and clinical significance. Am J Obstet Gynecol 2015;213(4):S29–52.

22. Venkatesh KK, Jackson W, Hughes BL, et al. Association of chorioamnionitis and its duration with neonatal morbidity and mortality. J Perinatol 2019;39(5):673–82.

23. Martinelli P, Sarno L, Maruotti GM, et al. Chorioamnionitis and prematurity: a critical review. J Maternal Fetal Neonatal Med 2012;25(sup4):21–3.

24. Andrews WW, Goldenberg RL, Faye-Petersen O, et al. The Alabama Preterm Birth study: polymorphonuclear and mononuclear cell placental infiltrations, other markers of inflammation, and outcomes in 23- to 32-week preterm newborn infants. Am J Obstet Gynecol 2006;195(3):803–8.

25. Been JV, Lievense S, Zimmermann LJ, et al. Chorioamnionitis as a risk factor for necrotizing enterocolitis: a systematic review and meta-analysis. J Pediatr 2013; 162(2):236–242 e2.
26. March MI, Gupta M, Modest AM, et al. Maternal risk factors for neonatal necrotizing enterocolitis. J Matern Fetal Neonatal Med 2015;28(11):1285–90.
27. Lee J-Y, Park K-H, Kim A, et al. Maternal and placental risk factors for developing necrotizing enterocolitis in very preterm infants. Pediatr Neonatal 2017;58(1): 57–62.
28. Duci M, Frigo AC, Visentin S, et al. Maternal and placental risk factors associated with the development of necrotizing enterocolitis (NEC) and its severity. J Pediatr Surg 2019;54(10):2099–102.
29. Rao SC, Basani L, Simmer K, et al. Peritoneal drainage versus laparotomy as initial surgical treatment for perforated necrotizing enterocolitis or spontaneous intestinal perforation in preterm low birth weight infants. Cochrane Database Syst Rev 2011;6:Cd006182.
30. Fricke EM, Elgin TG, Gong H, et al. Lipopolysaccharide-induced maternal inflammation induces direct placental injury without alteration in placental blood flow and induces a secondary fetal intestinal injury that persists into adulthood. Am J Reprod Immunol 2018;79(5):e12816.
31. Elgin TG, Fricke EM, Gong H, et al. Fetal exposure to maternal inflammation interrupts murine intestinal development and increases susceptibility to neonatal intestinal injury. Dis Models Mech 2019;12(10):dmm040808.
32. Wolfs TG, Kramer BW, Thuijls G, et al. Chorioamnionitis-induced fetal gut injury is mediated by direct gut exposure of inflammatory mediators or by lung inflammation. Am J Physiol Gastrointest Liver Physiol 2014;306(5):G382–93.
33. Wolfs TGAM, Buurman WA, Zoer B, et al. Endotoxin induced chorioamnionitis prevents intestinal development during gestation in fetal sheep. PLoS One 2009;4(6):e5837.
34. Yan X, Managlia E, Tan X-D, et al. Prenatal inflammation impairs intestinal microvascular development through a TNF-dependent mechanism and predisposes newborn mice to necrotizing enterocolitis. Am J Physiol Gastrointestinal Liver Physiol 2019;317(1):G57–66.
35. Lee SE, Romero R, Jung H, et al. The intensity of the fetal inflammatory response in intraamniotic inflammation with and without microbial invasion of the amniotic cavity. Am J Obstet Gynecol 2007;197(3):294.e1-6.
36. Higgins RD, Saade G, Polin RA, et al. Evaluation and management of women and newborns with a maternal diagnosis of chorioamnionitis: summary of a workshop. Obstet Gynecol 2016;127(3):426–36.
37. Jung E, Romero R, Yeo L, et al. The fetal inflammatory response syndrome: the origins of a concept, pathophysiology, diagnosis, and obstetrical implications. Semin Fetal Neonatal Med 2020;101146.
38. Combs CA, Gravett M, Garite TJ, et al. Amniotic fluid infection, inflammation, and colonization in preterm labor with intact membranes. Am J Obstet Gynecol 2014; 210(2):125.e1-.15.
39. Gayen nee' Betal S, Murthy S, Favara M, et al. Histological chorioamnionitis induces differential gene expression in human cord blood mononuclear leukocytes from term neonates. Sci Rep 2019;9(1):5862.
40. Sabic D, Koenig JM. A perfect storm: fetal inflammation and the developing immune system. Pediatr Res 2020;87(2):319–26.
41. Savasan ZA, Chaiworapongsa T, Romero R, et al. Interleukin-19 in fetal systemic inflammation. J Matern Fetal Neonatal Med 2012;25(7):995–1005.

42. Gomez-Lopez N, Romero R, Xu Y, et al. Are amniotic fluid neutrophils in women with intraamniotic infection and/or inflammation of fetal or maternal origin? Am J Obstet Gynecol 2017;217(6):693.e1-16.

43. Rito DC, Viehl LT, Buchanan PM, et al. Augmented Th17-type immune responses in preterm neonates exposed to histologic chorioamnionitis. Pediatr Res 2017; 81(4):639–45.

44. Luciano AA, Yu H, Jackson LW, et al. Preterm labor and chorioamnionitis are associated with neonatal T cell activation. PLoS One 2011;6(2):e16698.

45. Rueda CM, Wells CB, Gisslen T, et al. Effect of chorioamnionitis on regulatory T cells in moderate/late preterm neonates. Hum Immunol 2015;76(1):65–73.

46. Rueda CM, Presicce P, Jackson CM, et al. Lipopolysaccharide-induced chorioamnionitis promotes il-1-dependent inflammatory FOXP3+ CD4+ t cells in the fetal rhesus macaque. J Immunol 2016;196(9):3706–15.

47. Wu WL, Hsiao EY, Yan Z, et al. The placental interleukin-6 signaling controls fetal brain development and behavior. Brain Behav Immun 2017;62:11–23.

48. Franklin AL, Said M, Cappiello CD, et al. Are Immune Modulating Single Nucleotide Polymorphisms Associated with Necrotizing Enterocolitis? Sci Rep 2015;5: 18369.

49. Tian J, Liu Y, Jiang Y, et al. Association of single nucleotide polymorphisms of IL23R and IL17 with necrotizing enterocolitis in premature infants. Mol Cell Biochem 2017;430(1–2):201–9.

50. Cuna A, Sampath V. Genetic alterations in necrotizing enterocolitis. Semin Perinatology 2017;41(1):61–9.

51. Hackam DJ, Sodhi CP. Toll-like receptor-mediated intestinal inflammatory imbalance in the pathogenesis of necrotizing enterocolitis. Cell Mol Gastroenterol Hepatol 2018;6(2):229–38.e1.

52. Vaure C, Liu Y. A comparative review of toll-like receptor 4 expression and functionality in different animal species. Front Immunol 2014;5:316.

53. Heim VJ, Stafford CA, Nachbur U. NOD signaling and cell death. Front Cell Dev Biol 2019;7:208.

54. Sampath V, Bhandari V, Berger J, et al. A functional ATG16L1 (T300A) variant is associated with necrotizing enterocolitis in premature infants. Pediatr Res 2017; 81(4):582–8.

55. Zhou W, Yuan W, Huang L, Wang P, Rong X, Tang J. Association of neonatal necrotizing enterocolitis with myeloid differentiation-2 and GM2 activator protein genetic polymorphisms. Mol Med Rep 2015;12(1):974–80.

56. Sampath V, Menden H, Helbling D, et al. SIGIRR genetic variants in premature infants with necrotizing enterocolitis. Pediatrics 2015;135(6):e1530–4.

57. Sampath V, Mulrooney N, Patel AL, et al. A potential role for the NOD1 variant (rs6958571) in gram-positive blood stream infection in ELBW infants. Neonatology 2017;112(4):354–8.

58. Hartel C, Hartz A, Pagel J, et al. NOD2 loss-of-function mutations and risks of necrotizing enterocolitis or focal intestinal perforation in very low-birth-weight infants. Inflamm Bowel Dis 2016;22(2):249–56.

59. Frey HA, Klebanoff MA. The epidemiology, etiology, and costs of preterm birth. Semin Fetal Neonatal Med 2016;21(2):68–73.

60. Ahle M, Drott P, Elfvin A, et al. Maternal, fetal and perinatal factors associated with necrotizing enterocolitis in Sweden. A national case-control study. PLoS One 2018;13(3):e0194352.

61. Barros FC, Papageorghiou AT, Victora CG, et al. The distribution of clinical phenotypes of preterm birth syndrome implications for prevention. JAMA Pediatr 2015;169(3):220–9.
62. Garite TJ, Clark R, Thorp JA. Intrauterine growth restriction increases morbidity and mortality among premature neonates. Am J Obstet Gynecol 2004;191(2): 481–7.
63. Martins JG, Biggio JR, Abuhamad A. Society for maternal-fetal medicine consult series #52: diagnosis and management of fetal growth restriction: (replaces clinical guideline number 3, April 2012). Am J Obstet Gynecol 2020;223(4):B2–17.
64. Hackett GA, Campbell S, Gamsu H, et al. Doppler studies in the growth retarded fetus and prediction of neonatal necrotising enterocolitis, haemorrhage, and neonatal morbidity. Br Med J (Clin Res Ed 1987;294(6563):13–6.
65. Malcolm G, Ellwood D, Devonald K, et al. Absent or reversed end diastolic flow velocity in the umbilical artery and necrotising enterocolitis. Arch Dis Child 1991; 66(7 Spec No):805–7.
66. Kamoji VM, Dorling JS, Manktelow B, et al. Antenatal umbilical Doppler abnormalities: an independent risk factor for early onset neonatal necrotizing enterocolitis in premature infants. Acta Paediatr 2008;97(3):327–31.
67. Cetinkaya M, Ozkan H, Koksal N. Maternal preeclampsia is associated with increased risk of necrotizing enterocolitis in preterm infants. Early Hum Dev 2012;88(11):893–8.
68. Perger L, Mukhopadhyay D, Komidar L, et al. Maternal pre-eclampsia as a risk factor for necrotizing enterocolitis. J Matern Fetal Neonatal Med 2015;29(13): 2098–103.
69. Yang C-C, Tang P-L, Liu P-Y, et al. Maternal pregnancy-induced hypertension increases subsequent neonatal necrotizing enterocolitis risk. Medicine 2018; 97(31):e11739.
70. Bossung V, Fortmann MI, Fusch C, et al. Neonatal outcome after preeclampsia and HELLP syndrome: a population-based cohort study in Germany. Front Pediatr 2020;8(666):579293.
71. Fung CM, White JR, Brown AS, et al. Intrauterine growth restriction alters mouse intestinal architecture during development. PLoS One 2016;11(1):e0146542.
72. Bauer CR, Morrison JC, Poole WK, et al. A decreased incidence of necrotizing enterocolitis after prenatal glucocorticoid therapy. Pediatrics 1984;73(5):682–8.
73. Roberts D, Brown J, Medley N, et al. Antenatal corticosteroids for accelerating fetal lung maturation for women at risk of preterm birth. Cochrane Database Syst Rev 2017;(3):CD004454.
74. Israel EJ, Schiffrin EJ, Carter EA, et al. Prevention of necrotizing enterocolitis in the rat with prenatal cortisone. Gastroenterology 1990;99(5):1333–8.
75. Mercer BM, Miodovnik M, Thurnau GR, et al. Antibiotic therapy for reduction of infant morbidity after preterm premature rupture of the membranes: a randomized controlled trial. JAMA 1997;278(12):989–95.
76. Reed BD, Schibler KR, Deshmukh H, et al. The Impact of Maternal Antibiotics on Neonatal Disease. J Pediatr 2018;197:97–103.e3.
77. Kenyon SL, Taylor DJ, Tarnow-Mordi W. Broad-spectrum antibiotics for spontaneous preterm labour: the ORACLE II randomised trial. The Lancet 2001; 357(9261):989–94.
78. Weintraub AS, Ferrara L, Deluca L, et al. Antenatal antibiotic exposure in preterm infants with necrotizing enterocolitis. J Perinatology 2012;32(9):705–9.
79. Ehsanipoor RM, Chung JH, Clock CA, et al. A retrospective review of ampicillin-sulbactam and amoxicillin + clavulanate vs cefazolin/cephalexin and

erythromycin in the setting of preterm premature rupture of membranes: maternal and neonatal outcomes. Am J Obstet Gynecol 2008;198(5):e54–6.

80. Al-Sabbagh A, Moss S, Subhedar N. Neonatal necrotising enterocolitis and perinatal exposure to co-amoxyclav. Arch Dis Child Fetal Neonatal Ed 2004;89(2): F187.

81. Prelabor rupture of membranes: ACOG Practice Bulletin, Number 217. Obstet Gynecol 2020;135(3):e80–97.

82. Kamyar M, Clark EAS, Yoder BA, et al. Antenatal magnesium sulfate, necrotizing enterocolitis, and death among neonates < 28 weeks gestation. AJP Rep 2016; 6(1):e148–54.

83. Hong JY, Hong JY, Choi Y-S, et al. Antenatal magnesium sulfate treatment and risk of necrotizing enterocolitis in preterm infants born at less than 32 weeks of gestation. Sci Rep 2020;10(1):12826.

84. Mikhael M, Bronson C, Zhang L, et al. Lack of evidence for time or dose relationship between antenatal magnesium sulfate and intestinal injury in extremely preterm neonates. Neonatology 2019;115(4):371–8.

85. Li W, Wu X, Yu J, et al. Magnesium sulfate attenuates lipopolysaccharides-induced acute lung injury in mice. Chin J Physiol 2019;62(5):203–9.

86. Khatib N, Ginsberg Y, Shalom-Paz E, et al. Fetal neuroprotective mechanism of maternal magnesium sulfate for late gestation inflammation: in a rodent model. J Matern Fetal Neonatal Med 2020;33(22):3732–9.

87. Sood BG, Lulic-Botica M, Holzhausen KA, et al. The risk of necrotizing enterocolitis after indomethacin tocolysis. Pediatrics 2011;128(1):e54–62.

88. Rovers JFJ, Thomissen IJC, Janssen LCE, et al. The relationship between antenatal indomethacin as a tocolytic drug and neonatal outcomes: a retrospective cohort study. J Matern Fetal Neonatal Med 2019;9:1–7.

89. Hammers AL, Sanchez-Ramos L, Kaunitz AM. Antenatal exposure to indomethacin increases the risk of severe intraventricular hemorrhage, necrotizing enterocolitis, and periventricular leukomalacia: a systematic review with metaanalysis. Am J Obstet Gynecol 2015;212(4):505.e1-13.

90. Conde-Agudelo A, Rosas-Bermúdez A, Kafury-Goeta AC. Birth spacing and risk of adverse perinatal outcomes: a meta-analysis. JAMA 2006;295(15):1809–23.

91. Balogun OO, O'Sullivan EJ, McFadden A, et al. Interventions for promoting the initiation of breastfeeding. Cochrane Database Syst Rev 2016;(11):CD001688.

Post-infection Irritable Bowel Syndrome

Antonio Berumen, MD[a], Adam L. Edwinson, PhD[a], Madhusudan Grover, MD[a,b],*

KEYWORDS

- Infectious gastroenteritis • Diarrhea • Inflammation • Bacteria • Gut-brain axis
- Microbiome • Barrier function

KEY POINTS

- Acute infectious gastroenteritis is a strong risk factor for development of irritable bowel syndrome (IBS). Approximately, 90% of post-infection IBS (PI-IBS) is either mixed or diarrhea predominant.
- Younger age, female sex, infection severity, and psychological distress are associated with greater risk of PI-IBS. Risk also varies with pathogen type, protozoal having the highest prevalence, followed by bacterial, and lastly viral.
- Key pathophysiologic mechanisms in PI-IBS include microbial dysbiosis, mucosal barrier dysfunction, immune dysregulation, and neuronal hypersensitivity.
- Although some treatment strategies, such as mesalamine, corticosteroids, and glutamine, have been tested specifically for PI-IBS, current management recommendations for PI-IBS are extrapolated from routine IBS.

INTRODUCTION

With a worldwide prevalence ranging between 7% and 21%, irritable bowel syndrome (IBS) is one of the most commonly diagnosed gastrointestinal (GI) conditions.[1] It is characterized by chronic abdominal pain associated with bowel disturbances such as diarrhea, constipation, or both. Although the cause of IBS remains to be fully clarified, the heterogeneous pathophysiology involves peripheral (gut) and central (spinal, supraspinal) factors operating in a bidirectional manner. Growing literature has provided a deeper understanding of the alterations involving the mucosal barrier, immune function, gut microbiota, and enteroendocrine and visceral sensorimotor function.[2] In addition, genetics and environment (diet, infections, and psychosocial factors) seem to play a role in the predisposition and manifestations of IBS.[3,4]

[a] Division of Gastroenterology and Hepatology, Mayo Clinic, Rochester, MN 55905, USA;
[b] Department of Medicine and Physiology, Enteric NeuroScience Program, 200 First Street Southwest, Rochester, MN 55905, USA
* Corresponding author. Department of Medicine and Physiology, Enteric NeuroScience Program, 200 First Street Southwest, Rochester, MN 55905.
E-mail address: grover.madhusudan@mayo.edu

Gastroenterol Clin N Am 50 (2021) 445–461
https://doi.org/10.1016/j.gtc.2021.02.007
0889-8553/21/© 2021 Elsevier Inc. All rights reserved.

gastro.theclinics.com

Acute infectious gastroenteritis (bacterial, viral, and protozoal) has been shown to be one of the strongest risk factors for development of IBS,[5] a condition referred to as post-infection IBS (PI-IBS). Although described in literature on medical diseases of the war in 1917,[6] the first formal description of PI-IBS was made in 1962 by Chaudhary and Truelove.[7] Every year, 1 in 6 adults experience an episode of foodborne illness in the United States, placing a great number of individuals at risk of developing PI-IBS.[8] Conservative estimates through mathematical modeling suggest that PI-IBS prevalence in the community could be 9%, accounting for more than half the overall prevalence of IBS in the United States.[9]

DIAGNOSIS

Recently, the Rome Foundation Working Group proposed diagnostic criteria for PI-IBS based on Rome IV criteria (**Box 1**).[1] The symptoms typically develop immediately after resolution of acute infectious gastroenteritis. The gastroenteritis episode can be diagnosed either by a positive stool culture or clinically by the presence of greater than or equal to 2 of fever, vomiting, or diarrhea.[10] In order to aid diagnosis and management, PI-IBS is further classified into 4 subtypes by the predominant bowel pattern graded on the Bristol Stool Scale: diarrhea-predominant IBS (IBS-D), constipation-predominant (IBS-C), mixed bowel habits (IBS-M), and unclassified (IBS-U). A bowel pattern is considered predominant when it is present greater than or equal to one-quarter of the time as either hard/lumpy (IBS-C), loose/watery (IBS-D), or both (IBS-M). In a recent meta-analysis of studies from 1994 to 2015 including more than 21,000 patients that had an episode of infectious enteritis, IBS-M and IBS-D were the most common phenotypes, accounting for 46% and 40% of the cases, respectively.[5]

The burden of chronic GI symptoms post-infection may even be greater than what is captured by the Rome criteria. In a recent study, the authors showed that, in addition to 21% prevalence of PI-IBS following campylobacter enteritis, an additional 9% had new-onset abdominal pain, bowel disturbances, or both, without meeting the Rome criteria for IBS.[11] In addition to the development of new-onset IBS, a GI infection can also result in changes in preexisting IBS phenotype. Approximately 50% of IBS-C switched to either IBS-M or IBS-D after an episode of campylobacter enteritis

---

Box 1

Diagnostic criteria for post-infection irritable bowel syndrome based on Rome IV

1. Recurrent abdominal pain, on average, at least 1 d/wk in the last 3 months, with symptom onset at least 6 months before diagnosis, associated with 2 or more of the following[a]:
   a. Related to defecation
   b. A change in frequency of stool
   c. A change in form (appearance) of stool

Supportive criteria
1. Infectious gastroenteritis defined by either:
   a. A positive culture in a symptomatic individual
   b. Presence of at least 2 of the following acute symptoms: fever, vomiting, and diarrhea
2. Should not meet criteria for IBS before onset of acute illness
3. Symptom development either immediately after resolution of acute infectious gastroenteritis or within 30 days of resolution of acute symptoms

[a] Criteria fulfilled for the last 3 months with symptom onset at least 6 months before diagnosis.

in our study.[11] It is unclear whether the infection is causative in this switch because IBS subtypes have been known to switch over time.[12] Furthermore, 38% of the patients showed an increase in pain frequency post-infection.[11] Overall, these data suggest that GI infections can result in new onset of chronic GI symptoms as well as changes in preexisting chronic GI symptoms.

DIFFERENTIAL DIAGNOSIS

The diagnosis of PI-IBS should be primarily based on the clinical features, reserving diagnostic tests for when alarm features for an organic disease are present.[1] A positive diagnostic approach, rather than by exclusion, has been shown to reduce health care costs while increasing patient satisfaction.[13] Limited diagnostic testing, including complete blood count, C-reactive protein, celiac serology, and fecal calprotectin, may be considered based on clinical suspicion.[14]

Small intestinal bacterial overgrowth (SIBO) is a condition where an excessive growth of microorganisms occurs in the small intestine. Patients present with a variety of symptoms, including bloating, flatulence, abdominal discomfort, and diarrhea. It can be diagnosed with a jejunal aspirate showing more than 1×10^3 colony-forming units per milliliter or with carbohydrate breath testing. Patients with IBS have 3 times higher odds for SIBO than healthy individuals, as shown in 2 meta-analyses.[15,16] However, the prevalence of SIBO in PI-IBS is unknown and routine testing for SIBO in PI-IBS is not recommended. Tropical sprue also shares similarities with PI-IBS and is triggered by a GI infection.[17] In contrast with PI-IBS, enteropathy in tropical sprue predominantly involves the small bowel and results in malabsorption of carbohydrates, fat, folate, and vitamin B_{12}, which can be tested using specific assays (D-xylose, fecal fat, and vitamin B_{12} level), and enteropathy confirmed with histologic findings in a duodenal biopsy.[18] Interestingly, in the last 20 years, reports on tropical sprue have decreased, whereas they have increased for PI-IBS.[19] Given the similarities, some have hypothesized that, in certain geographic settings, these might reflect the spectrum of a disease process initiated by an infectious insult.[20] Prevalence of *Giardia* in PI-IBS ranged from 38% to 80%, although only 1 of the studies confirmed eradication.[21–23] Symptoms of giardiasis such as diarrhea, abdominal cramps, and flatulence can mimic those of PI-IBS. These symptoms are often caused by lactose malabsorption.[24] Hence, chronic giardiasis should be excluded in patients with suspected *Giardia* PI-IBS.

Celiac disease can have a clinical picture similar to PI-IBS. In a recent meta-analysis of 36 studies, patients with suspected IBS, regardless of the subtype, had 3 to 4 times the odds of having a positive celiac disease test (serologic or histologic) compared with asymptomatic individuals.[14] Another condition with potential overlap of symptoms with PI-IBS is microscopic colitis. A recent systematic review showed that, in individuals meeting criteria for IBS-D, the prevalence of microscopic colitis is 10%.[25] As of yet, no specific studies for PI-IBS exist, but, given the high prevalence of the diarrhea subtype in PI-IBS, it is an important differential diagnosis to take into consideration.[26] However, microscopic colitis usually presents at ages older than 50 years, whereas the rate of PI-IBS is higher in younger people. In addition, patients with microscopic colitis have painless chronic watery diarrhea (commonly with a Bristol Stool Scale score ≥ 6), whereas PI-IBS is accompanied by abdominal pain and Bristol Stool Scale score of 4 to 5. Random colonic biopsies may be warranted to diagnose microscopic colitis when clinical suspicion is high. According to a study that evaluated colonic biopsies in patients with non–IBS-C, the presence of inflammatory bowel disease (IBD) was 0.4%, similar to healthy controls.[27] However, acute enterocolitis has been associated with an increased risk of IBD. One study reported a hazard ratio of 1.9 in the first year after a salmonella or campylobacter infection, which increased to 2.9 over 7.5 years of follow-up.[28] Another study showed an odds ratio of 1.4 for development of IBD after an infectious enteritis (viral, bacterial, and protozoal). Risk was 5 times higher in patients with a preexisting IBS.[29] The authors do not recommend routine work-up for exclusion of IBD unless there are suggestive symptoms, such as weight loss, GI bleeding, fever, or tenesmus. The diagnostic approach for PI-IBS is outlined in **Fig. 1**.

EPIDEMIOLOGY AND NATURAL HISTORY

Viral (Norovirus, Rotavirus),[30,31] bacterial (*Campylobacter, Salmonella, Escherichia coli, Shigella, Clostridium difficile*),[11,32–35] and protozoal (*Giardia*)[21–23] enterocolitis have been associated with PI-IBS with varying degrees of risk. In our meta-analysis, the overall point prevalences of PI-IBS in studies of 12 months and greater than 12 months post-infection were 10% and 15%, respectively (**Fig. 2**).[5] Exposed individuals were 4.2 times more likely to develop PI-IBS than unexposed individuals within 12 months of infection. Risk decreased beyond 12 months; however, it remained significantly higher compared with individuals without history of infection.[5] There was no significant difference in prevalence comparing Rome I, II, and III.[5] None of the studies included have used Rome IV thus far, which may result in lower prevalence, as noted with general IBS.[36] It is hypothesized that, because of the high incidence of infectious gastroenteritis and poor recall of milder episodes, the true prevalence of PI-IBS may be underestimated.[10] Comparing different pathogens, protozoal enteritis shows the highest risk for PI-IBS development, followed by bacterial, and, lastly, viral. The significant decrease in PI-IBS prevalence from 19% to 4% 1 year after viral infection may be caused by the less invasive nature of the pathogen, perhaps avoiding a stronger host response.[5] Pathogen-based risk over time is summarized in **Fig. 2**.

Demographic, psychological, and clinical factors related to the acute infection have been associated with PI-IBS risk. Female and younger patients are more likely to develop PI-IBS.[5] Higher anxiety, depression, somatization, and neuroticism scores preceding or during acute enteritis increase the risk, possibly by altering host or pathogen responses.[5] Clinical characteristics of the acute enterocolitis, such as longer duration of diarrhea, presence of bloody stools, abdominal cramps, and hospitalization, significantly increase the risk.[4,5,11] Fever was not observed to be a risk factor.[5] In fact, our study showed that it might be protective,[11] possibly reflecting a protective host response to the injury. Antibiotic use has been shown to be a risk factor; however, most of those studies are from outside the United States where the overall use of antibiotics was considerably lower (5%–14%),[37,38] perhaps representing a bias between health care seeking and subsequent PI-IBS. In other studies, including those from the United States, where antibiotic use is higher (47%–77%), no association with PI-IBS risk was seen.[11,39] Understanding and modeling these clinical risk factors may allow identification of high-risk cohorts that are most suitable for strategies to prevent PI-IBS development.

Functional dyspepsia (FD) is another common functional GI disorder that causes epigastric pain, postprandial fullness, and early satiety. Its development after infectious gastroenteritis has been reported,[40] with a prevalence of ~9% and a relative risk (RR) of 2.5 in a systematic review of 19 studies.[41] An overlap between PI-IBS and PI-FD can exist, as shown after giardiasis, where 26% developed PI-FD, 85% of whom also met criteria for PI-IBS.[42]

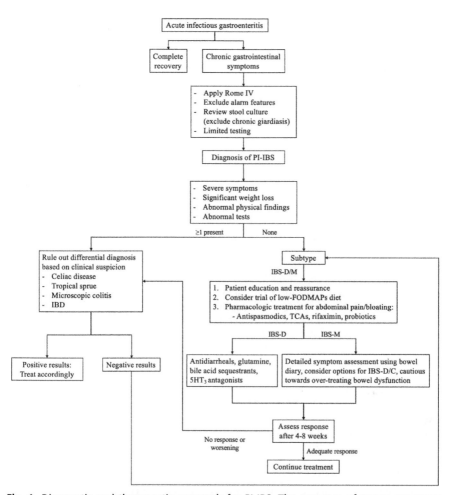

Fig. 1. Diagnostic and therapeutic approach for PI-IBS. The presence of severe symptoms, significant weight loss, or abnormal physical findings or testing when diagnosing PI-IBS, as well as lack of treatment response after 4 to 8 weeks, warrants considering for other causes. Further diagnostic tests should be selected based on clinical suspicion. Pharmacologic treatment recommendations include focus on IBS-M and IBS-D, which account for most patients with PI-IBS. Antispasmodics (peppermint oil, dicyclomine, hyoscine, pinaverium), tricyclic antidepressants (TCAs) (amitriptyline, imipramine, desipramine), probiotics (*Bifidobacterium* sp, *Lactobacillus plantarum*), antidiarrheals (loperamide, eluxadoline), bile acid sequestrants (cholestyramine, colesevelam, colestipol), and 5-hydroxytryptamine type 3 ($5HT_3$) antagonists (ondansetron, alosetron, ramosetron). In the case of IBS-C, the treatment recommendations for the altered bowel habit are soluble fibers (psyllium), osmotic laxatives (polyethylene glycol, lactulose), and intestinal secretagogues (linaclotide, lubiprostone, plecanatide). FODMAP, fermentable oligosaccharides, disaccharides, monosaccharides, and polyols. (*Modified from* Barbara G, Grover M, Bercik P, et al. Rome Foundation working team report on post-infection irritable bowel syndrome. Gastroenterology 2019;156:46-58 e7.)

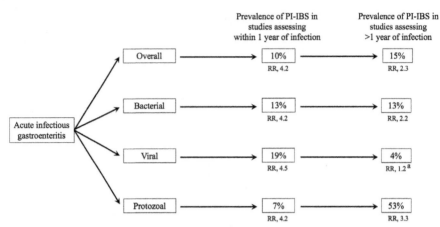

Fig. 2. Natural history of PI-IBS. Within 1 year after an acute gastrointestinal infection (bacterial, viral, parasitic, and overall), there is a 4-fold increase in risk for development of IBS compared with nonexposed individuals. Risk decreases beyond 1 year of infection but remains significantly increased, except in viral enteritis. [a]Nonsignificant. Relative risk (RR) is compared with unexposed derived from same population. Not all studies had unexposed controls; hence, prevalence and RR estimates are not from completely overlapping studies. (*Data from* Klem F, Wadhwa A, Prokop LJ, et al. Prevalence, risk factors, and outcomes of irritable bowel syndrome after infectious enteritis: A systematic review and meta-analysis. Gastroenterology 2017;152:1042-54 e1.)

PATHOPHYSIOLOGY

Next, this article highlights changes in the gut microbiome, epithelium, and neuronal excitation that have been either shown or postulated to play a role in PI-IBS pathophysiology (**Fig. 3**).

Gut Microbiome

A healthy microbiome, although difficult to characterize, is an interconnected community that serves a wide array of functions in the gut, including digestion and production of valuable nutrients, shaping host immunity, xenobiotic metabolism, and protection from pathogens and exogenous antigens. The microbiome is resilient to external stressors such as GI infection, antibiotic exposure, and dietary changes.[43] Firmicutes, Bacteroidetes, and Actinobacteria are the dominant microbial taxa; however, in infectious enteritis and subsequently in PI-IBS, significant disruption to the core microbiome has been shown.[44] Patients with PI-IBS showed a 12-fold increase in Bacteroidetes, and decrease in Firmicutes and Clostridiales, compared with healthy individuals.[45] Patients with travelers' diarrhea also showed a decrease in the Firmicutes/Bacteroidetes ratio and changes in β diversity compared with healthy controls.[46] Similarly, studies from both The United Kingdom and Sweden found a significant increase in *Bacteroides* and decrease in *Clostridiales*.[47,48] Moreover, an individual's susceptibility to developing acute infection as well as PI-IBS may also depend on microbiota composition before infection. In abattoir workers, increased abundance of *Bacteroides* in preemployment stool samples predicted a greater risk of *Campylobacter jejuni* infection during employment.[49] Further work needs to be done to understand how the microbiome before infection may shift after acute gastroenteritis and whether it can serve as a biomarker or predictor for PI-IBS development.

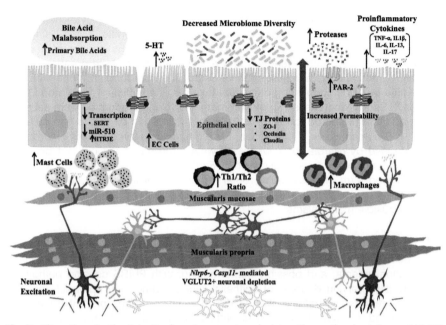

Fig. 3. Alterations in the intestinal environment underlying the pathophysiology of PI-IBS. The development of PI-IBS after acute infectious enterocolitis may be caused by several changes in intestinal microbiome or mucosal, immune, or neuronal function. Microbiota changes include decreased diversity and increased Firmicutes/Bacteroides ratio. These changes may affect luminal milieu by altering composition of bile acids, bile salts, and proteases. Epithelial changes, such as increased density of enteroendocrine cells and increased serotonin availability may increase intestinal motility. An altered mucosal barrier function can contribute to immune dysregulation and neuronal hypersensitivity. Furthermore, immunophenotypic changes, such as increased mast cell density, increased T-helper (Th) 1/Th2 cell ratio, and expression of proinflammatory cytokines, can mediate chronic gut dysfunction as well as neuronal excitability. Lastly, inflammasome-mediated depletion of neurons and nervous remodeling can affect motility and secretion. 5-HT, 5-hydroxytryptamine; EC, enterochromaffin; HTRE3E, 5-hydroxytryptamine receptor 3E; IL, interleukin; PAR-2, protease activated receptor-2; SERT, serotonin transporter; TJ, tight junction; TNF-α, tumor necrosis factor alpha; VGLUT2, vesicular glutamate transporter 2; ZO-1, zonula occludens-1.

An example of how microbiota changes may influence host physiology is by altering the intestinal protease milieu. Proteases are important mediators of intestinal barrier dysfunction and visceral hypersensitivity, both robustly associated with IBS.[50,51] Higher fecal proteolytic activity (PA) associates with greater symptom severity and lower microbial diversity in patients with C jejuni PI-IBS.[52] Moreover, microbiota changes can also mediate changes in bile salts as well as cause bile acid malabsorption in patients with PI-IBS, which can induce diarrhea.[53] These observations highlight some plausible mechanisms by which changes in intestinal microbiome can mediate the pathophysiology of PI-IBS.

One of the most commonly used models is inducing *Trichinella spiralis* infection in rodents. Many of the pathophysiologic mechanisms associated with PI-IBS in humans, such as immune dysfunction,[54–56] hypersensitivity,[57] and changes in colonic motility,[58] have been shown in this model. *Lactobacillus* and *Bifidobacterium* administration caused a reduction in visceral sensitivity, an increase in tight junction protein expression, and suppression of proinflammatory cytokines (interleukin [IL]-6 and IL-17) compared with control treated animals.[54,55,59] Using the same model, daily fecal microbial transplant (FMT) over the course of a week resulted in improved barrier function and a higher pain threshold compared with controls.[60] Interestingly, administration of *Bifidobacterium longum* alone was just as effective as FMT, suggesting individual taxa may be sufficient for restoring gut function.[60] Similar decreases in proinflammatory cytokine production were seen after the addition of *Lactobacillus* in both ileum and colonic ex vivo organ cultures from PI-IBS human tissue.[61] In addition, FMT in humans proved effective in treating PI-IBS caused by *Giardia* for 7 weeks; however, the effect did not last because symptoms recurred at 1-year follow-up.[62] Further studies investigating the short-term and long-term efficacy of microbial replenishment in PI-IBS are needed to determine the specific taxa or consortium of taxa that can induce an effect as well as plausible mechanisms.

Epithelial Changes

Acute gastroenteritis has immediate effects on the intestinal epithelium, such as inflammation, edema, and possibly hemorrhaging, with PI-IBS causing pathogens known to illicit varying degrees of epithelial injury.[10] Long-term epithelial changes have been reported in patients with PI-IBS. Small noncoding, microRNA-510 was downregulated in mucosal biopsies of patients with PI-IBS, which correlated with increased proinflammatory cytokine levels.[63] Gene expression changes have been seen in the serotonin reuptake transporter (SERT), a critical transporter for the metabolism of serotonin (5-HT), with patients with PI-IBS having significantly lower expression, which increases luminal availability of 5-HT[64] where stimulation of 5-HT receptors on nerve endings by ligands triggers neural stimuli. Experimental PI-IBS rats administered *Lactobacillus rhamnosus* supernatant had an increase in colonic SERT messenger RNA and protein expression, indicating microbial modulation can restore serotonergic imbalance.[65] Enterochromaffin (EC) cells release 5-HT and have chemosensory and mechanosensory roles. In both *Shigella* and *Campylobacter* PI-IBS, there is an increase in density of colonic EC cells (up to 25%).[66–68] In contrast, patients with post-*Giardia* IBS had lower EC cell counts compared with controls but increased cholecystokinin immunoreactive enteroendocrine cells.[69] Patients with *Shigella* PI-IBS also have increased ileal and rectal IL-1β expression, as well as ileal mast cell infiltration.[70] In cases of PI-IBS attributable to viral infection, the effect on the GI epithelium remains less clear.

Mucosal permeability

Four human studies assessing intestinal permeability found evidence of greater permeability in PI-IBS.[67,71–73] One study showed 5 of 10 patients with *Campylobacter* PI-IBS had increased permeability[67]; however, a much larger study from the Walkerton outbreak reported an increase in permeability in only 16% of the patients with PI-IBS studied.[72] Epithelial barrier integrity depends on cell-to-cell adhesion, which is regulated by the presence of tight junctions. Genetic variations in E-cadherin (*CDH1*) were associated with PI-IBS risk in the Walkerton cohort.[3] In rodent models, barrier disruption and bacterial translocation correlated with occludin and claudin-4 degradation, along with decreased zona occludens and increased myosin light chain kinase (MLCK) expression, a mediator of barrier dysfunction.[74,75] Moreover, patients with PI-IBS with high fecal PA have shown increased in vivo and ex vivo distal gut permeability, which depended on the level of fecal PA.[52]

Immune responses

Acute infectious gastroenteritis results in the recruitment of immune cells to the gut. Cytokines IL-1β, IL-10, IL-13, and interferon gamma (IFNγ) are increased in patients with PI-IBS compared with controls long after acute infection.[70,76,77] Compared with healthy controls, colonic biopsies from patients with PI-IBS release proinflammatory cytokines when exposed to commensal bacteria ex vivo.[76] This observation suggests colonic mucosa from PI-IBS may inappropriately respond to commensal bacteria, thereby creating a milieu of prolonged immune dysregulation. Mast cells, macrophages, and monocytes[34,67] along with T lymphocytes and intraepithelial lymphocytes (IEL) have all been found to be increased in PI-IBS up to 5 years after infection.[66,67] Colonic supernatants from patients with PI-IBS can activate mast cells, which are an established mediator of visceral hypersensitivity in IBS.[78,79] Unspecified infections resulting in PI-IBS have reported an increase in EC and T cells, but no changes in IEL cells.[66] Significantly increased proportions of cluster of differentiation (CD) 4+ T cells and double-positive CD4/CD8+ cells have been reported in the lamina propria of mucosal biopsies from patients with PI-IBS.[80] CD3+ and CD8+ lymphocytes, IELs, and CD68+ macrophages are increased in patients with *Shigella* PI-IBS compared with controls as well.[68]

Patients with PI-IBS seem to have a shift in the T-helper (Th) response with an increased ratio of Th1/Th2 with increased IFNγ and decreased IL-10 levels, respectively.[77] In a perpetual state of disequilibrium, increased Th1 cells may mediate pain through effects on intestinal permeability. In a PI-IBS mouse model, inhibition of MLCK caused significant decreases in the production of Th1 cytokines, decreased visceral hypersensitivity, and restoration of intestinal barrier function, suggesting a mechanistic link between barrier and sensory dysfunction.[75] In contrast, some studies have found no differences in mast cell or IEL counts in PI-IBS cases compared with control biopsies.[64,79] This finding indicates that more needs to be done to understand immune dysfunction in PI-IBS beyond simplistic assessment of cell counts.

Neuronal Activation

Commensal microbes as well as enteric pathogens have been shown to influence the excitability of enteric-associated neurons (EANs), neurons critical for monitoring and maintaining homeostasis within the gut by facilitating nutrient absorption and colonic motility,[81] as well as the activation of immune cells.[82] A recent study showed that, through NLRP6 inflammasome and caspase 11 activation, acute infections in mice caused a 20% to 30% reduction in intrinsic ileocolonic EANs 7 days after infection, with neuronal loss persisting up to 126 days after infection. This finding was associated with delayed intestinal transit time.[83] This loss was only seen for the excitatory vesicular glutamate transporter (VGLUT2+) neurons and not for the neuronal nitric oxide synthase (nNOS) or somatostatin-positive inhibitory neurons. Interestingly, restoration of a healthy microbiome in these mice resulted in the recovery of EANs; however, it was not reported whether transit time normalized. In addition, *B longum* has recently been shown to reduce visceral hypersensitivity in mice infected with *T spiralis* by specifically inhibiting the NLRP3 inflammasome.[84] Extensive nerve remodeling was reported in rats infected with *Nippostrongylus brasiliensis*,[85] accompanied by recruitment and activation of mast cells.[86] Activated mast cells surrounding nerve fibers in the ileum have been reported in patients with PI-IBS,[70] and released tryptase can mediate neuronal excitation through cleavage of protease-activated receptor-2 (PAR-2).[87] Activation of PAR-2 is known to increase permeability and visceral sensitivity.[51] In a mouse model of PI-IBS, visceral hypersensitivity was reduced after the administration of a PAR-2 antagonist.[88] This finding is further supported by the observation that excitability of dorsal root ganglion neurons is absent in PAR-2 knockout mice after incubation with colonic supernatants from patients with IBS-D.[89] A pro-nociceptive change was reported in the rectal biopsies of patients with PI-IBS as a result of sensitization of the ion channel, transient receptor potential vanilloid 1 (TRPV1). Submucosal neuronal activation was significantly increased in patients with PI-IBS compared with healthy controls, even 2 years after initial infection was cleared.[90] Recently, EphrinB2/ephB2 receptor tyrosine kinase, an enzyme important for regulating neuronal activation and excitation, was found to be upregulated in the colonic muscularis of rats infected with *T spiralis*. Colonic hypersensitivity and hypercontractility were ameliorated on administration of ephB2Fc, an ephB2 blocker, indicating a critical role for ephrinB2/ephB2 signaling in facilitating neuronal maturation and potentiation in the gut.[91]

MANAGEMENT

Currently, treatment options for PI-IBS are limited, with no specific US Food and Drug Administration–approved agents. Therefore, current management strategies of PI-IBS are based on expert opinion. As with IBS in general, treatment should be guided based on phenotype and predominant symptoms.[10]

Patient Education and Reassurance

Effective doctor-patient relationship and communication are essential in the management of PI-IBS. The first step involves educating the patients about the link between the infection and the development of chronic GI symptoms. Patients should be reassured that PI-IBS tends to have a more benign course and symptoms tend to improve and sometimes disappear over time in many patients, especially when the cause is viral.[5,92]

Dietary Modifications

Given that a large proportion of patients with PI-IBS have IBS-D or IBS-M, a reasonable initial approach is a trial of 4 to 8 weeks of low fermentable oligosaccharides, disaccharides, monosaccharides, and polyols (FODMAPs), because it has been shown to improve symptoms in IBS-D.[93] A gluten-free diet in patients with IBS without celiac disease has not been found to be effective. However, 1 randomized controlled trial showed that reintroduction of gluten led to rebound of symptoms in patients with IBS previously symptomatically controlled on a gluten-free diet.[94] Given that wheat contains fructans, which are oligosaccharides, a trial comparing gluten-free with a low-FODMAPs diet alone found no difference in response, suggesting that the benefit from the gluten-free diet is likely caused by the lower ingestion of oligosaccharides.[95]

Pharmacologic Agents

A summary of recommended pharmacologic treatments is included in **Fig. 1**. One of the few treatment strategies that has been tested specifically for PI-IBS is glutamine. A randomized controlled trial studying patients with PI-IBS-D with increased in vivo intestinal permeability found 80% of patients reporting a greater than or equal to 50-point reduction in the IBS symptom severity score, compared with only 6% in the placebo group. Other significant findings were an improvement of bowel movement frequency and consistency, as well as a normalization of intestinal permeability.[96] If replicated, this could serve as a key therapeutic option for patients with PI-IBS. A randomized, placebo-controlled trial of mesalazine 4 g/d showed no benefit in symptom relief of patients with IBS-D. However, in a small subgroup that met criteria for PI-IBS (n = 13), a significant improvement in abdominal pain, urgency, and stool consistency was observed.[97] In another double-blind controlled trial including 17 patients with diarrhea-predominant PI-IBS, mesalamine failed to show improvement of symptoms and quality of life.[98] However, in an uncontrolled study evaluating 389 patients affected in a large outbreak of hemorrhagic enterocolitis by Shiga-like toxin–producing E coli in Germany, the use of mesalazine intended to reduce intestinal inflammation during the acute infection seemed to significantly protect against PI-IBS development.[99] A randomized controlled trial of prednisone focused primarily on evaluating changes in rectal biopsies in PI-IBS observed a significant reduction of T-lymphocyte counts; however, no changes were observed in EC count and overall symptom improvement.[100]

SUMMARY

Intestinal infections can significantly increase the risk of IBS, a chronic and morbid GI disorder with high health care use. Epidemiologic and mechanistic studies in humans as well as animal models point toward specific host-pathogen interactions that may lead to the development of this chronic sequel after infection. These advancements in understanding will be helpful in triaging individuals who are at high risk as well as designing targeted pharmacotherapy. Microbial restoration, augmentation of barrier function, and targeting visceral hypersensitivity remain the most promising areas for therapeutic intervention. From a clinical standpoint, recognition and communication of this condition by physicians will result in better patient outcomes and lower costs. Much needs to be done in expanding the implications of the findings seen in human biopsies and models of PI-IBS, as well as designing proof-of-concept clinical trials specific to the PI-IBS population. The information gained from this will help target this chronic complication of intestinal infections and will also have broader implications for understanding and treating IBS, one of the commonest GI diagnoses.

CLINICS CARE POINTS

- Acute infectious gastroenteritis leads to development of IBS in approximately 1 in 10 individuals. Risk is highest with parasitic infections, followed by bacterial, and lastly viral.
- Main risk factors are younger age, female sex, psychological distress, and a greater severity of infection. Identifying patients at risk is important to give appropriate follow-up and treatment.
- Follow a positive diagnostic approach rather than reaching diagnosis by exclusion. Reserve limited testing (complete blood count, C-reactive protein, celiac serology, and fecal calprotectin) for cases where clinical suspicion of another diagnosis is high.
- Patient education regarding a GI infection acting as a trigger of IBS, as well as reassurance that PI-IBS symptoms tend to resolve in a subset of patients, is the first step in management.
- Although some treatment strategies have been tested specifically in PI-IBS, current management recommendations are extrapolated from routine IBS.
- Glutamine may be an effective therapy for patients with PI-IBS; however, currently it can only be used in off-label settings.
- Lack of response to initial treatment after 4 to 8 weeks, worsening symptoms, or severe symptoms may warrant the need to rule out other causes.

DISCLOSURE

This work was supported by NIH DK 103911 and 120745 to Dr M. Grover. Dr M. Grover reports grants from Takeda and Dong-A Pharmaceuticals.

REFERENCES

1. Mearin F, Lacy BE, Chang L, et al. Bowel disorders. Gastroenterology 2016; 150(6):1393–407.
2. Enck P, Aziz Q, Barbara G, et al. Irritable bowel syndrome. Nat Rev Dis Primers 2016;2:16014.
3. Villani AC, Lemire M, Thabane M, et al. Genetic risk factors for post-infectious irritable bowel syndrome following a waterborne outbreak of gastroenteritis. Gastroenterology 2010;138:1502–13.
4. Marshall JK, Thabane M, Garg AX, et al. Incidence and epidemiology of irritable bowel syndrome after a large waterborne outbreak of bacterial dysentery. Gastroenterology 2006;131:445–50.
5. Klem F, Wadhwa A, Prokop LJ, et al. Prevalence, risk factors, and outcomes of irritable bowel syndrome after infectious enteritis: a systematic review and meta-analysis. Gastroenterology 2017;152:1042–10454.e1.
6. Hurst AF. Medical diseases of the war. London: Arnold; 1917.
7. Chaudhary NA, Truelove SC. The irritable colon syndrome. A study of the clinical features, predisposing causes, and prognosis in 130 cases. Q J Med 1962;31: 307–22.
8. Scallan E, Hoekstra RM, Angulo FJ, et al. Foodborne illness acquired in the United States–major pathogens. Emerg Infect Dis 2011;17:7–15.
9. Shah ED, Riddle MS, Chang C, et al. Estimating the contribution of acute gastroenteritis to the overall prevalence of irritable bowel syndrome. J Neurogastroenterol Motil 2012;18:200–4.
10. Barbara G, Grover M, Bercik P, et al. Rome Foundation working team report on post-infection irritable bowel syndrome. Gastroenterology 2019;156:46–58.e7.
11. Berumen A, Lennon R, Breen-Lyles M, et al. Characteristics and risk factors of post-infection irritable bowel syndrome following *Campylobacter* enteritis. Clin Gastroenterol Hepatol 2020. https://doi.org/10.1016/j.cgh.2020.07.033. S1542-3565(20)30995-2.
12. Halder SL, Locke GR 3rd, Schleck CD, et al. Natural history of functional gastrointestinal disorders: a 12-year longitudinal population-based study. Gastroenterology 2007;133:799–807.
13. Begtrup LMB, Engsbro AL, Kjeldsen J, et al. A positive diagnostic strategy is noninferior to a strategy of exclusion for patients with irritable bowel syndrome. Clin Gastroenterol Hepatol 2013;11:956–62.e1.
14. Irvine AJ, Chey WD, Ford AC. Screening for celiac disease in irritable bowel syndrome: an updated systematic review and meta-analysis. Am J Gastroenterol 2017;112:65–76.
15. Ford AC, Spiegel BM, Talley NJ, et al. Small intestinal bacterial overgrowth in irritable bowel syndrome: systematic review and meta-analysis. Clin Gastroenterol Hepatol 2009;7:1279–86.
16. Shah ED, Basseri RJ, Chong K, et al. Abnormal breath testing in IBS: a meta-analysis. Dig Dis Sci 2010;55:2441–9.
17. McCarroll MG, Riddle MS, Gutierrez RL, et al. Infectious gastroenteritis as a risk factor for tropical sprue and malabsorption: a case-control study. Dig Dis Sci 2015;60:3379–85.
18. Rahman MM, Ghoshal UC, Sultana S, et al. Long-term gastrointestinal consequences are frequent following sporadic acute infectious diarrhea in a tropical country: a prospective cohort study. Am J Gastroenterol 2018;113:1363–75.

19. Ghoshal UC, Gwee KA. Post-infectious IBS, tropical sprue and small intestinal bacterial overgrowth: the missing link. Nat Rev Gastroenterol Hepatol 2017; 14:435–41.

20. Ghoshal UC, Srivastava D, Verma A, et al. Tropical sprue in 2014: the new face of an old disease. Curr Gastroenterol Rep 2014;16:391.

21. Hanevik K, Dizdar V, Langeland N, et al. Development of functional gastrointestinal disorders after Giardia lamblia infection. BMC Gastroenterol 2009;9:27.

22. Wensaas KA, Langeland N, Hanevik K, et al. Irritable bowel syndrome and chronic fatigue 3 years after acute giardiasis: historic cohort study. Gut 2012; 61:214–9.

23. Hanevik K, Wensaas KA, Rortveit G, et al. Irritable bowel syndrome and chronic fatigue 6 years after giardia infection: a controlled prospective cohort study. Clin Infect Dis 2014;59:1394–400.

24. Singh KD, Bhasin DK, Rana SV, et al. Effect of Giardia lamblia on duodenal disaccharidase levels in humans. Trop Gastroenterol 2000;21:174–6.

25. Guagnozzi D, Arias A, Lucendo AJ. Systematic review with meta-analysis: diagnostic overlap of microscopic colitis and functional bowel disorders. Aliment Pharmacol Ther 2016;43:851–62.

26. Gudsoorkar VS, Quigley EM. Distinguishing microscopic colitis from irritable bowel syndrome. Clin Gastroenterol Hepatol 2016;14:669–70.

27. Chey WD, Nojkov B, Rubenstein JH, et al. The yield of colonoscopy in patients with non-constipated irritable bowel syndrome: results from a prospective, controlled US trial. Am J Gastroenterol 2010;105:859–65.

28. Gradel KO, Nielsen HL, Schonheyder HC, et al. Increased short- and long-term risk of inflammatory bowel disease after salmonella or campylobacter gastroenteritis. Gastroenterology 2009;137:495–501.

29. Porter CK, Tribble DR, Aliaga PA, et al. Infectious gastroenteritis and risk of developing inflammatory bowel disease. Gastroenterology 2008;135:781–6.

30. Zanini B, Ricci C, Bandera F, et al. Incidence of post-infectious irritable bowel syndrome and functional intestinal disorders following a water-borne viral gastroenteritis outbreak. Am J Gastroenterol 2012;107:891–9.

31. Porter CK, Faix DJ, Shiau D, et al. Postinfectious gastrointestinal disorders following norovirus outbreaks. Clin Infect Dis 2012;55:915–22.

32. Scallan Walter EJ, Crim SM, Bruce BB, et al. Postinfectious irritable bowel syndrome after Campylobacter infection. Am J Gastroenterol 2019;114:1649–56.

33. Mearin F, Perez-Oliveras M, Perello A, et al. Dyspepsia and irritable bowel syndrome after a Salmonella gastroenteritis outbreak: one-year follow-up cohort study. Gastroenterology 2005;129:98–104.

34. Ji S, Park H, Lee D, et al. Post-infectious irritable bowel syndrome in patients with Shigella infection. J Gastroenterol Hepatol 2005;20:381–6.

35. Wadhwa A, Al Nahhas MF, Dierkhising RA, et al. High risk of post-infectious irritable bowel syndrome in patients with Clostridium difficile infection. Aliment Pharmacol Ther 2016;44:576–82.

36. Palsson OS, Whitehead W, Tornblom H, et al. Prevalence of Rome IV functional bowel disorders among adults in the United States, Canada, and the United Kingdom. Gastroenterology 2020;158:1262–73.e3.

37. Stermer E, Lubezky A, Potasman I, et al. Is traveler's diarrhea a significant risk factor for the development of irritable bowel syndrome? A prospective study. Clin Infect Dis 2006;43:898–901.

38. Tornblom H, Holmvall P, Svenungsson B, et al. Gastrointestinal symptoms after infectious diarrhea: a five-year follow-up in a Swedish cohort of adults. Clin Gastroenterol Hepatol 2007;5:461–4.
39. Nielsen HL, Engberg J, Ejlertsen T, et al. Psychometric scores and persistence of irritable bowel after Campylobacter concisus infection. Scand J Gastroenterol 2014;49:545–51.
40. Tack J, Demedts I, Dehondt G, et al. Clinical and pathophysiological characteristics of acute-onset functional dyspepsia. Gastroenterology 2002;122:1738–47.
41. Futagami S, Itoh T, Sakamoto C. Systematic review with meta-analysis: post-infectious functional dyspepsia. Aliment Pharmacol Ther 2015;41:177–88.
42. Wensaas KA, Hanevik K, Hausken T, et al. Postinfectious and sporadic functional gastrointestinal disorders have different prevalences and rates of overlap: results from a controlled cohort study 3 years after acute giardiasis. Neurogastroenterol Motil 2016;28:1561–9.
43. Karl JP, Hatch AM, Arcidiacono SM, et al. Effects of psychological, environmental and physical stressors on the gut microbiota. Front Microbiol 2018;9:2013.
44. Barman M, Unold D, Shifley K, et al. Enteric salmonellosis disrupts the microbial ecology of the murine gastrointestinal tract. Infect Immun 2008;76:907–15.
45. Jalanka J, Salonen A, Fuentes S, et al. Microbial signatures in post-infectious irritable bowel syndrome – toward patient stratification for improved diagnostics and treatment. Gut Microbes 2015;6:364–9.
46. Youmans BP, Ajami NJ, Jiang Z-D, et al. Characterization of the human gut microbiome during travelers' diarrhea. Gut Microbes 2015;6:110–9.
47. Jalanka-Tuovinen J, Salojärvi J, Salonen A, et al. Faecal microbiota composition and host-microbe cross-talk following gastroenteritis and in postinfectious irritable bowel syndrome. Gut 2014;63:1737–45.
48. Sundin J, Rangel I, Fuentes S, et al. Altered faecal and mucosal microbial composition in post-infectious irritable bowel syndrome patients correlates with mucosal lymphocyte phenotypes and psychological distress. Aliment Pharmacol Ther 2015;41:342–51.
49. Dicksved J, Ellstrom P, Engstrand L, et al. Susceptibility to Campylobacter infection is associated with the species composition of the human fecal microbiota. mBio 2014;5:e01212–4.
50. Tooth D, Garsed K, Singh G, et al. Characterisation of faecal protease activity in irritable bowel syndrome with diarrhoea: origin and effect of gut transit. Gut 2014;63:753–60.
51. Annaházi A, Ferrier L, Bézirard V, et al. Luminal cysteine-proteases degrade colonic tight junction structure and are responsible for abdominal pain in constipation-predominant IBS. Am J Gastroenterol 2013;108:1322–31.
52. Edogawa S, Edwinson AL, Peters SA, et al. Serine proteases as luminal mediators of intestinal barrier dysfunction and symptom severity in IBS. Gut 2020;69:62.
53. Niaz SK, Sandrasegaran K, Renny FH, et al. Postinfective diarrhoea and bile acid malabsorption. J R Coll Physicians Lond 1997;31:53–6.
54. Hong K-B, Seo H, Lee J-s, et al. Effects of probiotic supplementation on post-infectious irritable bowel syndrome in rodent model. BMC Complement Altern Med 2019;19:195.
55. Wang H, Gong J, Wang W, et al. Are there any different effects of Bifidobacterium, Lactobacillus and Streptococcus on intestinal sensation, barrier function and intestinal immunity in PI-IBS mouse model? PLoS One 2014;9:e90153.

56. Galeazzi F, Haapala EM, Van Rooijen N, et al. Inflammation-induced impairment of enteric nerve function in nematode- infected mice is macrophage dependent. Am J Physiol Gastrointest Liver Physiol 2000;278:G259–65.

57. Bercík P, Wang L, Verdú EF, et al. Visceral hyperalgesia and intestinal dysmotility in a mouse model of postinfective gut dysfunction. Gastroenterology 2004;127: 179–87.

58. Der T, Bercik P, Donnelly G, et al. Interstitial cells of Cajal and inflammation-induced motor dysfunction in the mouse small intestine. Gastroenterology 2000;119:1590–9.

59. Chen Q, Ren Y, Lu J, et al. A novel prebiotic blend product prevents irritable bowel syndrome in mice by improving gut microbiota and modulating immune response. Nutrients 2017;9:1341.

60. Bai T, Zhang L, Wang H, et al. Fecal microbiota transplantation is effective in relieving visceral hypersensitivity in a postinfectious model. Biomed Res Int 2018;2018:3860743.

61. Compare D, Rocco A, Coccoli P, et al. Lactobacillus casei DG and its postbiotic reduce the inflammatory mucosal response: an ex-vivo organ culture model of post-infectious irritable bowel syndrome. BMC Gastroenterol 2017;17:53.

62. Morken MH, Valeur J, Norin E, et al. Antibiotic or bacterial therapy in post-giardiasis irritable bowel syndrome. Scand J Gastroenterol 2009;44:1296–303.

63. Zhang Y, Wu X, Wu J, et al. Decreased expression of microRNA-510 in intestinal tissue contributes to post-infectious irritable bowel syndrome via targeting PRDX1. Am J Transl Res 2019;11:7385–97.

64. Dunlop SP, Jenkins D, Neal KR, et al. Relative importance of enterochromaffin cell hyperplasia, anxiety, and depression in postinfectious IBS. Gastroenterology 2003;125:1651–9.

65. Cao Y-N, Feng L-J, Liu Y-Y, et al. Effect of Lactobacillus rhamnosus GG supernatant on serotonin transporter expression in rats with post-infectious irritable bowel syndrome. World J Gastroenterol 2018;24:338–50.

66. Dunlop SP, Jenkins D, Spiller RC. Distinctive clinical, psychological, and histological features of postinfective irritable bowel syndrome. Am J Gastroenterol 2003;98:1578–83.

67. Spiller R, Jenkins D, Thornley J, et al. Increased rectal mucosal enteroendocrine cells, T lymphocytes, and increased gut permeability following acute Campylobacter enteritis and in post-dysenteric irritable bowel syndrome. Gut 2000;47: 804–11.

68. Kim HS, Lim JH, Park H, et al. Increased immunoendocrine cells in intestinal mucosa of postinfectious irritable bowel syndrome patients 3 years after acute shigella infection - An observation in a small case control study. Yonsei Med J 2010;51:45–51.

69. Dizdar V, Spiller R, Singh G, et al. Relative importance of abnormalities of CCK and 5-HT (serotonin) in Giardia-induced post-infectious irritable bowel syndrome and functional dyspepsia. Aliment Pharmacol Ther 2010;31:883–91.

70. Wang LH, Fang XC, Pan GZ. Bacillary dysentery as a causative factor of irritable bowel syndrome and its pathogenesis. Gut 2004;53:1096–101.

71. Dunlop SP, Hebden J, Campbell E, et al. Abnormal intestinal permeability in subgroups of diarrhea-predominant irritable bowel syndromes. Am J Gastroenterol 2006;101:1288–94.

72. Marshall JK, Thabane M, Garg AX, et al. Intestinal permeability in patients with irritable bowel syndrome after a waterborne outbreak of acute gastroenteritis in Walkerton, Ontario. Aliment Pharmacol Ther 2004;20:1317–22.

73. Swan C, Duroudier NP, Campbell E, et al. Identifying and testing candidate genetic polymorphisms in the irritable bowel syndrome (IBS): association with TNFSF15 and TNFalpha. Gut 2013;62:985–94.

74. Halliez MC, Motta JP, Feener TD, et al. Giardia duodenalis induces paracellular bacterial translocation and causes postinfectious visceral hypersensitivity. Am J Physiol Gastrointest Liver Physiol 2016;310:G574–85.

75. Long Y, Du L, Kim JJ, et al. MLCK-mediated intestinal permeability promotes immune activation and visceral hypersensitivity in PI-IBS mice. Neurogastroenterol Motil 2018;30:e13348.

76. Sundin J, Rangel I, Repsilber D, et al. Cytokine response after stimulation with key commensal bacteria differ in post-infectious irritable bowel syndrome (PI-IBS) patients compared to healthy controls. PLoS One 2015;10:e0134836.

77. Chen J, Zhang Y, Deng Z. Imbalanced shift of cytokine expression between T helper 1 and T helper 2 (Th1/Th2) in intestinal mucosa of patients with post-infectious irritable bowel syndrome. BMC Gastroenterol 2012;12:91.

78. Han W, Lu X, Jia X, et al. Soluble mediators released from PI-IBS patients' colon induced alteration of mast cell: involvement of reactive oxygen species. Dig Dis Sci 2012;57:311–9.

79. Han W, Wang Z, Lu X, et al. Protease activated receptor 4 status of mast cells in post infectious irritable bowel syndrome. Neurogastroenterol Motil 2012;24:113-e82.

80. Sundin J, Rangel I, Kumawat AK, et al. Aberrant mucosal lymphocyte number and subsets in the colon of post-infectious irritable bowel syndrome patients. Scand J Gastroenterol 2014;49:1068–75.

81. Veiga-Fernandes H, Mucida D. Neuro-immune interactions at barrier surfaces. Cell 2016;165:801–11.

82. Muller PA, Schneeberger M, Matheis F, et al. Microbiota modulate sympathetic neurons via a gut–brain circuit. Nature 2020;583:441–6.

83. Matheis F, Muller PA, Graves CL, et al. Adrenergic signaling in muscularis macrophages limits infection-induced neuronal loss. Cell 2020;180:64–78.e16.

84. Gu Q-Y, Zhang J, Feng Y-C. Role of NLRP3 inflammasome in Bifidobacterium longum-regulated visceral hypersensitivity of postinfectious irritable bowel syndrome. Artif Cells Nanomed Biotechnol 2016;44:1933–7.

85. Gay J, Fioramonti J, Garcia-Villar R, et al. Alterations of intestinal motor responses to various stimuli after Nippostrongylus brasiliensis infection in rats: role of mast cells. Neurogastroenterol Motil 2000;12:207–14.

86. McLean PG, Picard C, Garcia-Villar R, et al. Role of kinin B1 and B2 receptors and mast cells in post intestinal infection-induced hypersensitivity to distension. Neurogastroenterol Motil 1998;10:499–508.

87. Boitano S, Hoffman J, Flynn AN, et al. The novel PAR2 ligand C391 blocks multiple PAR2 signalling pathways in vitro and in vivo. Br J Pharmacol 2015;172:4535–45.

88. Du L, Long Y, Kim JJ, et al. Protease activated receptor-2 induces immune activation and visceral hypersensitivity in post-infectious irritable bowel syndrome mice. Dig Dis Sci 2019;64:729–39.

89. Valdez-Morales EE, Overington J, Guerrero-Alba R, et al. Sensitization of peripheral sensory nerves by mediators from colonic biopsies of diarrhea-predominant irritable bowel syndrome patients: a role for PAR2. Am J Gastroenterol 2013;108:1634–43.

90. Balemans D, Mondelaers SU, Cibert-Goton V, et al. Evidence for long-term sensitization of the bowel in patients with post-infectious-IBS. Sci Rep 2017;7: 13606.
91. Zhang L, Wang R, Bai T, et al. EphrinB2/ephB2-mediated myenteric synaptic plasticity: mechanisms underlying the persistent muscle hypercontractility and pain in postinfectious IBS. FASEB J 2019;33:13644-59.
92. Schmulson MJ, Ortiz-Garrido OM, Hinojosa C, et al. A single session of reassurance can acutely improve the self-perception of impairment in patients with IBS. J Psychosom Res 2006;61:461-7.
93. Halmos EP, Power VA, Shepherd SJ, et al. A diet low in FODMAPs reduces symptoms of irritable bowel syndrome. Gastroenterology 2014;146:67-75.e5.
94. Biesiekierski JR, Newnham ED, Irving PM, et al. Gluten causes gastrointestinal symptoms in subjects without celiac disease: a double-blind randomized placebo-controlled trial. Am J Gastroenterol 2011;106:508-14 [quiz: 515].
95. Biesiekierski JR, Peters SL, Newnham ED, et al. No effects of gluten in patients with self-reported non-celiac gluten sensitivity after dietary reduction of fermentable, poorly absorbed, short-chain carbohydrates. Gastroenterology 2013;145: 320-8.e1-3.
96. Zhou Q, Verne ML, Fields JZ, et al. Randomised placebo-controlled trial of dietary glutamine supplements for postinfectious irritable bowel syndrome. Gut 2019;68:996-1002.
97. Lam C, Tan W, Leighton M, et al. A mechanistic multicentre, parallel group, randomised placebo-controlled trial of mesalazine for the treatment of IBS with diarrhoea (IBS-D). Gut 2016;65:91-9.
98. Tuteja AK, Fang JC, Al-Suqi M, et al. Double-blind placebo-controlled study of mesalamine in post-infective irritable bowel syndrome–a pilot study. Scand J Gastroenterol 2012;47:1159-64.
99. Andresen V, Lowe B, Broicher W, et al. Post-infectious irritable bowel syndrome (PI-IBS) after infection with Shiga-like toxin-producing Escherichia coli (STEC) O104:H4: a cohort study with prospective follow-up. United Eur Gastroenterol J 2016;4:121-31.
100. Dunlop SP, Jenkins D, Neal KR, et al. Randomized, double-blind, placebo-controlled trial of prednisolone in post-infectious irritable bowel syndrome. Aliment Pharmacol Ther 2003;18:77-84.

Small Intestinal Bacterial Overgrowth

Daniel Bushyhead, MD*, Eamonn M. Quigley, MD, FRCP, MACG, FRCPI, MWGO

KEYWORDS

- Small intestinal bacterial overgrowth • Breath test • Small bowel aspirate
- Microbiome • Microbiota • Antibiotics • Malabsorption syndrome

KEY POINTS

- Small intestinal bacterial overgrowth (SIBO) is a disease in which the small bowel is abnormally colonized by an increased number and abnormal types of microorganisms.
- The clinical spectrum of SIBO is quite broad and ranges from a malabsorption syndrome to irritable bowel syndrome–like symptoms.
- Abnormalities in gastric acid secretion, small bowel motility, pancreaticobiliary secretions, anatomy, and immune function are risk factors for SIBO.
- There is no "gold standard" for the diagnosis of SIBO, and both culture of small bowel aspirate and breath tests have significant limitations as diagnostic tests.
- Treatment of SIBO entails risk factor modification, correction of nutritional deficiencies, and oral antibiotics.

INTRODUCTION

Small intestinal bacterial overgrowth (SIBO) is a clinical disorder that results from the colonization of the small bowel by increased numbers and/or abnormal types of microorganisms. SIBO often entails colonization with anaerobic bacteria that normally reside in the colon. As one of the earliest descriptions of "blind-loop syndrome" in 1939, wherein macrocytic anemia and steatorrhea were noted in patients with altered postsurgical gastrointestinal (GI) tract anatomy,[1] the concept of SIBO has undergone significant change and challenges in light of further clinical studies and advances in technology that have increased our understanding of the gut microbiome. The diagnosis and overall conception of SIBO has, thereby, become mired in uncertainty and controversy, as there remains a lack of consensus or "gold standard" for diagnosis. The purpose of this review is to discuss current views on the pathophysiology,

Division of Gastroenterology and Hepatology, Lynda K and David M Underwood Center for Digestive Disorders, Houston Methodist Hospital, 6550 Fannin Street Suite 1201, Houston, TX 77030, USA
* Corresponding author.
E-mail address: dwbushyhead@houstonmethodist.org

Gastroenterol Clin N Am 50 (2021) 463–474
https://doi.org/10.1016/j.gtc.2021.02.008
0889-8553/21/© 2021 Elsevier Inc. All rights reserved.

diagnosis, and management of SIBO and to explore recent controversies surrounding diagnosis of SIBO and the purported association between SIBO and irritable bowel syndrome (IBS).

PATHOPHYSIOLOGY OF SMALL INTESTINAL BACTERIAL OVERGROWTH

The gut microbiota and microbiome—the former referring to all of the gut microorganisms and the latter rereferring to the genomes of all of the gut microorganisms, but which herein be used interchangeably—begins to develop at and soon after birth in humans. Despite such all-encompassing terminology, the microbiota of different segments of the GI tract are distinct.

In healthy hosts, microorganism counts increase distally along the GI tract. The proximal small bowel normally contains bacterial counts up to 10^3 colony-forming units per milliliter (CFU/mL), whereas the colon can harbor up to 10^{11} CFU/ml.[2] Bacteria found in proximal small bowel cultures are typically gram-positive aerobic or facultative anaerobic bacteria such as *Enterococcus* and *Streptococcus*; the latter thought to originate in the oral cavity. As the primary site of nutrient digestion and absorption, such small bacterial counts ensure that the small bowel does not face competition for nutrients following the ingestion of a meal.

In the more densely populated colon, typical coliforms include anaerobes such as *Bacteroides*, *Lactobacillus*, and *Clostridia*.[3,4] The colon uses these bacteria to accomplish tasks such as bile acid deconjugation[5] and the production of short-chain fatty acids (SCFAs), a substrate for the colonic mucosa formed from otherwise unabsorbed carbohydrates.[6] Colonocytes use SCFAs as a primary energy source and to maintain homeostasis.[7]

A healthy small bowel uses several different protective mechanisms to avoid colonization and maintain relatively low bacterial numbers. Gastric acid, bile, and pancreatic secretions inhibit the growth of both ingested and oropharyngeal bacteria that may migrate distally. Small bowel antegrade motor patterns, including peristalsis and phase III of the interdigestive migrating motor complex, reduce stasis and bacterial growth.[8] The ileocecal valve prevents retrograde movement of anaerobic colonic bacteria, and ileocecal valve dysfunction has been associated with the development of SIBO.[9,10] Native host immunity, including an important role for locally secreted immunoglobulin A (IgA), helps eliminate pathogens.

Given the variety of mechanisms preventing small bowel microbial colonization, it is no surprise that risk factors for SIBO are just as varied (**Table 1**). These include disorders of decreased gastric acid production such as atrophic gastritis—the association between proton-pump inhibitor (PPI) use and SIBO is, however, controversial.[11,12] Pancreaticobiliary disorders such as chronic pancreatitis[13] and cirrhosis[14] compromise pancreatic and biliary secretions. Disorders that disrupt motility such as scleroderma, chronic intestinal pseudo-obstruction,[15] amyloidosis,[16] and hypothyroidism[17] impair the small bowel's ability to clear bacteria. Anatomic anomalies such as strictures, fistulas, and blind loops promote bacterial stasis. Immunodeficiency syndromes such as IgA deficiency may allow unchecked proliferation of bacteria that would otherwise be eliminated by the host's immune system.[18]

When pathologic microbial colonization does occur, it results in numerous and varied pathologic disturbances that result in the signs and symptoms of SIBO. Direct mucosal injury by bacteria may cause malabsorption and protein-losing enteropathy.[19] Carbohydrate maldigestion resulting from decreased brush border enzyme activity may lead to bloating, flatulence, and diarrhea consequent on the fermentation of undigested carbohydrates by bacteria generating such biologically active metabolites

Table 1
Proposed risk factors for small intestinal bacterial overgrowth

Hypochlorhydria	Pancre-aticobiliary	Motility Disorders	Anatomic Disorders	Immune Disorders
Atrophic gastritis	Chronic pancreatitis	Connective tissue diseases	Adhesion	Acquired immunodeficiency syndrome
Proton-pump inhibitor use	Cirrhosis	Chronic intestinal pseudo-obstruction	Stricture	Common variable immune deficiency
	Cystic fibrosis	Amyloidosis	Fistula	IgA deficiency
		Diabetes	Crohn disease	Celiac disease
		Hypothyroidism	Malignancy	
		Myelopathy	Small bowel diverticulosis	
		Neuropathy	Blind intestinal loops	
			Loss of the ileocecal valve/ ileocolonic junctional region	
			Gastric bypass	

as SCFAs, hydrogen, and methane gas. Although direct injury by bacterial toxins may result in villous blunting, most small bowel biopsies from patients with SIBO reveal normal morphology.[20] Bacterial bile acid deconjugation can cause fat malabsorption and result in steatorrhea, weight loss, fat-soluble vitamin deficiencies, and osteoporosis. Bacterial utilization of cobalamin and production of cobalamin analogues may lead to B12 deficiency, associated with megaloblastic anemia and peripheral neuropathy. Bacterial production of folate that can be used by the host may result in elevated folate levels.

DIAGNOSIS OF SMALL INTESTINAL BACTERIAL OVERGROWTH

Although there is no pathognomonic symptom of SIBO, patients most commonly report abdominal pain and distension, bloating, flatulence, and diarrhea.[21] Because these symptoms are neither exclusive to nor predictive of SIBO, a diagnosis must rely on objective evidence of pathologically abnormal numbers and types of microorganisms in the small bowel. And given that SIBO is, in part, treated with antibiotics, which carry their own risks, there is a need to accurately identify patients who would truly benefit from this treatment. However, despite recent advances in the scientific community's understanding of the microbiome, the diagnosis of SIBO remains uncertain, as there is no universally acknowledged or validated "gold standard" for diagnosis.

The most obvious method to assess for SIBO would seem to involve a microbial analysis of the small bowel to identify and quantify culprit organisms. Early studies of SIBO primarily composed of postsurgical patients with blind intestinal loops, which established the diagnostic criterion of bacterial counts in excess of 10^5 CFU/mL cultured from jejunal aspirate. However, the limitations of this historical standard were exposed by Khoshini and colleagues (2008)[22] in a landmark systematic review to determine the validity of bacterial overgrowth diagnostic testing. The investigators found that this cutoff level has not in fact been adequately validated nor has any other cutoff level from small bowel aspirate culture. The patient population from the 71 included studies varied significantly and included patients with a range of comorbidities including cirrhosis, cystic fibrosis, celiac disease, diabetes, surgically altered GI tract anatomy, small bowel diverticulosis, systemic sclerosis, rheumatoid arthritis, and IBS. The actual technique of aspiration and culture in terms of sample location (duodenum vs proximal jejunum), acquisition, volume, and culture techniques was also highly variable. The investigators did find that in healthy adults without any GI symptoms who were used as controls, small bowel bacterial counts rarely exceeded 10^3 CFU/mL. Given this finding, a lower cutoff of greater than 10^3 CFU/ml has been proposed and adopted by some in the diagnosis of SIBO.[23]

As this study[22] suggested, culturing aspirated jejunal fluid as the test of choice for diagnosing SIBO has numerous limitations. The procedure is invasive, costly, and entails the risks of endoscopy and sedation. Fluoroscopic jejunal aspiration may be performed but carries the risks of radiation exposure. There is a risk of contamination by oropharyngeal flora, limiting culture specificity, although there have been advances in endoscopic biopsy that have attempted to mitigate this.[24] Sensitivity may be limited if SIBO is patchily distributed throughout the small bowel or located in the distal small bowel, which is not sampled during duodenal/jejunal aspiration. Sampling only the proximal small bowel may also miss "early" SIBO in instances where bacterial translocation begins in the distal small bowel and progresses proximally. Certain anatomic areas such as blind intestinal loops may not be easily accessible. Sample processing and culture techniques must be adequate to identify anaerobic bacteria. Lastly, although microbial research has rapidly progressed beyond culture to high-throughput sequencing, metagenomics, and metabolomics, the normal microbiome along the length of the gut remains to be completely and accurately cataloged and the normal small intestinal microbiome remains to be defined.[25]

Given the aforementioned difficulties in identifying and quantifying small bowel flora, breath tests have supplanted jejunal culture as more popular through indirect methods for diagnosing SIBO. Breath tests for SIBO operate on the principle that the metabolism of carbohydrate substrates such as lactulose or glucose by microorganisms results in the production of hydrogen or methane that are then absorbed and exhaled as gas in an exhaled breath sample. Human cells are incapable of producing these gases, so their measurement allows one to make inferences on the status of the gut microbiome. Breath testing also has the practical advantages of being inexpensive, readily available, potentially administered at home, and noninvasive. Measuring another microbially produced gas, hydrogen sulfide, has a theoretic role in diagnosing SIBO that has yet to reach clinical relevance.[26]

Lactulose is not normally absorbed in the small intestine and is, instead, metabolized by coliforms to release hydrogen and methane gas. Patients with SIBO may thus have an early peak in exhaled hydrogen or methane due to lactulose metabolism by an abnormal small bowel flora. Conversely, glucose is normally absorbed in the proximal small bowel and also metabolized by bacteria to hydrogen. Patients with SIBO may thus have elevated levels of exhaled hydrogen.

Per the North American Consensus statement on hydrogen and methane breath testing,[27] an increase of greater than or equal to 20 parts per million (ppm) from baseline in hydrogen by 90 minutes is considered a positive test to diagnose SIBO. A level of greater than or equal to 10 ppm in methane is considered positive for methanogenic overgrowth. Although hydrogen is only produced by anaerobic bacteria normally found in the colon, methanogens such as *Methanobrevibacter smithii* are not in fact bacteria but Archaea. Thus, instead of SIBO, the term intestinal methanogen overgrowth (IMO) was proposed in the setting of a positive methane breath test, which has been associated with constipation due to methane's inhibitory effect on intestinal transit.[28,29] Because up to 30% of the population does not produce exhaled hydrogen on breath tests, which may be due to the presence of methanogenic microbes using hydrogen, both hydrogen and methane should be measured during breath testing.[30]

Breath tests require the application of several stringent criteria for participating patients. These include avoidance of antibiotics for 4 weeks before testing; stopping prokinetics and laxatives for 1 week before testing; avoiding complex carbohydrates, which may elevate basal hydrogen levels, for 12 hours before testing; and avoiding smoking and strenuous exercise on the day of the test, as the former may increase and the latter may decrease breath hydrogen levels.

An importing factor that may confound the interpretation of lactulose breath tests is orocecal transit time. If lactulose were to reach the cecum before 90 minutes due to accelerated transit, this could account for a positive lactulose breath test rather than imply SIBO.[31] It is also possible that glucose malabsorption could lead to a positive glucose breath test.[32] Moreover, when compared with jejunal aspirate cultures, the sensitivity and specificity for breath testing is poor, which may in part be due to the heterogeneity of current studies.[16] For glucose breath tests, sensitivity ranges from 20% to 93% and specificity from 30% to 86%; for lactulose breath tests, sensitivity ranges from 31% to 68% and specificity from 44% to 100%.

Given the limitations of breath tests for diagnosing SIBO—including the fact there is no gold standard for diagnosing the disease, rendering calculations of sensitivity and specificity moot—the utility of this testing modality has generated substantial controversy.[33] One wonders if we presently have the ability to accurately define what is and what is not SIBO. Not only is there no accepted gold standard but there is a paucity of data on the value of aspirate and culture or any breath test in predicting clinical outcome, including response to antibiotic therapy. Clinical context is all important— in a patient with one or more of the aforementioned risk factors for SIBO and symptoms that suggest maldigestion/malabsorption and/or chronic diarrhea these tests will be largely confirmatory.

When we stray into less certain territory and begin to search for SIBO among those with less specific and "functional" symptoms, diagnostic certainty evaporates, and we are liable to overdiagnose SIBO and overtreat. For now, pending the development of a true gold standard for the definition of SIBO, we will remain reliant on breath testing as the first-line diagnostic modality for SIBO,[34] and, mindful of all their limitations, results should be interpreted according to the North American Consensus statement.

MANAGEMENT OF SMALL INTESTINAL BACTERIAL OVERGROWTH

When a diagnosis of SIBO is suspected or established by diagnostic testing, consideration should first be given to whether a putative cause for SIBO can be detected and corrected (**Fig. 1**). Although this may be easier said than done for challenging diseases such as connective tissue disorders, chronic pancreatitis, and cirrhosis, the presence of SIBO should lead clinicians to address as many modifiable risk factors as possible. These risk factors may include stopping PPIs, achieving deep remission in patients

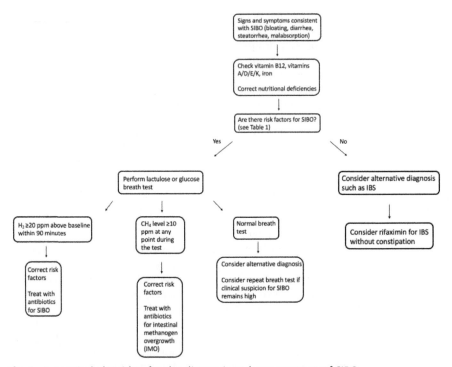

Fig. 1. A practical algorithm for the diagnosis and management of SIBO.

with Crohn disease, or aggressively controlling diabetes. Consideration may be given to using prokinetics to stimulate motility in patients with GI motility disorders.[35]

Secondly, nutritional deficiencies in vitamin B_{12}, the fat-soluble vitamins A/D/E/K, and iron should be identified and treated.

Although there are no Food and Drug Administration–approved medications to treat SIBO, the mainstay of treatment of SIBO has been oral antibiotics to eliminate culprit bacteria. Given the risks of antibiotic therapy—medication side effects, promoting drug-resistant bacteria and *Clostridium difficile* colitis—it would be hoped that data on the efficacy of antibiotics for SIBO are sufficiently rigorous. Unfortunately, antibiotic regimens for SIBO have, in general, been poorly studied, given small numbers of patients and lack of placebo controls.

The most widely studied antibiotic for the treatment of SIBO is rifaximin. As a well-tolerated,[36] nonsystemic antibiotic with poor oral bioavailability,[37] and whose antimicrobial effects may be increased in the presence of bile acids,[38] this may be an ideal candidate for the treatment of SIBO. A systematic review and meta-analysis of rifaximin for SIBO, which included doses ranging from 600 mg to 1600 mg daily with durations ranging from 5 to 28 days, demonstrated that the overall eradication rate according to intention-to-treat analysis was 70.8%.[39] However, these investigators noted that the quality of included studies was generally poor, as only 1 study was placebo-controlled.

Other antibiotics that have been studied for the treatment of SIBO include ciprofloxacin, norfloxacin, metronidazole, trimethoprim/sulfamethoxazole, doxycycline, amoxicillin-clavulanic acid, tetracycline, and neomycin (**Table 2**). For IMO, there are some data to suggest that neomycin-based antibiotic regimens may be effective.[40,41]

Table 2 Proposed antibiotic treatment regimens for small intestinal bacterial overgrowth and intestinal methanogen overgrowth (typically given as a 7–10 d course)	
SIBO	IMO
Rifaximin (800–1200 mg once daily)	Neomycin (500 mg 2 times daily)
Ciprofloxacin (250 mg 2 times daily)	Neomycin (500 mg 2 times daily) and rifaximin (400 mg 3 times daily)
Norfloxacin (800 mg once daily)	
Metronidazole (250 mg 3 times daily)	
Trimethoprim/sulfamethoxazole (160/800 mg 2 times daily)	
Doxycycline (100 mg 2 times daily)	
Amoxicillin-clavulanic acid (500 mg 3 times daily)	
Tetracycline (250 mg 4 times daily)	
Neomycin (500 mg 2 times daily)	

A surprising consequence of antibiotic treatment of SIBO may be ethanol production, as there have been case reports of alcohol intoxication from endogenous ethanol production by intestinal yeast following therapy.[42]

Other treatment modalities that may have a theoretic benefit in restoring healthy GI flora such as dietary modification, probiotics,[43] prebiotics, and even fecal microbiota transplantation (FMT) have not been adequately studied for the treatment of SIBO. In fact, FMT for *C difficile* colitis has been implicated in causing iatrogenic IMO.[44]

Recurrence rates for SIBO following treatment with antibiotics are reported to be high but, given the myriad of uncertainties surrounding diagnosis and treatment efficacy, the accuracy of these rates of disease recurrence is unclear. Was the successful treatment of SIBO supported by symptom resolution alone or repeat breath testing with subsequent normalization? Were there any objective signs of remission of SIBO, such as weight gain, resolution of steatorrhea, or normalization of nutritional deficiencies? Was the initial diagnosis of SIBO supported by clear risk factors and evidence of malabsorption/maldigestion? In order to avoid the risks of cyclic antibiotics[45] for what may ultimately represent a short-lived placebo response, it is necessary to tailor the decision to treat a patient with recurrent SIBO with antibiotics to the individual patient following a robust discussion of the limitations of testing for SIBO and the risks of repeat antibiotic therapy.

A NEW NAME FOR AN OLD DIAGNOSIS

The most controversial claim relating SIBO has been its implication in the pathogenesis of IBS. An early study demonstrating both a higher prevalence of positive lactulose breath tests in patients with IBS in comparison to healthy controls and significant improvement in IBS symptoms following normalization of breath tests with antibiotic therapy suggested a very strong association between IBS and SIBO.[40] Further research clarifying the microbial changes of IBS brought further credence to a potential association with SIBO.[46]

A systematic review and meta-analysis of SIBO in IBS challenged the validity of this association.[47] Although the pooled prevalence of a positive lactulose breath test was 54%, the prevalence of a positive jejunal aspirate and culture with a cutoff of greater than 10^5 CFU/mL was only 4% and no higher than controls, suggesting that the association depends on test choice. Significant study heterogeneity and funnel plot asymmetry, which indicate publication bias, were also evident. Some have suggested that finding evidence of SIBO in patients with IBS may be confounded by PPI use.[48] And as previously mentioned, a positive lactulose breath test for elevated hydrogen may simply signify an abnormally fast orocecal transit time.

A more recent systematic review and meta-analysis of case-control studies found a higher prevalence of SIBO in patients with IBS when compared with controls. These findings were seen when using either culture-based (at both 10^3 and 10^5 CFU/mL cutoffs) or breath test diagnostic criteria.[49] The investigators also found no association between PPI use and SIBO. However, as with the prior systematic review and meta-analysis, these findings were tempered by low-quality evidence and study heterogeneity, and it remains theoretically plausible that PPI use predisposes to SIBO; this would accord with findings that long-term PPI use is associated with an increased risk for enteric infections—the only long-term PPI side effect supported by high-quality, prospective data.[50]

The efficacy of rifaximin in IBS has also been used to support an association between SIBO and IBS; a systematic review and meta-analysis demonstrated that rifaximin is more effective than placebo for global IBS symptoms.[51] As there is some suggestion that the pathophysiology of IBS entails abnormal colonic rather than small bowel fermentation,[52] it is possible that the efficacy of rifaximin in IBS is due to an impact on colonic rather than small bowel bacterial populations. Indeed, the precise mode of action of rifaximin in SIBO remains poorly understood, as impacts on bacterial numbers may be minimal and effects may be related more to perturbations of bacterial metabolism rather than actual suppression of bacterial species or strains.

The association between SIBO and IBS remains controversial.[53] Whether SIBO is associated with IBS, and whether such an association is causative or merely an effect of IBS, has yet to be definitively adjudicated. Because SIBO lacks a gold standard for diagnosis, and IBS is a diagnosis of exclusion based on symptomatology that lacks a validated biomarker, it is impossible to come to firm conclusions about any putative association or lack thereof. From a pragmatic perspective, however, such research has been fruitful in leading to the addition of rifaximin to the therapeutic armamentarium for IBS and in promoting microbial analyses of the proximal small bowel in patients with IBS.[54,55] One hopes that future research on the association between these 2 diseases will continue to result in novel findings and productive discussions.

SUMMARY

Because of its original utility in explaining malabsorption in patients with postsurgical GI anatomy, the concept of SIBO has been challenged by more recent clinical studies and our understanding of the gut microbiome. Although the concept of classic signs and symptoms of maldigestion and malabsorption, as the result of disruptions in the protective mechanisms of the small bowel to maintain relative sterility, continues to offer clinical utility, the limitations of currently available diagnostic tests pose challenges to developing a gold standard for diagnosis. Absent such a benchmark, it is unclear how far the reach of SIBO should extend beyond its historical context to diseases such as IBS. Future research focused on defining the normal small bowel microbiome with novel genomic and metabolomic technologies, and on the clinical utility of breath tests in predicting response to treatment, that are needed to ensure that the concept of SIBO continues to offer benefit in patient care.

CLINICS CARE POINTS

- There is no validated "gold standard" for the diagnosis of SIBO.
- Sensitivity and specificity for breath testing for the diagnosis of SIBO is poor.
- Future research on defining the normal small bowel microbiome with novel genomic and metabolomic technologies are needed.

DISCLOSURE

D. Bushyhead reports no relevant commercial or financial conflicts of interest or any funding sources. E.M. Quigley reports that he is a consultant for Alimentary Health, Allergan, Axon Pharma, Biocodex, Salix, and Vibrant and has research support from 4D Pharma, Biomerica, and Vibrant.

REFERENCES

1. Barker WH, Hummel LE. Macrocytic anemia in association with intestinal strictures and anastomoses: review of literature and report of 2 new cases. Bull Johns Hopkins Hosp 1939;64:215–56.
2. Sender R, Fuchs S, Milo R. Revised Estimates for the Number of Human and Bacteria Cells in the Body. PLoS Biol 2016;14:e1002533.
3. Eckburg PB, Bik EM, Bernstein CN, et al. Microbiology: Diversity of the human intestinal microbial flora. Science 2005;308:1635–8.
4. Bouhnik Y, Alain S, Attar A, et al. Bacterial populations contaminating the upper gut in patients with small intestinal bacterial overgrowth syndrome. Am J Gastroenterol 1999;94:1327.
5. Molinero N, Ruiz L, Sanchez B, et al. Intestinal Bacteria Interplay With Bile and Cholesterol Metabolism: Implications on Host Physiology. Front Physiol 2019;10:185.
6. Wong JM, de Souza R, Kendall CW, et al. Colonic health: fermentation and short chain fatty acids. J Clin Gastroenterol 2006;40:235–43.
7. Parada Venegas D, De la Fuente MK, Landskron G, et al. Short Chain Fatty Acids (SCFAs)-Mediated Gut Epithelial and Immune Regulation and Its Relevance for Inflammatory Bowel Diseases. Front Immunol 2019;10:277.
8. Vantrappen G, Janssens J, Coremans G, et al. Gastrointestinal motility disorders. Dig Dis Sci 1986;31:5S–25S.
9. Miller LS, Vegesna AK, Sampath AM, et al. Ileocecal valve dysfunction in small-intestinal bacterial overgrowth: a pilot study. World J Gastroenterol 2012;18:6801–8.
10. Roland BC, Ciarleglio MM, Clarke JO, et al. Low ileocecal valve pressure is significantly associated with small intestinal bacterial overgrowth (SIBO). Dig Dis Sci 2014;59:1269–77.
11. Lombardo L, Foti M, Ruggia O, et al. Increased incidence of small intestinal bacterial overgrowth during proton pump inhibitor therapy. Clin Gastroenterol Hepatol 2010;8:504–8.
12. Ratuapli SK, Ellington TG, O'Neill MT, et al. Proton pump inhibitor therapy use does not predispose to small intestinal bacterial overgrowth. Am J Gastroenterol 2012;107:730–5.

13. Capurso G, Signoretti M, Archibugi L, et al. Systematic review and meta-analysis: small intestinal bacterial overgrowth in chronic pancreatitis. United European Gastroenterol J 2016;4:697–705.

14. Bonnel AR, Bunchorntavakul C, Reddy KR. Immune dysfunction and infections in patients with cirrhosis. Clin Gastroenterol Hepatol 2011;9:727–38.

15. De Giorgio R, Cogliandro RF, Barbara G, et al. Chronic intestinal pseudo-obstruction: clinical features, diagnosis, and therapy. Gastroenterol Clin North Am 2011;40:787–807.

16. Matsumoto T, Iida M, Hirakawa M, et al. Breath hydrogen test using water-diluted lactulose in patients with gastrointestinal amyloidosis. Dig Dis Sci 1991;36: 1756–60.

17. Ebert EC. The thyroid and the gut. J Clin Gastroenterol 2010;44:402–6.

18. Pignata C, Budillon G, Monaco G, et al. Jejunal bacterial overgrowth and intestinal permeability in children with immunodeficiency syndromes. Gut 1990;31: 879–82.

19. Braamskamp MJ, Dolman KM, Tabbers MM. Clinical practice. Protein-losing enteropathy in children. Eur J Pediatr 2010;169:1179–85.

20. Lappinga PJ, Abraham SC, Murray JA, et al. Small intestinal bacterial overgrowth: histopathologic features and clinical correlates in an underrecognized entity. Arch Pathol Lab Med 2010;134:264–70.

21. Rao SSC, Bhagatwala J. Small Intestinal Bacterial Overgrowth: Clinical Features and Therapeutic Management. Clin Transl Gastroenterol 2019;10:e00078.

22. Khoshini R, Dai SC, Lezcano S, et al. A systematic review of diagnostic tests for small intestinal bacterial overgrowth. Dig Dis Sci 2008;53:1443e54.

23. Erdogan A, Rao SS, Gulley D, et al. Small intestinal bacterial overgrowth: duodenal aspiration vs glucose breath test. Neurogastroenterol Motil 2015;27: 481–9.

24. Shanahan ER, Zhong L, Talley NJ, et al. Characterisation of the gastrointestinal mucosa-associated microbiota: a novel technique to prevent cross-contamination during endoscopic procedures. Aliment Pharmacol Ther 2016; 43:1186–96.

25. Fraher MH, O'Toole PW, Quigley EMM. Techniques used to characterize the intestinal microbiota: A guide for the clinician. Nat Rev Gastroenterol Hepatol 2012;9: 312–22.

26. Singh SB, Lin HC. Hydrogen sulfide in physiology and diseases of the digestive tract. Microorganisms 2015;3:866–89.

27. Rezaie A, Buresi M, Lembo A, et al. Hydrogen and methane-based breath testing in gastrointestinal disorders: the north american consensus. Am J Gastroenterol 2017;112:775–84.

28. Kunkel D, Basseri RJ, Makhani MD, et al. Methane on breath testing is associated with constipation: a systematic review and meta-analysis. Dig Dis Sci 2011;56: 1612–8.

29. Pimentel M, Lin HC, Enayati P, et al. Methane, a gas produced by enteric bacteria, slows intestinal transit and augments small intestine contractile activity. Am J Physiol Gastrointest Liver Physiol 2006;290:G1089–95.

30. Saad RJ, Chey WD. Breath testing for small intestinal bacterial overgrowth: maximizing test accuracy. Clin Gastroenterol Hepatol 2014;12:1964–72.

31. Yu D, Cheesman F, Vanner S. Combined oro-cecal scintigraphy and lactulose hydrogen breath testing demonstrate that breath testing detects oro-cecal transit, not small intestinal bacterial overgrowth in patients with IBS. Gut 2011; 60:334–40.

32. Sundin O, Mendoza-Ladd A, Morales E, et al. Does glucose-based hydrogen and methane breath test detect bacterial overgrowth in the jejunum? Neurogastroenterol Motil 2018;30:e13350Q.

33. Rezaie A, Buresi M, Rao S. Response to Paterson et al. Am J Gastroenterol 2017; 112:1889–92.

34. Pimentel M, Saad RJ, Long MD, et al. ACG clinical guideline: small intestinal bacterial overgrowth. Am J Gastroenterol 2020;115:165–78.

35. Soudah HC, Hasler WL, Owyang C. Effect of octreotide on intestinal motility and bacterial overgrowth in scleroderma. N Engl J Med 1991;325:1461–7.

36. Pimentel M, Lembo A, Chey WD, et al. Rifaximin therapy for patients with irritable bowel syndrome without constipation. N Engl J Med 2011;364:22–32.

37. Descombe JJ, Dubourg D, Picard M, et al. Pharmacokinetic study of rifaximin after oral administration in healthy volunteers. Int J Clin Pharmacol Res 1994; 14:51–6.

38. Darkoh C, Lichtenberger LM, Ajami N, et al. Bile acids improve the antimicrobial effect of rifaximin. Antimicrob Agents Chemother 2010;54:3618–24.

39. Gatta L, Scarpignato C. Systematic review with meta-analysis: Rifaximin is effective and safe for the treatment of small intestine bacterial overgrowth. Aliment Pharmacol Ther 2017;45:604–16.

40. Pimentel M, Chow EJ, Lin HC. Normalization of lactulose breath testing correlates with symptom improvement in irritable bowel syndrome: A double-blind, randomized, placebo-controlled study. Am J Gastroenterol 2003;98:412–9.

41. Low K, Hwang L, Hua J, et al. A combination of rifaximin and neomycin is most effective in treating irritable bowel syndrome patients with methane on lactulose breath test. J Clin Gastroenterol 2010;44:547–50.

42. Spinucci G, Guidetti M, Lanzoni E, et al. Endogenous ethanol production in a patient with chronic intestinal pseudo-obstruction and small intestinal bacterial overgrowth. Eur J Gastroenterol Hepatol 2006;18:799–802.

43. Zhong C, Qu C, Wang B, et al. Probiotics for preventing and treating small intestinal bacterial overgrowth: A meta-analysis and systematic review of current evidence. J Clin Gastroenterol 2017;51:300–11.

44. Chang BW, Rezaie A. Irritable bowel syndrome-like symptoms following fecal microbiota transplantation: A possible donor-dependent complication. Am J Gastroenterol 2017;112:186–7.

45. Meropol SB, Chan KA, Chen Z, et al. Adverse events associated with prolonged antibiotic use. Pharmacoepidemiol Drug Saf 2008;17:523–32.

46. Pittayanon R, Lau JT, Yuan Y, et al. Gut Microbiota in Patients With Irritable Bowel Syndrome-A Systematic Review. Gastroenterology 2019;157:97–108.

47. Ford AC, Spiegel BM, Talley NJ, et al. Small intestinal bacterial overgrowth in irritable bowel syndrome: Systematic review and meta-analysis. Clin Gastroenterol Hepatol 2009;7:1279–86.

48. Spiegel BM, Chey WD, Chang L. Bacterial overgrowth and irritable bowel syndrome: Unifying hypothesis or a spurious consequence of proton pump inhibitors? Am J Gastroenterol 2008;103:2972–6.

49. Shah A, Talley NJ, Jones M, et al. Small Intestinal Bacterial Overgrowth in Irritable Bowel Syndrome: A Systematic Review and Meta-Analysis of Case-Control Studies. Am J Gastroenterol 2020;115:190–201.

50. Moayyedi P, Eikelboom JW, Bosch J, et al. Safety of proton pump inhibitors based on a large, multi-year, randomized trial of patients receiving rivaroxaban or aspirin. Gastroenterology 2019;157:682–91.

51. Menees SB, Maneerattannaporn M, Kim HM, et al. The efficacy and safety of rifaximin for the irritable bowel syndrome: a systematic review and meta-analysis. Am J Gastroenterol 2012;107:28.
52. Ringel-Kulka T, Choi CH, Temas D, et al. Altered colonic bacterial fermentation as a potential pathophysiological factor in irritable bowel syndrome. Am J Gastroenterol 2015;110:1339–46.
53. Spiegel BM. Questioning the bacterial overgrowth hypothesis of irritable bowel syndrome: An epidemiologic and evolutionary perspective. Clin Gastroenterol Hepatol 2011;9:461–9.
54. Giamarellos-Bourboulis E, Tang J, Pyleris E, et al. Molecular assessment of differences in the duodenal microbiome in subjects with irritable bowel syndrome. Scand J Gastroenterol 2015;50:1076–87.
55. Shah A, Morrison M, Holtmann GJ. Gastroduodenal "dysbiosis": a new clinical entity. Curr Treat Options Gastroenterol 2018;16:591–604.

Intra-abdominal and Anorectal Abscesses

Dakota T. Thompson, MD, Jennifer E. Hrabe, MD*

KEYWORDS

- Intra-abdominal abscess • Anorectal abscess • Crohn's disease • Phlegmon

KEY POINTS

- The diagnosis and treatment of abscesses depends on their size, location, and etiology.
- Multimodal treatment including antibiotics, percutaneous drainage, and occasionally surgery, are key to abscess treatment. Without drainage (source control), abscesses pose high morbidity and mortality.
- Intra-abdominal and anorectal abscesses have numerous etiologies, including benign, malignant, and inflammatory conditions.
- Anorectal abscesses are characterized by location and trajectory relative to the internal and external sphincters and are common even in patients without predisposing diseases.
- Inflammatory bowel diseases, particularly Crohn's disease, increase the likelihood of developing intra-abdominal and anorectal abscesses and subject patients to increased rates of recurrence.

INTRODUCTION

Intra-abdominal and anorectal abscesses are seen in both inpatient and outpatient settings by general practitioners, gastroenterologists, emergency medicine physicians, and surgeons. Establishing a diagnosis can be challenging but is necessary because these abscesses can carry high morbidity and mortality.[1] It is essential to diagnose and, when possible, drain the sepsis promptly, and to identify and manage any underlying cause to prevent recurrence and complications. With this article, the aim is to provide an overview of these abscesses, describe their diagnosis and treatment options, and discuss additional considerations when managing these patients.

INTRA-ABDOMINAL ABSCESS DIAGNOSIS

Intra-abdominal abscesses are collections of purulent fluid surrounded by a fibrin matrix. They may be further sequestered by adhesions, intestine, and omentum. As the

Funding Support: D.T. Thompson was supported by the NIH grant T32CA148062.
Department of Surgery, University of Iowa Hospitals & Clinics, Iowa City, IA, USA
* Corresponding author. Division of Colorectal Surgery, University of Iowa Hospital and Clinics, 200 Hawkins Drive, Iowa City, IA 52242.
E-mail address: jennifer-hrabe@uiowa.edu

abdomen isolates the infection to form an abscess cavity, it creates a hypoxic, acidotic, and stationary environment, leading to impaired abscess resolution despite appropriate systemic antimicrobial therapy.[2] As a result, multiple treatment modalities may be needed to control these collections adequately, including antimicrobials and a drainage procedure.

Diagnosing an intra-abdominal abscess can be challenging without imaging. Patients may present with nonspecific systemic signs of infection, including fever, tachycardia, anorexia, pain, ileus, diarrhea, constipation, and a palpable abdominal mass; however, the symptoms are variable depending on abscess location and size (**Fig. 1**). Leukocytosis and increased inflammatory markers typically manifest as well. Physical examination findings depend on the abscess location and size, as well as patient characteristics. Patients may have no tenderness on examination, tenderness to palpation, or focal peritonitis. Diffuse peritonitis, including guarding, rebound tenderness, or a rigid abdomen, signals gross contamination and warrants urgent surgical evaluation. Radiological imaging is necessary for intra-abdominal abscess confirmation, usually

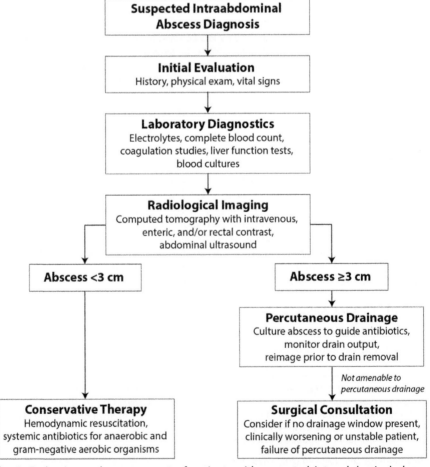

Fig. 1. Evaluation and management of patients with suspected intra-abdominal abscess based on abscess size.

computed tomography (CT) scan, MRI, and, in select conditions, ultrasound imaging.[3] Endoscopy may later be useful in defining the underlying pathology, such as a colorectal malignancy or inflammatory bowel disease, but it is unnecessary for the diagnosis of the abscess itself.

Overall, a CT scan is the best imaging modality to confirm the diagnosis, and abscesses will appear as a region of low density with a surrounding rim.[4,5] Intravenous contrast enhances the abscess rim, which assists in localizing and confirming the diagnosis. The most specific imaging finding is air within the abscess cavity from gas-producing bacteria such as *Escherichia coli*, *Clostridium* species, and anaerobic streptococci; however, this finding is absent 50% of the time.[4,6] Noncontrast CT scans are of limited value in defining abscesses and preference should be given to performing a CT scan with intravenous contrast when at all possible. The addition of enteric or rectal contrast may help to reveal contributing pathology, such as a perforation of hollow viscera.

INTRA-ABDOMINAL ABSCESS CAUSES AND TREATMENT

Most commonly, abscesses are polymicrobial with both aerobic and anaerobic bacteria from the gastrointestinal tract. The 3 most common anaerobes encountered in intra-abdominal infections are *Bacteroides fragilis*, *Clostridia* species, and anaerobic cocci.[7] In particular, *B fragilis* is the most common anaerobe isolated in intra-abdominal sepsis despite being less than 1% to 2% of colonic flora.[7,8] This prevalence is likely due to its complex polysaccharide capsule, which increases its virulence and the host–bacteria response, leading to abscess formation.[2] Based on previous studies, one of the underlying mechanisms is believed to be the host polysaccharide/T-cell interaction evoking an intraperitoneal T-cell–dependent defense against unique, oppositely charged polysaccharide structural motifs.[9] Peritoneal $CD4^+/CD8^+$ T cells induce abscess formation as part of the local immune response, and 4 to 5 days after infection, capsular polysaccharide-primed $CD8^+$ T cells then target bacteria for lysis.[10] Other bacteria, including *Streptococcus pneumoniae*, with similarly charged capsular polysaccharides lead to abscess formation as well.

Frequent sources of micro-organism translocation and abscess formation include the stomach, small and large intestines, appendix, and rectum.[11] The underlying pathology for intra-abdominal seeding most commonly includes iatrogenic, inflammatory, infectious, neoplastic, and traumatic causes. Recent intra-abdominal surgery is implicated as the most common cause of abscess formation and carries a significant risk of morbidity and mortality.[12] Postoperative infections may be related to gross contamination at time of surgery, missed enteric injuries, or anastomotic leak. Clinical suspicion and a knowledge of recent surgical history are beneficial in the diagnosis of these abscesses. Typically, abscesses form no sooner than 3 to 5 days postoperatively. Imaging has been controversial for postoperative abscess diagnosis.[4] Historically, the benefit of imaging within the first postoperative week was low, because it may be difficult to differentiate between a benign fluid collection and a pathologic abscess.[13] However, advances in CT technology and imaging resolution have changed this and a CT scan with intravenous contrast is now the preferred diagnostic tool when an intra-abdominal abscess is suspected.[4] Early percutaneous drainage can be considered if an adequate drainage window is present. Reoperation is to be avoided if possible owing to increased perioperative complications, although this decision is tailored to each patient's clinical course.

After iatrogenic causes, appendicitis and diverticulitis are 2 of the most common causes of perforation and bacterial seeding of the peritoneal cavity. CT imaging is essential and will show appendicular or colonic inflammation accompanied by an abscess or a phlegmon, which is an acute inflammation of soft tissue without a drainable fluid component. Treating the infection with antibiotics and percutaneous drainage instead of operating immediately has been shown to have fewer complications and reoperation rates.[14] Abscess size and location influences treatment options, with nonoperative management being appropriate for small (<3 cm) abscesses in adults (see **Fig. 1**).[15,16] Larger abscesses (≥3–4 cm), patients who fail nonoperative management, and systemically ill adult patients will likely benefit from abscess drainage.[17,18] The Hinchey and modified Hinchey classification systems help to classify diverticular disease and its treatment options (**Table 1**).[19–21] However, diverticular sepsis treatment depends on numerous factors, including Hinchey class, the patient's clinical status, abscess size, and whether the abscess is located where it can be drained percutaneously.[22]

Gastrointestinal malignancy needs to be considered in patients with intra-abdominal abscess formation, including in young patients, particularly because the rate of colorectal cancer in patients under 50 years of age is increasing.[23] The perforation site is commonly at the tumor, with the second most common location being proximal to the lesion owing to distal obstruction from the malignancy.[24] Abscesses localized to the tumor site are likely explained by a slow leakage of enteric contents that become sequestered.[25] Evaluation requires a tissue diagnosis to confirm the neoplastic process, as well as appropriate staging studies. The involvement of multidisciplinary oncological specialists also helps to guide subsequent steps.

Mechanical perforation from foreign bodies and traumatic events may result in abscess formation as well. This rare cause only occurs at a rate of 3.6 per 100,000 person-years and perforation of the gastrointestinal tract is seen in 1% of cases.[26,27] Commonly ingested foreign bodies include fish bones, chicken bones, and toothpicks. Unfortunately, radiologic imaging is not sensitive for locating the object unless it is radiopaque. Establishing an accurate diagnosis may be difficult because the patient

Table 1		
Modified Hinchey classification for diverticulitis and associated CT imaging findings		
Classification	**Disease Characteristics**	**CT Findings**
Stage 0	Mild diverticulitis	No confirmation via imaging Diverticula with or without wall thickening
Stage Ia	Pericolic inflammation and/or phlegmon formation	Diverticular wall thickening with pericolic inflammation
Stage Ib	Small (<5 cm) pericolic abscess formation in location of diverticulitis	Pericolic inflammation with associated an abscess <5 cm
Stage II	Abscess distant from diverticulitis, for example, pelvic, intra-abdominal, or retroperitoneal abscess formation	Pericolic inflammation with distant abscess formation
Stage III	Purulent peritonitis	Extraluminal air and/or free fluid, possible peritoneal wall thickening, and no communication with bowel lumen
Stage IV	Feculent peritonitis	Free perforation with bowel communication

Data from Kaiser, A.M., et al., *The management of complicated diverticulitis and the role of computed tomography.* Am J Gastroenterol, 2005. 100(4): p. 910-7.[21]

often does not recall foreign body ingestion. To treat the abscess, the foreign body needs to be removed, which requires operative exploration. Both blunt and penetrating abdominal trauma can lead to intra-abdominal abscess formation, with an incidence ranging from 3.3% to 45.0% of cases.[28]

Regardless of the etiology, intra-abdominal abscesses in the clinically stable patient should be first treated with antibiotics and, for abscesses greater than 3 cm, percutaneous drainage. The benefits of percutaneous drainage are controlling the sepsis with a less invasive intervention and allowing time to stabilize the patient and identify the underlying etiology. Although patients may ultimately require surgery, operations performed at a time of maximum inflammation and in an unprepped bowel are associated with greater morbidity. Occasionally, the abscess may evolve and require additional drain placement or require drain repositioning and upsizing. For abscesses near the parietal peritoneum, Akinci and colleagues[1] have shown a 91% success rate with percutaneous drainage. Previously reported technical reasons for percutaneous drainage failure include an inappropriate route, a too small catheter size, suboptimal drain positioning, and inadequate duration of treatment.[29] Multiloculated abscesses, thick effluent, and an associated fistula also increase failure rates. Operative drainage may be considered after percutaneous drainage failure, especially if the patient's clinical status worsens owing to inadequate source control.

ANORECTAL ABSCESS CAUSES, CLASSIFICATION, AND DIAGNOSIS

Anorectal abscesses occur in patients with and without underlying conditions such as Crohn's disease. These abscesses are typically seen in an outpatient setting, are diagnosed more commonly in men, and occur at a median age of 40 years.[30,31] Men are twice as likely to be diagnosed as women and it is estimated that there are between 68,000 and 100,000 anorectal abscesses per year. However, the true incidence is not known because many spontaneously drain and go unreported.[32,33]

The currently accepted understanding of spontaneous anorectal abscess formation is that they are secondary to outlet obstruction of the mucus-secreting anal gland. Obstruction can be secondary to trauma or fecal material impaction, leading to inflammation and abscess formation.[34] The cryptoglandular theory developed by Eisenhammer in 1956 claimed that almost all anal fistulae were due to an intermuscular anal gland infection that then extends in different directions. Most obstructed glands drain spontaneously and do not cause infection, but glands terminating deeper between the internal and external sphincters are less likely to drain back into the anus. Besides cryptoglandular etiologies, additional causes of perianal and perirectal abscesses include inflammatory and infectious proctitides, trauma, stercoral ulceration, and ischemia. Crohn's disease is one such inflammatory cause and is discussed elsewhere in this article. In extreme cases, ulcerative colitis may result in a full-thickness perforation of the rectum with resultant abscesses.

The classification of anorectal abscesses is based on their location relative to the anal sphincters (**Fig. 2, Table 2**). Infection spreads in 1 of 3 directions relative to the intersphincteric plane—that is, downwards, outwards, and upwards. Perianal abscesses are the most common and characterized by downwards spread in the intersphincteric plain to the anal verge. Ischiorectal abscesses penetrate outwards through the external anal sphincter and terminate in the ischiorectal fatty tissue surrounding the anorectum. If low, they are characterized by buttock swelling, redness, and tenderness. High ischiorectal abscesses may lack these external findings. Supralevator abscesses, which are the least common, have penetration above the levator muscles and into the pelvic floor. Clinical findings can be less discrete, and imaging is

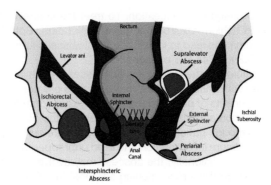

Fig. 2. Potential locations for anorectal abscesses in relation to normal anorectal anatomy.

usually required to distinguish supralevator from high ischiorectal infections. Intersphincteric abscesses are located between the internal and external sphincters without penetration into the surrounding tissue. They have no visible abnormality, but patients have pain and rectal fullness, painful defecation, and may not be able to tolerate digital rectal examination. MRI or examination under anesthesia can diagnose. Horseshoe abscesses are characterized by a deep posterior anal abscess with a lateral extension to 1 or both of the ischiorectal fossa.[35]

Patients with an anorectal abscess are diagnosed based on perianal pain, bulging, redness, and fluctuance. Less common symptoms include changes of bowel habits such as diarrhea or constipation. Symptoms are variable based on the location of the anorectal abscess. For perianal abscesses, patients have pain and perianal swelling.[32] In high-lying abscesses, such as supralevator abscesses, patients are more likely present with vague symptoms and systemic signs of infection including

Table 2
Location, symptoms, and treatment for common anorectal abscesses

Type	Location	Typical Symptoms	Treatment
Perianal	Downward extension to subcutaneous tissue adjacent to anus	Redness, swelling, pain, and tenderness near the anal verge	Drainage via the perianal skin
Ischiorectal	Extension outwards through the external anal sphincter and into surrounding fat and fibrous tissue	Perianal pain, systemic signs of infection, variable redness or swelling	Drainage via the perianal skin, evaluate for horseshoe abscess
Supralevator	Extension cephalad in the rectal wall above the levators	Perianal pain, systemic signs of infection Potential difficulty with urination, no redness or swelling	Complex, staged surgical drainage
Intersphincteric	Confined between the internal and external anal sphincter	Perianal pain, variable systemic signs of infection, no redness or swelling, fullness and painful defecation	Internal sphincterotomy

fever and anorexia. It is important to consider additional pathology in the differential, such as an anal fissure, thrombosed hemorrhoid, cancer, Crohn's disease or ulcerative proctitis, and prostatitis when evaluating a patient with a suspected anorectal abscess.[36] MRI or a CT scan can be beneficial to identify and localize the lesion, but they are not essential.[36] Surgical evaluation including examination under anesthesia is sometimes necessary, particularly in patients who cannot tolerate an awake examination. Ultimately, whether imaging or examination under anesthesia is performed first may best be decided by a surgeon.

Anorectal abscesses are commonly caused by enteric flora, specifically *B fragilis* and *E coli*, but *S aureus* and *Streptococcus* are also common.[37] There are other rare causes of perianal abscesses reported in the literature. For example, parasites including schistosomiasis should be considered as a cause for recurrent perirectal abscesses in patients from endemic areas.[38] Methicillin-resistant *S aureus* is an under-recognized cause of abscess formation, with previous reports showing its presence in 19% of perirectal abscesses despite only 33% of those patients receiving adequate antimicrobial coverage.[39] Actinomycosis is another rare cause for recurrent perianal abscess and resultant fistula formation.[40,41] Perianal tuberculosis can lead to abscess formation, even in immunocompetent patients without a prior history of tuberculosis.[42] Cultures of anorectal abscesses may help to tailor the treatment and should be obtained in atypical presentations of disease.

Hidradenitis suppurativa, a disease characterized by chronic, recurrent, purulent, and painful inflammation in apocrine gland regions, should be considered when evaluating patients for perianal abscess. Most commonly, patients with hidradenitis suppurativa have axillary disease, but approximately one-third of patients with hidradenitis suppurativa have perineal involvement.[43] Hidradenitis suppurativa is most frequently diagnosed in females; however, perianal hidradenitis suppurativa is twice as likely to be seen in males.[44] Additionally, 1 in 6 patients with hidradenitis suppurativa have perianal involvement and 1 in 13 cases have solely perianal involvement. Early perianal hidradenitis suppurativa may be misleading because it can resemble cellulitis or formation of furuncles. Late-stage perianal hidradenitis suppurativa results in the formation of abscesses, fistulae, and sinuses. Owing to the association between hidradenitis suppurativa and Crohn's disease, patients should be evaluated for Crohn's disease.[45,46] Unlike typical anorectal abscesses, patients with hidradenitis suppurativa have abscesses that are not associated with the anal sphincters. When patients have a diminished quality of life owing to painful and deep nodules, incision and drainage can be used to help mitigate symptoms and manage disease. Unfortunately, perianal hidradenitis suppurativa can recur despite adequate excision. Patients need to be aware of the high likelihood of recurrence, because the disease is not well-understood and difficult to cure.

ANORECTAL ABSCESS TREATMENT

The goal in anorectal abscess treatment is to control sepsis and inflammation while preserving continence and quality of life. Patients should be offered early surgical consultation for potential incision and drainage. These abscesses should be drained within 1 day of diagnosis; however, patients with immunosuppression, preoperative diabetes, or evidence of a systemic inflammatory response or sepsis require urgent drainage to minimize the risk of worsening infection, necrotizing soft tissue infection, and septic shock.[30] Drainage can occur with either local anesthesia for superficial, palpable, accessible abscesses, or under monitored anesthesia care or general anesthesia, which allows for a more thorough examination of the perineum and anorectum. A stab incision of the abscess is insufficient, because it can lead to premature wound closure and abscess recurrence. Completing an elliptical incision or cruciate with excision of the corners spanning the width of the abscess cavity allows for drainage while decreasing recurrence (**Fig. 3**). If a fistula is found at the time of examination under anesthesia, a seton may be placed to facilitate drainage, although one should avoid aggressive exploration for fistula owing to the risk of iatrogenic fistula formation. After drainage, the wound heals via secondary intention, which is from the base upward. Drain placement or packing the wound may be used to help keep the overlying skin open.[47] In a retrospective consecutive case series of 500 patients who required urgent drainage of their perirectal abscess, 7.6% of patients needed reoperation within the first 10 days.[48] The need for reoperation is commonly owing to incomplete drainage or premature closure of the abscess cavity. Fecal diversion can be considered for patients who have perianal disease from abscesses or fistulae that are refractory to treatment or that require advanced surgical repair. In general, the diversion is temporary.

ANORECTAL ABSCESS COMPLICATIONS

The most common complication after perianal abscess drainage is a fistula. However, some investigators consider abscesses and fistulae 2 phases of the same disease, because almost all fistulae result from an abscess, but not all abscesses lead to fistula formation. Previous studies report the incidence of fistula formation after abscess drainage to be between 26% and 37%.[49–51] Unfortunately, many of the predisposing factors to fistula formation are not currently known.

A dreaded complication of anorectal abscess is progression to Fournier's gangrene. It is an acute surgical emergency that is a form of necrotizing fasciitis involving the genital, perineal, or perianal area. Previously, Fournier's gangrene was believed to be idiopathic, although now, urinary or perianal infection is suspected to cause

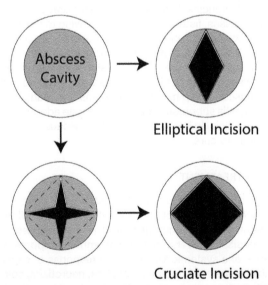

Fig. 3. Incision techniques to ensure adequate drainage of underlying abscess. Elliptical incisions and cruciate incisions with excision of the skin edges both prevent recurrence by removing the roof of the abscess.

most cases.[52] It can progress rapidly from a localized to a life-threatening infection, especially in immunosuppressed patients. These patients present with metabolic derangements, hemodynamic instability, and perineal cellulitis, and have characteristic crepitations between the skin and fascia if gas-forming organisms are present. Bullae and pain out of proportion to the localized findings may also be present. The use of the Laboratory Risk Indicator for Necrotizing Fasciitis score can help to detect early cases of necrotizing fasciitis and to determine its severity.[53] Early diagnosis, hemodynamic stabilization, intravenous antibiotics, and extensive surgical debridement are necessary, because mortality can range between 13% and 45%.[52] Previous reports show that fecal diversion has been used in 50% of patients with Fournier's gangrene to help improve postoperative perineal wound healing.[54]

ADDITIONAL CONSIDERATION: CROHN'S DISEASE

Crohn's disease predisposes patients to both intra-abdominal and anorectal abscess development. Crohn's disease is characterized by transmural inflammation and there are 3 main phenotypes: inflammatory, stricturing, and penetrating.[55] Fibrostenotic disease can lead to bowel perforation and thus abscesses secondary to obstruction. With penetrating Crohn's disease, enteric fistulae can form with adjacent structures including the bowel, ureters, bladder, and the muscles around the abdominal cavity. Incomplete fistulization with adjacent structures may lead to the formation of an intra-abdominal abscess after enteric content seeding. Symptoms vary depending on the abscess characteristics. These patients develop symptoms concerning for an infection including peritonitis, fever, chills, and anorexia. However, symptoms may be nonspecific and mild, making it difficult to confirm. The most common presenting symptoms of an abscess in Crohn's patients are abdominal pain (83%), fever (40%), and diarrhea (27%).[56] The historical incidence of Crohn's-related abscesses was approximately 20% based on previous reports with no difference noted between patient sexes. However, recent studies show fewer than 10% of patients developing an abscess, possibly owing to improvements in Crohn's disease therapeutic management.[56,57]

Crohn's-related fistulas no longer mandate surgery; biologics have demonstrated efficacy in promoting fistula healing.[58,59] However, determining the appropriate intervention for Crohn's-related intra-abdominal abscesses can be challenging. Successful treatment has a variable definition, but generally it is viewed as resolution of symptoms and the abscess while avoiding surgery within 30 to 60 days.[60] Because the vast majority of intra-abdominal abscesses are polymicrobial, antibiotics targeting both gram-negative and anaerobic bacteria are necessary.[61] Metronidazole with or without ciprofloxacin has been shown to be beneficial in multiple studies for treatment of active Crohn's disease, perianal fistula disease, and preventing relapse in quiescent disease.[62] However, based on retrospective studies, between 37% and 50% of patients managed with antibiotics alone had abscess recurrence necessitating surgery.[63] Percutaneous drainage is considered a first-line treatment option and it allows opportunity to determine which patients will require surgical intervention, while nutritionally and medically optimizing the patient (**Fig. 4**).[63] Factors influencing recurrence include spontaneously formed (vs postoperative) abscesses, fistulous connection, and active perianal and ileal disease.[56,64] Retrospective analyses have been conducted showing no difference in recurrence between percutaneously and surgically drained abscesses (31.2% vs 20.3%; $P = .25$).[65] Fecal diversion with or without resection should be considered in patients with difficult to manage disease.

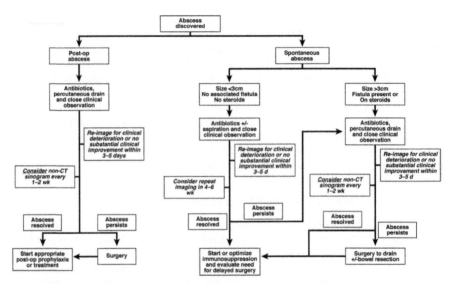

Fig. 4. Treatment algorithm suggested by Feagins and colleagues for intra-abdominal abscesses in Crohn's disease. (*From* Feagins, L.A., et al., Current strategies in the management of intra-abdominal abscesses in Crohn's disease. Clin Gastroenterol Hepatol, 2011. 9(10): p. 842-50.[63])

Crohn's disease increases the likelihood of perianal abscess formation owing to several factors: an underlying inflammatory state, chronic immunosuppressive medication use, poor wound healing, and loose stools. Crohn's disease is often the cause of complex, recurrent, multifocal perianal abscesses. Patients with Crohn's disease and concern for anorectal sepsis necessitate a prompt evaluation by specialists in proctology because of nuanced surgical decision-making and an inherently higher complication risk. One study showing complication rates for Crohn's-associated perianal abscess of 24.0% versus 4.8% in patients without Crohn's disease.[66] Like patients with cryptoglandular disease, incisional drainage of the abscess with or without drain placement is the accepted treatment. However, an awareness of the potential for repeated drainage procedures and the potential for sphincter injury must guide judicious surgical decision making. These patients should be monitored postoperatively, because persistent pain and inflammation represent incomplete drainage or worsening sepsis and may necessitate repeat examination under anesthesia.[67] Patients need to be cautioned that abscess recurrence is seen in approximately 50%.[68] Fecal diversion improves symptoms in approximately two-thirds of patients with perianal Crohn's disease refractory to medical therapy.[69] For the majority of those patients, bowel continuity is not able to be restored. If fecal diversion does not resolve symptoms, proctectomy may be indicated to improve quality of life. Approximately 20% of patients with anorectal Crohn's disease will need proctectomy owing to recurrent abscesses, fistulae, anal stenosis, and severe proctitis.[70,71]

CLINICS CARE POINTS

- Intra-abdominal and anorectal abscesses require timely evaluation and treatment. Drainage for source control is critical to preventing worsening of patient condition.

- Radiographic imaging facilitates diagnosis and guides treatment. CT with IV contrast is most appropriate in intraabdominal abscesses, whereas MRI of the pelvis provides optimal delineation of anorectal abscesses.

- Abscess etiology varies, and adjunctive studies including endoscopy with biopsy may be necessary to help define cause of abscesses.

DISCLOSURE

D.T. Thompson and J.E. Hrabe have no relevant conflicts of interest or financial ties to disclose.

REFERENCES

1. Akinci D, Akhan O, Ozmen MN, et al. Percutaneous drainage of 300 intraperitoneal abscesses with long-term follow-up. Cardiovasc Intervent Radiol 2005;28(6): 744–50.
2. Broche F, Tellado JM. Defense mechanisms of the peritoneal cavity. Curr Opin Crit Care 2001;7(2):105–16.
3. Berg DF, Bahadursingh AM, Kaminski DL, et al. Acute surgical emergencies in inflammatory bowel disease. Am J Surg 2002;184(1):45–51.
4. Antevil JL, Egan JC, Woodbury RO, et al. Abdominal computed tomography for postoperative abscess: is it useful during the first week? J Gastrointest Surg 2006;10(6):901–5.
5. Fry DE. Noninvasive imaging tests in the diagnosis and treatment of intra-abdominal abscesses in the postoperative patient. Surg Clin North Am 1994; 74(3):693–709.
6. Callen PW. Computed tomographic evaluation of abdominal and pelvic abscesses. Radiology 1979;131(1):171–5.
7. Gorbach SL, Bartlett JG. Anaerobic infections. 1. N Engl J Med 1974;290(21): 1177–84.
8. Tilg H, Adolph TE, Gerner RR, et al. The intestinal microbiota in colorectal cancer. Cancer Cell 2018;33(6):954–64.
9. Tzianabos AO, Onderdonk AB, Zaleznik DF, et al. Structural characteristics of polysaccharides that induce protection against intra-abdominal abscess formation. Infect Immun 1994;62(11):4881–6.
10. Crabb JH, Finberg R, Onderdonk AB, et al. T cell regulation of Bacteroides fragilis-induced intraabdominal abscesses. Rev Infect Dis 1990;12(Suppl 2):S178–84.
11. Goldstein EJ, Snydman DR. Intra-abdominal infections: review of the bacteriology, antimicrobial susceptibility and the role of ertapenem in their therapy. J Antimicrob Chemother 2004;53(Suppl 2):ii29–36.
12. Connell TR, Stephens DH, Carlson HC, et al. Upper abdominal abscess: a continuing and deadly problem. AJR Am J Roentgenol 1980;134(4):759–65.
13. Norwood SH, Civetta JM. Abdominal CT scanning in critically ill surgical patients. Ann Surg 1985;202(2):166–17575.
14. Simillis C, Symeonides P, Shorthouse AJ, et al. A meta-analysis comparing conservative treatment versus acute appendectomy for complicated appendicitis (abscess or phlegmon). Surgery 2010;147(6):818–29.
15. Collins G, Allaway MGR, Eslick GD, et al. Non-operative management of small post-appendicectomy intra-abdominal abscess is safe and effective. ANZ J Surg 2020;90(10):1979–83.

16. Ambrosetti P, Chautems R, Soravia C, et al. Long-term outcome of mesocolic and pelvic diverticular abscesses of the left colon: a prospective study of 73 cases. Dis Colon Rectum 2005;48(4):787–91.
17. Andeweg CS, Mulder IM, Felt-Bersma RJ, et al. Guidelines of diagnostics and treatment of acute left-sided colonic diverticulitis. Dig Surg 2013;30(4-6):278–92.
18. Hall J, Hardiman K, Lee S, et al. The American Society of colon and rectal surgeons clinical practice guidelines for the treatment of left-sided colonic diverticulitis. Dis Colon Rectum 2020;63(6):728–47.
19. Hinchey EJ, Schaal PG, Richards GK. Treatment of perforated diverticular disease of the colon. Adv Surg 1978;12:85–109.
20. Wasvary H, Turfah F, Kadro O, et al. Same hospitalization resection for acute diverticulitis. Am Surg 1999;65(7):632–5, discussion 636.
21. Kaiser AM, Jiang JK, Lake JP, et al. The management of complicated diverticulitis and the role of computed tomography. Am J Gastroenterol 2005;100(4):910–7.
22. Tochigi T, Kosugi C, Shuto K, et al. Management of complicated diverticulitis of the colon. Ann Gastroenterol Surg 2018;2(1):22–7.
23. Siegel RL, Fedewa SA, Anderson WF, et al. Colorectal cancer incidence patterns in the United States, 1974-2013. J Natl Cancer Inst 2017;109(8):djw322.
24. Kelley WE, Brown PW, Lawrence W, et al. Penetrating, obstructing, and perforating carcinomas of the colon and rectum. Arch Surg 1981;116(4):381–4.
25. Crowder VH, Cohn I. Perforation in cancer of the colon and rectum. Dis Colon Rectum 1967;10(6):415–20.
26. Budnick LD. Toothpick-related injuries in the United States, 1979 through 1982. JAMA 1984;252(6):796–7.
27. Henderson CT, Engel J, Schlesinger P. Foreign body ingestion: review and suggested guidelines for management. Endoscopy 1987;19(2):68–71.
28. Goins WA, Rodriguez A, Joshi M, et al. Intra-abdominal abscess after blunt abdominal trauma. Ann Surg 1990;212(1):60–5.
29. Gerzof SG, Robbins AH, Johnson WC, et al. Percutaneous catheter drainage of abdominal abscesses: a five-year experience. N Engl J Med 1981;305(12):653–7.
30. Sahnan K, Adegbola SO, Tozer PJ, et al. Perianal abscess. BMJ 2017;356:j475.
31. Ommer A, Herold A, Berg E, et al. German S3 guideline: anal abscess. Int J Colorectal Dis 2012;27(6):831–7.
32. Abcarian H. Anorectal infection: abscess-fistula. Clin Colon Rectal Surg 2011;24(1):14–21.
33. Sho S, Dawes AJ, Chen FC, et al. Operative incision and drainage for perirectal abscesses: what are risk factors for prolonged length of stay, reoperation, and readmission? Dis Colon Rectum 2020;63(8):1127–33.
34. Gosselink MP, van Onkelen RS, Schouten WR. The cryptoglandular theory revisited. Colorectal Dis 2015;17(12):1041–3.
35. Rosen SA, Colquhoun P, Efron J, et al. Horseshoe abscesses and fistulas: how are we doing? Surg Innov 2006;13(1):17–21.
36. Klein JW. Common anal problems. Med Clin North Am 2014;98(3):609–23.
37. Brook I, Frazier EH. The aerobic and anaerobic bacteriology of perirectal abscesses. J Clin Microbiol 1997;35(11):2974–29766.
38. Sandhu G, Georgescu A, Korniyenko A, et al. Recurrent perirectal abscess. Am J Med 2010;123(9):e13–4.
39. Brown SR, Horton JD, Davis KG. Perirectal abscess infections related to MRSA: a prevalent and underrecognized pathogen. J Surg Educ 2009;66(5):264–6.

40. Ferreira Cardoso M, Carneiro C, Carvalho Lourenço L, et al. Actinomycosis causing recurrent perianal fistulae. ACG Case Rep J 2017;4:e82.
41. Magdeburg R, Grobholz R, Dornschneider G, et al. Perianal abscess caused by Actinomyces: report of a case. Tech Coloproctol 2008;12(4):347–9.
42. Mosena G, Della Giustina A, Matos D'Almeida Santos JC, et al. Perianal tuberculosis in an immunocompetent patient. J Eur Acad Dermatol Venereol 2018;32(6): e229–30.
43. Kawak S. Hidradenitis Suppurativa. Dis Colon Rectum 2019;62(11):1278–80.
44. Anderson MJ, Dockerty MB. Perianal hidradenitis suppurativa; a clinical and pathologic study. Dis Colon Rectum 1958;1(1):23–31.
45. Kamal N, Cohen BL, Buche S, et al. Features of patients with Crohn's disease and hidradenitis suppurativa. Clin Gastroenterol Hepatol 2016;14(1):71–9.
46. Burrows NP, Jones RR. Crohn's disease in association with hidradenitis suppurativa. Br J Dermatol 1992;126(5):523.
47. Zhu DA, Houlihan LM, Mohan HM, et al. Packing versus mushroom catheters following incision and drainage in anorectal abscess. Ir J Med Sci 2019;188(4): 1343–8.
48. Onaca N, Hirshberg A, Adar R. Early reoperation for perirectal abscess: a preventable complication. Dis Colon Rectum 2001;44(10):1469–73.
49. Ramanujam PS, Prasad ML, Abcarian H, et al. Perianal abscesses and fistulas. A study of 1023 patients. Dis Colon Rectum 1984;27(9):593–7.
50. Scoma JA, Salvati EP, Rubin RJ. Incidence of fistulas subsequent to anal abscesses. Dis Colon Rectum 1974;17(3):357–9.
51. Vasilevsky CA, Gordon PH. The incidence of recurrent abscesses or fistula-in-ano following anorectal suppuration. Dis Colon Rectum 1984;27(2):126–30.
52. Chen Y, Wang X, Lin G, et al. Successful treatment following early recognition of a case of Fournier's scrotal gangrene after a perianal abscess debridement: a case report. J Med Case Rep 2018;12(1):193.
53. Wong CH, Khin LW, Heng KS, et al. The LRINEC (Laboratory Risk Indicator for Necrotizing Fasciitis) score: a tool for distinguishing necrotizing fasciitis from other soft tissue infections. Crit Care Med 2004;32(7):1535–41.
54. Villanueva-Sáenz E, Martínez Hernández-Magro P, Valdés Ovalle M, et al. Experience in management of Fournier's gangrene. Tech Coloproctol 2002;6(1):5–13.
55. Feuerstein JD, Cheifetz AS. Crohn disease: epidemiology, diagnosis, and management. Mayo Clin Proc 2017;92(7):1088–103.
56. Bermejo F, Garrido E, Chaparro M, et al. Efficacy of different therapeutic options for spontaneous abdominal abscesses in Crohn's disease: are antibiotics enough? Inflamm Bowel Dis 2012;18(8):1509–14.
57. Ribeiro MB, Greenstein AJ, Yamazaki Y, Aufses AH. Intra-abdominal abscess in regional enteritis. Ann Surg 1991;213(1):32–6.
58. Sands BE, Anderson FH, Bernstein CN, et al. Infliximab maintenance therapy for fistulizing Crohn's disease. N Engl J Med 2004;350(9):876–85.
59. Colombel JF, Sandborn WJ, Reinisch W, et al. Infliximab, azathioprine, or combination therapy for Crohn's disease. N Engl J Med 2010;362(15):1383–95.
60. Richards RJ. Management of abdominal and pelvic abscess in Crohn's disease. World J Gastrointest Endosc 2011;3(11):209–12.
61. Mazuski JE. Antimicrobial treatment for intra-abdominal infections. Expert Opin Pharmacother 2007;8(17):2933–45.
62. Khan KJ, Ullman TA, Ford AC, et al. Antibiotic therapy in inflammatory bowel disease: a systematic review and meta-analysis. Am J Gastroenterol 2011;106(4): 661–73.

63. Feagins LA, Holubar SD, Kane SV, et al. Current strategies in the management of intra-abdominal abscesses in Crohn's disease. Clin Gastroenterol Hepatol 2011; 9(10):842–50.
64. Golfieri R, Cappelli A, Giampalma E, et al. CT-guided percutaneous pelvic abscess drainage in Crohn's disease. Tech Coloproctol 2006;10(2):99–105.
65. Nguyen DL, Sandborn WJ, Loftus EV, et al. Similar outcomes of surgical and medical treatment of intra-abdominal abscesses in patients with Crohn's disease. Clin Gastroenterol Hepatol 2012;10(4):400–4.
66. Causey MW, Nelson D, Johnson EK, et al. An NSQIP evaluation of practice patterns and outcomes following surgery for anorectal abscess and fistula in patients with and without Crohn's disease. Gastroenterol Rep (Oxf) 2013;1(1):58–63.
67. Pogacnik JS, Salgado G. Perianal Crohn's Disease. Clin Colon Rectal Surg 2019; 32(5):377–85.
68. Makowiec F, Jehle EC, Becker HD, et al. Perianal abscess in Crohn's disease. Dis Colon Rectum 1997;40(4):443–50.
69. Singh S, Ding NS, Mathis KL, et al. Systematic review with meta-analysis: faecal diversion for management of perianal Crohn's disease. Aliment Pharmacol Ther 2015;42(7):783–92.
70. Rius J, Nessim A, Nogueras JJ, et al. Gracilis transposition in complicated perianal fistula and unhealed perineal wounds in Crohn's disease. Eur J Surg 2000; 166(3):218–22.
71. Basu A, Wexner SD. Perianal Crohn's Disease. Curr Treat Options Gastroenterol 2002;5(3):197–206.

Moving?

Make sure your subscription moves with you!

To notify us of your new address, find your **Clinics Account Number** (located on your mailing label above your name), and contact customer service at:

Email: journalscustomerservice-usa@elsevier.com

800-654-2452 (subscribers in the U.S. & Canada)
314-447-8871 (subscribers outside of the U.S. & Canada)

Fax number: 314-447-8029

Elsevier Health Sciences Division
Subscription Customer Service
3251 Riverport Lane
Maryland Heights, MO 63043

*To ensure uninterrupted delivery of your subscription, please notify us at least 4 weeks in advance of move.

Printed and bound by CPI Group (UK) Ltd, Croydon, CR0 4YY

13/10/2024

01773588-0002